# Ankylosing Spondylitis: Diagnosis and Management

# Ankylosing Spondylitis: Diagnosis and Management

Editor: Sharlton Pierce

www.fosteracademics.com

www.fosteracademics.com

Cataloging-in-Publication Data

Ankylosing spondylitis : diagnosis and management / edited by Sharlton Pierce.
    p. cm.
Includes bibliographical references and index.
ISBN 978-1-63242-489-1
1. Ankylosing spondylitis. 2. Ankylosing spondylitis--Diagnosis. 3. Ankylosing spondylitis--Treatment.
4. Spondylitis. 5. Arthritis. 6. Rheumatoid arthritis. I. Pierce, Sharlton.
RD771.A5 A55 2017
616.73--dc23

© Foster Academics, 2017

Foster Academics,
118-35 Queens Blvd., Suite 400,
Forest Hills, NY 11375, USA

ISBN 978-1-63242-489-1 (Hardback)

Printed and bound in the United States of America.

# Contents

# Preface

Ankylosing Spondylitis is a debilitating ailment that causes inflammation in the joints of the spine. It is a popular type of arthritis. This book on ankylosing spondylitis discusses the pathophysiology and treatment of this disease. Chronic pain is a symptom of this disease and pain management is one of the most common treatments that persons suffering from spondylitis undergo. The book aims to shed light on some of the unexplored aspects of ankylosing spondylitis and the recent researches in this field. It will help new researchers by foregrounding their knowledge in this branch. For someone with an interest and eye for detail, this book covers the most significant topics in the field of ankylosing spondylitis.

After months of intensive research and writing, this book is the end result of all who devoted their time and efforts in the initiation and progress of this book. It will surely be a source of reference in enhancing the required knowledge of the new developments in the area. During the course of developing this book, certain measures such as accuracy, authenticity and research focused analytical studies were given preference in order to produce a comprehensive book in the area of study.

This book would not have been possible without the efforts of the authors and the publisher. I extend my sincere thanks to them. Secondly, I express my gratitude to my family and well-wishers. And most importantly, I thank my students for constantly expressing their willingness and curiosity in enhancing their knowledge in the field, which encourages me to take up further research projects for the advancement of the area.

**Editor**

# Global Metabolite Profiling of Synovial Fluid for the Specific Diagnosis of Rheumatoid Arthritis from Other Inflammatory Arthritis

**Sooah Kim[1]◉, Jiwon Hwang[2]◉, Jinhua Xuan[1], Young Hoon Jung[1], Hoon-Suk Cha[2]\*, Kyoung Heon Kim[1]\***

**1** Department of Biotechnology, Korea University Graduate School, Seoul, Republic of Korea, **2** Samsung Medical Center, Sungkyunkwan University School of Medicine, Seoul, Republic of Korea

## Abstract

Currently, reliable biomarkers that can be used to distinguish rheumatoid arthritis (RA) from other inflammatory diseases are unavailable. To find possible distinctive metabolic patterns and biomarker candidates for RA, we performed global metabolite profiling of synovial fluid samples. Synovial fluid samples from 38 patients with RA, ankylosing spondylitis, Behçet's disease, and gout were analyzed by gas chromatography/time-of-flight mass spectrometry (GC/TOF MS). Orthogonal partial least-squares discriminant and hierarchical clustering analyses were performed for the discrimination of RA and non-RA groups. Variable importance for projection values were determined, and the Wilcoxon-Mann-Whitney test and the breakdown and one way analysis of variance were conducted to identify potential biomarkers for RA. A total of 105 metabolites were identified from synovial fluid samples. The score plot of orthogonal partial least squares discriminant analysis showed significant discrimination between the RA and non-RA groups. The 20 metabolites, including citrulline, succinate, glutamine, octadecanol, isopalmitic acid, and glycerol, were identified as potential biomarkers for RA. These metabolites were found to be associated with the urea and TCA cycles as well as fatty acid and amino acid metabolism. The metabolomic analysis results demonstrated that global metabolite profiling by GC/TOF MS might be a useful tool for the effective diagnosis and further understanding of RA.

**Editor:** Yong-Sun Bahn, Yonsei University, Republic of Korea

**Funding:** This work was supported by the Advanced Biomass R&D Center of Korea (2011-0031353) and the National Foundation of Research (2013059103), both funded by the Korean Government. Experiments were performed by using the facilities of the Institute of Biomedical Science and Food Safety at the Korea University Food Safety Hall. The funders had no role in study design, data collection and analysis, decision to publish, or preparation of the manuscript.

**Competing Interests:** The authors have declared that no competing interests exist.

\* E-mail: hoonsuk.cha@samsung.com (HSC); khekim@korea.ac.kr (KHK)

◉ These authors contributed equally to this work.

## Introduction

Rheumatoid arthritis (RA) is a chronic autoimmune disease characterized by synovial proliferation and damage of the affected joints. In spite of current treatment advances including the use of tumor necrosis factor-$\alpha$ (TNF-$\alpha$) inhibitors, early diagnosis of RA using reliable biomarkers is important for early intervention. Rheumatoid factor (RF), a well-known biomarker for RA, is not useful for specific diagnosis of RA because RF is also detected in various other rheumatic (other than RA) and nonrheumatic disorders such as infection and malignancy, and even in normal individuals [1,2]. Anti-citrullinated protein antibodies (ACPA) have recently received much attention as a valuable tool to differentiate RA from other kinds of arthritis in the 2010 American College of Rheumatology/European League Against Rheumatism (ACR/EULAR) classification criteria [3,4]. However, not all RA patients are seropositive for ACPA, and the 2010 ACR/EULAR classification criteria does not satisfactorily rule in RA for patients with seronegative arthritis, especially involving only one joint. Therefore, more reliable biomarkers with diagnostic capabilities are still needed for RA.

Recently, omics technologies such as genomics, transcriptomics, proteomics, and metabolomics have been increasingly exploited for the discovery of disease biomarkers, including those for RA. Genomics has clearly revealed differences between ACPA-positive and ACPA-negative diseases [5]. In addition, transcriptomics has been used to discover immunity and defense-related genes in RA patients and to predict the efficacy of the anti-TNF-$\alpha$ biologic agent, infliximab, in RA patients [6,7]. Metabolomics, which is a non-targeted analysis of global changes of the complete set of metabolites in organisms [8], has shown its potential in the discovery in disease biomarkers [9–12]. Because metabolite profile changes can be indicative of a disease state [13–15], metabolomics may be a powerful tool for discovering new biomarkers for diseases. Recently, the application of metabolomics to plasma samples was successful in finding metabolic discrimination and potential biomarkers for RA by using nuclear magnetic resonance spectroscopy (NMR) [16], gas chromatography/mass spectrometry (GC/MS), and liquid chromatography/mass spectrometry (LC/MS) [17]. However, to date, reliable biomarkers of RA that discriminate RA from other inflammatory arthritis have not been identified using metabolomics.

Synovial fluid is a body fluid that provides nutrition and lubrication to the articular cartilage. In the pathological joint, the amount of synovial fluid is higher than normal, and a high number of inflammatory cytokines and immune cells are present in the synovial fluid [7]. Thus far, although synovial fluid is the direct medium for the pathological products of RA, no study has examined the changes in metabolism of RA synovial fluid, and biomarkers for RA have not been discovered using synovial fluid. In the present study, in order to find potential biomarkers for RA, discriminating from other kinds of inflammatory arthritis except for septic arthritis (i.e., ankylosing spondylitis (AS), Behçet's disease (BD), and gout), metabolite profiling of synovial fluid from the patients with inflammatory arthritis was performed using gas chromatography/time-of-flight mass spectrometry (GC/TOF MS). These biomarker candidates were verified by multivariate statistical analyses in comparison with other kinds of inflammatory arthritis.

## Materials and Methods

### Human synovial fluid collection and patients

Among patients visiting the rheumatology clinic at the Samsung Medical Center in Seoul, Korea between July 2000 and September 2007, 77 patients who received arthrocentesis were retrospectively screened. Patients with osteoarthritis or a septic condition were excluded from the screening, and thus 38 patients who were diagnosed with RA, ankylosing spondylitis (AS), Behçet's disease (BD), and gout were enrolled in our study. Medical records of the 38 patients were reviewed for age, gender, duration of disease, and laboratory data along with the disease category such as RF, ACPA, fluorescent anti-nuclear antibody, and human leukocyte antigen B27 (HLA-B27). Fulfillment of the above criteria was assessed following the 1987 ACR and 2010 ACR/EULAR classification criteria for RA, the 1984 modified New York criteria, the Assessment of SpondyloArthritis international Society (ASAS) classification criteria for axial spondyloarthritis, and the criteria of the 1990 International Study Group for BD. For gout, the presence of monosodium urate (MSU) crystals was examined in joint fluid. Radiographic findings for the involvement of sacroiliac joints in AS and BD were evaluated, and bony erosion with overhanging edges was checked for gout patients. Following disease categorization, treatment data were obtained for previous uses of non-steroidal anti-inflammatory drugs (NSAIDs) and disease-modifying anti-rheumatic drugs (DMARDs) or uric acid lowering treatment (ULT). In addition, the history of intraarti-cular steroid injection was investigated.

Synovial fluid samples were obtained from arthrocentesis for the sake of the clinical diagnosis of arthritis. This aspirated synovial fluid was routinely analyzed by examining the white blood cell count, polarizing microscopy, the Gram staining and culture, fungus culture, and acid-fast bacteria staining and culture. The final diagnosis was made by experienced rheumatologists. Synovial fluid samples were collected and stored at −80°C. To identify presumed biomarkers for RA, samples were divided into 2 groups: RA versus non-RA including AS, BD, and gout. The study was carried out in accordance with the Helsinki Declaration and approved by the Institutional Review Board of Samsung Medical Center, Seoul, Korea. All subjects were provided with written informed consent prior to study enrollment.

### Patient characteristics

Synovial fluid samples from 38 patients with inflammatory arthritis were analyzed as RA (13 samples), AS (7 samples), BD (5 samples), and gout (13 samples), and their baseline characteristics are summarized in Table 1. The ages of patients with RA (44.2±10.7) and non-RA (42.1±10.3) did not significantly differ at a significance level of 0.05. Among them, 10 samples were obtained through diagnostic arthrocentesis, whereas other samples were obtained for therapeutic purposes. None of the diagnostic samples were positive for microbial culture. Sacroiliac joints were affected in all AS patients. Five patients with gout had typical erosive lesions as determined from the radiographs, and MSU crystals were confirmed in synovial fluid samples of 7 patients. All RA patients had a history of receiving DMARDs except one patient who was enrolled during the initial presentation of RA. Five of 7 AS patients and 2 of 5 BD patients were prescribed DMARDs before arthrocentesis. Of the 13 patients with gout, 9 had ULT and 10 had received colchicines before enrollment.

### Metabolite sample preparation

Metabolite extraction from synovial fluid was conducted using 80% (v/v) methanol at −20°C according to a previously described procedure with a slight modification [18]. Synovial fluid samples were thawed on ice for 3 min and then centrifuged at $500 \times g$ at 4°C for 5 min to remove cells and debris. The supernatant from the centrifuged synovial fluid was mixed with 80% (v/v) methanol at −20°C for metabolite extraction, and this mixture was vortexed for 3 min and then centrifuged at $16100 \times g$ for 5 min at 4°C. The supernatant was then completely dried in a vacuum concentrator (Labconco, Kansas City, MO). To eliminate lipids and waxes, the metabolite extract was re-extracted with 500 μL of an aqueous acetonitrile solution (acetonitrile:water = 1:1, v/v) at 0°C. After centrifugation at $16100 \times g$ for 5 min, the supernatant was collected and concentrated to dryness. The dried metabolite was derivatized with 5 μL of methoxyamine hydrochloride in pyridine (40 mg/mL; Pierce, Rockford, IL) for 90 min at 30°C and 45 μL of N-methyl-N-(trimethylsilyl) trifluoroacetamide (Fluka, Buchs, Switzerland) was added for 30 min and 37°C. Subsequently, a mixture of fatty acid methyl esters as retention index markers was added to the derivatized sample.

### Metabolite analysis

An Agilent 7890A GC (Hewlett-Packard, Atlanta, GA) coupled to a Pegasus HT TOF MS (Leco, St. Joseph, MI) was used for the analysis of derivatized metabolite samples. The derivatized extract (1 μL) was injected into the GC in splitless mode. An RTX-5Sil MS capillary column (30 m length, 25 mm inner diameter, and 0.25 mm film thickness; Restek, Bellefonte, PA) and an additional 10-m long integrated guard column were used for GC separation. The sample was initially held at a constant temperature of 50°C for 1 min, after which it was ramped to 330°C at 20°C/min and then finally held for 5 min. The transfer line temperature was set at 280°C. Mass spectra were acquired in a scanning range of 85–500 $m/z$ at an acquisition rate of 10 spectra/sec. The ionization mode was subjected to electron impact at 70 eV with an ion source temperature set at 250°C. GC/TOF MS data were preprocessed by Leco ChromaTOF software (version 3.34; Leco) by using automated peak detection and mass spectral deconvolution. Preprocessed MS data were processed using BinBase, an in-house programmed database for the identification of metabolites, as described previously [19,20]. The abundance of each identified metabolite was obtained by normalizing the peak intensity of each metabolite using the median of sums of peak intensities of all the identified metabolites in each sample [21,22].

**Table 1.** Baseline characteristics of RA and non-RA groups.

| | RA (n = 13) | Non-RA (n = 25) | | |
| --- | --- | --- | --- | --- |
| | | AS (n = 7) | BD (n = 5) | Gout (n = 13) |
| Age, mean ± SD years | 44.2±10.7 | 35.4±10.7 | 41.6±12.5 | 45.9±7.9 |
| Female, no. (%) | 13 (100) | 3 (42.9) | 2 (40.0) | 0 (0.0) |
| Disease duration, years | 6.5±6.3 | 3.1±3.3 | 6.3±7.9 | 7.9±2.7 |
| RF, no. of positive/tested (%) | 13 (100) | 0/5 (0.0) | 1/3 (33.3) | 0/7 (0.0) |
| ACPA, no. of positive/tested (%) | 3/3 (100) | n.a. | n.a. | n.a. |
| FANA, no. of positive/tested (%) | n.a. | 0/3 (0.0) | 0/2 (0.0) | 0/2 (0.0) |
| HLA-B27, no. of positive/tested (%) | n.a. | 6/6 (100.0) | n.a. | n.a. |
| Fulfillment of criteria, no. of positive/tested (%) | | | | |
| 　1987 ACR | 12/13 (92.3) | n.a. | n.a. | n.a. |
| 　1984 modified NY | n.a. | 7/7 (100.0) | 1/5 (20.0) | n.a. |
| 　2010 ACR/EULAR | 13/13 (100.0) | n.a. | n.a. | n.a. |
| 　ASAS axial | n.a. | 7/7 (100.0) | n.a. | n.a. |
| Previous NSAID, no. of positive/tested (%) | 12/13 (92.3) | 22/25 (88.0) | 2/5 (40.0) | 13/13 (100.0) |
| Previous intraarticular steroid injection, no. or no. of positive/tested (%) | 10/13 (76.9) | 4/7 (57.1) | 3/5 (60.0) | 3/13 (23.1) |

ACPA, anti-CCP antibody; ACR, The American College of Rheumatology classification criteria of RA; ACR/EULAR, The American College of Rheumatology/European League Against Rheumatism classification criteria for RA; AS, ankylosing spondylitis; ASAS axial, Assessment of SpondyloArthritis international Society classification criteria for axial spondyloarthritis; BD, Behçet's disease; FANA, fluorescent anti-nuclear antibody; HLA-B27, human leukocyte antigen B27; modified NY, Modified New York criteria for the diagnosis of AS; n.a, not applicable; non-RA, non-rheumatoid arthritis including ankylosing spondylitis, Behçet's disease, and gout; Previous NSAID, previously use of non-steroidal anti inflammatory drug; RA, rheumatoid arthritis; RF, rheumatoid factor.

## Statistical analyses and validation

As the statistical analyses of metabolite profiles of synovial fluid from the RA and non-RA (AS, BD, and gout) groups, univariate analysis [19,20,23], orthogonal partial least squares discriminant analysis (OPLS-DA), hierarchical clustering analysis (HCA) [24], and receiver operating characteristic (ROC) curve analysis were performed. To obtain maximal covariance between the measured data and the response variable, OPLS-DA was performed using SIMCA-P+ (version 12.0; Umetric AB, Umea, Sweden). Seven-fold internal cross validation and external validation were also conducted using SIMCA-P+. For the external validation, RA patients and non-RA patients were randomly collected from another cohort. The mean age of 6 RA patients (five female and one male) was 66.5 years, and that of 11 non-RA patients (one female and ten male) consisting of 4 AS patients, 4 BD patients and 3 gout patients was 32.5 years. Hierarchical clustering analysis (HCA) was performed using MultiExperiment Viewer for visualization and organization of metabolite profiles [24]. Statistica (version 7.1; StatSoft, Tulsa, OK) was used for univariate analysis [19,20,23]. A further diagnostic property was deduced by receiver operating characteristic (ROC) curve analysis using MedCalc software (Broekstraat, Mariakerke, Belgium).

## Results

### Metabolite profiles of RA and non-RA groups

A total of 38 synovial fluid samples of inflammatory arthritis including RA, AS, BD, and gout were analyzed by GC/TOF MS. After deconvolution, 105 metabolites were identified across the synovial fluid samples of 38 patients, which were classified into the following chemical classes: sugars and sugar alcohols (25%), amino acids (21%), fatty acids (16%), organic acids (16%), amines (9%), phosphates (8%), and miscellaneous (Table S1).

Since principal component analysis (PCA) showed only slight discrimination between RA and non-RA groups ($R^2X = 0.34$, $Q^2 = 0.20$) in a preliminary study (data not shown), OPLS-DA was employed in this study. OPLS-DA successfully minimized the possible contribution of intergroup variability and further increased the discrimination between the RA and non-RA groups compared to the results obtained by the PCA. As shown in Figure 1a, metabolite profiles of the RA and non-RA groups were distinctively separated on the score plot of OPLS-DA. The OPLS-DA model established with one predictive component and two orthogonal components generated the explained variation values: 0.36 of $R^2X$ and 0.99 of $R^2Y$ and the predictive capability: $Q^2$ of 0.97. These high value parameters indicated the excellence in modeling and prediction with good discrimination between the RA and non-RA groups since OPLS-DA models with the parameters higher than 0.5 are considered to be satisfactory in explanatory and predictive capabilities [25]. To validate the OPLS-DA model, the PLS-DA model with the same number of components was used. All permuted $R^2$ values to the left were lower than the original point to the right, and the $Q^2$ regression line had a negative intercept (Figure S1-a). These results strongly indicated that the OPLS-DA models were statistically validated without overfitting of the original model since the intercept of $Q^2$ was less than 0.05. In addition, 6 RA patients and 11 non-RA patients collected from another cohort were predicted to be in correct classes (Figure S1-b).

A total of 105 identified metabolites were clustered and visualized by the HCA using the Euclidean distance and the average linkage method to determine possible variations in the metabolite profiling of the RA and non-RA groups. The normalized peak intensity of each metabolite was transformed by unit variance scaling and loaded into a clustered heat map (Figure 2). The higher the abundance of the metabolites, the more

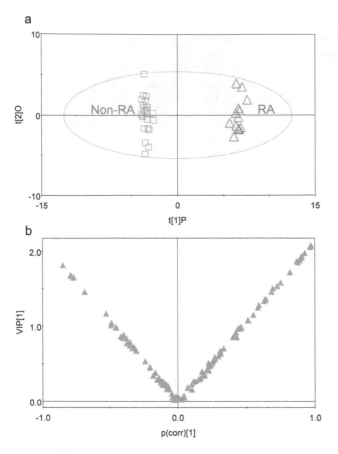

**Figure 1. OPLS-DA of the metabolite profiles of RA and non-RA groups.** (a) Score plot of the OPLS-DA model for RA and non-RA groups (t[1]P, score of the non-orthogonal component; t[2]O, score of the orthogonal component). (b) V-plot with p(corr) and VIP values of 105 metabolites. The metabolites with p(corr) <0 were those decreased in RA groups while the metabolites with p(corr) >0 were those increased in RA groups.

yellow in the heat map, and the lower the abundance of the metabolites, the more blue in the heat map. Clustering of the metabolites led to good separation between the RA and non-RA groups. The discrimination of metabolite profiles between the two groups was mainly caused by certain metabolites as shown in Figure 2.

## Identification of biomarkers for RA

Identification of potential biomarker candidates that account for the differentiation of diseases is a necessary step not only for diagnosis but also for better understanding of the functional metabolism in clinical diseases. To screen putative biomarkers for RA, the variable importance for projection (VIP) values from the OPLS-DA model were obtained. Then, the nonparametric Wilcoxon-Mann-Whitney test and the breakdown and one-way analysis of variance (ANOVA) with post hoc Tukey's honestly significant difference (HSD) test led to further testing of the selected metabolites with high VIP values as biomarker candidates for RA.

VIP values were used to rank the contribution of metabolites to the discrimination between the RA and non-RA groups, which are based on weighted coefficients of the OPLS-DA model [25]. Using the p(corr) and VIP values of the 105 metabolites in synovial fluid, a V-plot was constructed (Figure 1b). VIP values and correlation

coefficients (i.e., p(corr)) of each metabolites were shown in the V-plot. Metabolites in both terminals of V represented a high contribution to the discrimination of the RA and non-RA groups. In a VIP analysis, VIP values above 1 are considered important since the influence of variables with a VIP >1.0 on the explanation of the Y matrix is above average [25]. In this study, 33 metabolites were found to have VIP values higher than 1, of which 23 metabolites were higher in the RA group, whereas 10 metabolites were higher in the non-RA group.

Next, the Wilcoxon-Mann-Whitney test was employed to evaluate significant differences ($p<0.01$) of metabolite candidates and to eliminate variables without significant differences between the two groups. Because the abundance of ornithine between the RA and non-RA groups was not significantly different at the 99% significance level, ornithine was ruled out from the 33 biomarker candidates. Among the 32 metabolites that passed the Wilcoxon-Mann-Whitney test, the abundances of 22 metabolites, including succinate, octadecanol, asparagine, and terephthalate, were higher in the RA group than in the non-RA group. Meanwhile, the abundances of 10 metabolites, including isopalmitic acid, glycerol, myristic acid, and palmitoleic acid, were lower in the RA group than in the non-RA group.

One-way ANOVA was conducted to select putative biomarkers for the RA group only in comparison with the non-RA group representing other inflammatory arthritis including AS, BD, and gout. A post-hoc Tukey's HSD test at the 99% significance level was then performed to compare the mean values between groups. The following metabolites did not significantly differ in abundance between the RA group and each disease group of AS, BD, and gout in ANOVA and HSD tests: adipate, asparagine dehydrated, 2,5-dihydroxypyrazine NIST, lanosterol, lignoceric acid, $N$-methylalanine, palmitic acid, phosphoric acid, proline, pyrophosphate, serine, and stearic acid. All of these metabolites were eliminated from the putative biomarkers for RA.

The fold changes of the 20 metabolites selected as potential biomarkers to discriminate RA from non-RA are shown in Figure S2. The abundances of succinate, octadecanol, asparagine, terephthalate, salicylaldehyde, glutamine, citrulline, tyrosine, uracil, lysine, ribitol, tryptophan, xylose, and ribose were higher in the RA group than those in the non-RA group. However, the abundances of isopalmitic acid, glycerol, myristic acid, palmitoleic acid, hydroxylamine, and ethanolamine were lower in the RA group than those in the non-RA group. Notably, the fold change of succinate was highest in the RA group, and the fold changes of salicylaldehyde and glutamine were much higher than those of other metabolites in the RA group. The fold changes of the metabolite abundances increased in the RA group ranged from 1.7 to 73.6.

## ROC analysis

Twenty putative biomarkers of the RA group were selected after employing multiple statistical analyses as described earlier. Prior to clinical utility of the 20 putative biomarkers, validation of the biomarkers is needed. For disease diagnosis, the ROC curve and the area under the ROC curve (AUC) provide a numerical value of the relationship between the specificity and sensitivity of a biomarker. These sensitivity and specificity indicate the probably tests for correctly identifying patients with the disease and without the disease, respectively [26]. An AUC value of 0.5 or less for a biomarker indicates no information and discrimination within the test, thus implying no diagnostic utility of the biomarker, whereas an AUC value of 1.0 indicates perfect prediction of the diagnostic test [27-29]. Figure 3 shows the ROC curve analysis for the predictive power of the 20

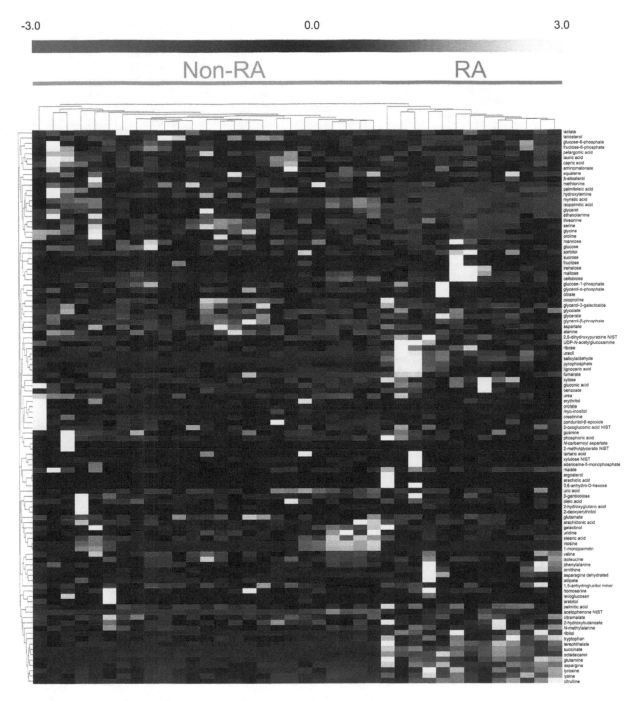

**Figure 2. HCA of 105 metabolites from synovial fluid samples of RA and non-RA patients.** Each column and row represents a disease and an individual metabolite, respectively.

combined biomarkers of the RA group to discriminate RA from non-RA. A sensitivity of 92.3% and a specificity of 68.0% were obtained from the ROC curve, and the value of AUC was 0.812. Since the 20 putative biomarkers showed the AUC value of greater than 0.8, they were selected as biomarkers of RA (Table 2).

## Discussion

Recently, the importance of metabolomics for the study of disease biomarkers and metabolism is rapidly increasing [30–32].

Zahi et al. reported the branched-chain amino acids to histidine ratio as a novel serum biomarker of osteoarthritis using a metabolomics approach [33]. However, only a few studies have performed non-targeted metabolite profiling of RA on a global scale by using plasma or synovial fluid [16,17,34]. Especially, reliable biomarkers of RA distinguished from other inflammatory arthritis such as AS, BD, and gout have not been identified using metabolite profiling in synovial fluids, which is the direct medium showing the state of disease. For example, in a previous study of metabolite profiling of synovial fluid from RA, AS, and gout patients using [1]H-NMR identifying 35 metabolites, no differences

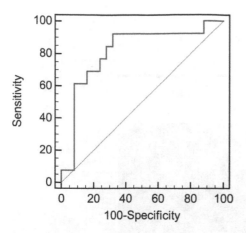

**Figure 3. ROC analysis of the predictive power of the 20 combined biomarkers for distinguishing RA and non-RA groups.** A sensitivity and specificity were 92.3% and 68.0%, respectively, and the value of AUC was 0.812.

metabolomics. The metabolite profiles of synovial fluid obtained from RA patients were distinguishable from those of other inflammatory arthritis, in which 20 metabolites were selected and validated as potential biomarkers with the capability of discriminating RA from the non-RA diseases like AS, BD, and gout with 92.3% sensitivity and 68.0% specificity. This is the first report of the discovery of potential biomarkers for RA, which discriminate RA from other inflammatory arthritis, by GC/TOF MS-based metabolomic analysis of synovial fluid.

In the present study, 105 metabolites classified into various chemical classes such as amines, amino acids, fatty acids, organic acids, phosphates, and sugars and sugar alcohols were identified by an in-house library. These metabolites are major intermediates of various metabolic pathways, including glycolysis, the TCA cycle, as well as pathways involving amino acid and fatty acid metabolism. The number of metabolites identified from synovial fluid of RA in this study was much higher than that in previous studies [34]. In this study, the metabolite profiles of synovial fluid from RA and non-RA groups were considerably discriminated by OPLS-DA. Following various statistical analyses, 20 metabolites of synovial fluid, including succinate, octadecanol, asparagine, terephthalate, salicylaldehyde, glutamine, citrulline, tyrosine, uracil, lysine, ribitol, tryptophan, xylose, ribose, isopalmitic acid, glycerol, myristic acid, palmitoleic acid, hydroxylamine, and ethanolamine were selected and validated as putative biomarkers for RA, which discriminated from non-RA diseases such as AS, BD, and gout.

in metabolite profiles were shown between those diseases [34]. In this study, GC/TOF MS was used to find possible biomarkers among metabolites in the synovial fluid of patients with inflammatory arthritis in order to differentiate RA from other – inflammatory arthritis such as AS, BD, and gout by using

**Table 2.** VIP and AUC values of the metabolites that significantly contribute to the discrimination between the RA and non-RA groups.

| Metabolite | VIP value (rank) | p-value[a] | AUC[b] |
|---|---|---|---|
| **Metabolites with higher abundances in the RA group than in the non-RA group** | | | |
| succinate | 2.09 (1) | <0.0001 | 1.000 |
| octadecanol | 2.07 (2) | <0.0001 | 1.000 |
| asparagine | 1.98 (3) | <0.0001 | 1.000 |
| terephthalate | 1.94 (4) | <0.0001 | 1.000 |
| salicylaldehyde | 1.93 (5) | <0.0001 | 1.000 |
| glutamine | 1.92 (6) | <0.0001 | 0.997 |
| citrulline | 1.91 (7) | <0.0001 | 1.000 |
| tyrosine | 1.89 (8) | <0.0001 | 1.000 |
| uracil | 1.87 (9) | <0.0001 | 0.997 |
| lysine | 1.86 (10) | <0.0001 | 0.994 |
| ribitol | 1.72 (12) | <0.0001 | 0.985 |
| tryptophan | 1.59 (17) | <0.0001 | 0.883 |
| xylose | 1.54 (18) | <0.0001 | 0.92 |
| ribose | 1.51 (19) | <0.0001 | 0.969 |
| **Metabolites with lower abundances in the RA group than in the non-RA group** | | | |
| isopalmitic acid | 1.82 (11) | <0.0001 | 0.994 |
| glycerol | 1.68 (13) | <0.0001 | 1.000 |
| myristic acid | 1.68 (14) | <0.0001 | 0.985 |
| palmitoleic acid | 1.66 (15) | <0.0001 | 1.000 |
| hydroxylamine | 1.65 (16) | <0.0001 | 1.000 |
| ethanolamine | 1.46 (20) | <0.0001 | 0.963 |

[a]p-values were determined using the Wilcoxon-Mann-Whitney test.
[b]Area under the receiver operator characteristics curve.

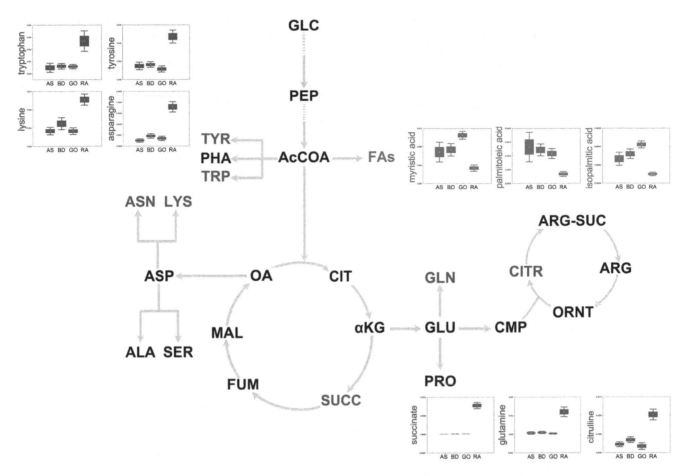

**Figure 4. Schematic comparison of the primary metabolisms of RA vs. non-RA groups (AS, BD, and GO).** The box and whisker plots indicate the intracellular metabolite levels for each disease group (red, increased in RA; green, increased in non-RA). *AcCOA*, acetyl-CoA; *ALA*, alanine; *ARG*, arginine; *ARG-SUC*, arginine-succinate; *ASN*, asparagine; *ASP*, aspartate; *CIT*, citrate; *CITR*, citrulline; *CMP*, carbamoyl phosphate; *FAs*, fatty acids; *FUM*, fumarate; *GLC*, glucose; *GLN*, glutamine; *GLU*, glutamate; *αKG*, α-ketoglutarate; *LYS*, lysine; *MAL*, malate; *OA*, oxalate; *ORNT*, ornithine; *PEP*, phosphoenolpyruvate; *PHA*, phenylalanine; *PRO*, proline; *SER*, serine; *SUCC*, succinate; *TRP*, tryptophan; *TYR*, tyrosine.

These metabolites are the major intermediates of the TCA cycle, urea cycle, and fatty acid and amino acid metabolism (Figure 4).

In particular, citrulline synthesized from ornithine and carbamoyl phosphate is a key intermediate of the urea cycle. It is also generated by posttranslational modification of arginine residues by peptidylarginine deiminase [35]. Because citrulline is a major antigenic determinant recognized by RA, ACPAs have been used for the diagnosis of RA and have been established as a useful tool to discriminate RA from other arthritic diseases [36]. Moreover, in this study, the abundances of citrulline and ornithine were significantly higher in the RA group than those in the non-RA group. In the TCA cycle, α-ketoglutarate is a precursor to such amino acids as glutamate, glutamine, proline, and arginine. Oxaloacetate, which is converted from succinate, fumarate, and malate, is also a precursor to such amino acids as asparagine, methionine, threonine, isoleucine, and lysine [37]. The abundances of asparagine, glutamine, tyrosine, lysine, and tryptophan were higher in the RA group than those in non-RA group. Although α-ketoglutarate and oxaloacetate from the TCA cycle were not identified as metabolites in the present study, the abundances of succinate and fumarate in the TCA cycle were higher in the RA group, as were their derivative amino acids asparagine, lysine, and glutamine. These results

indicate that the urea and TCA cycles as well as amino acid metabolism were highly activated in the RA group compared with the non-RA group consisting of AS, BD, and gout patients. In addition to citrulline, succinate, asparagine, glutamine, and lysine can be considered as major biomarkers for RA diagnosis.

Fatty acids are synthesized from acetyl-CoA and play important roles in cellular metabolism. RA is known to be affected by n-3 and n-6 fatty acids. For example, n-3 fatty acids suppress inflammation by reducing TNF-α and interleukin-1β levels in RA patients by competitively inhibiting the production of leukotriene B4 from arachidonic acid [38]. In our study, arachidonic acid (an n-6 fatty acid) was identified, but the level of arachidonic acid between the RA and non-RA groups did not significantly differ at the 99% significance level. Other than arachidonic acid, major fatty acids such as isopalmitic acid, myristic acid, and palmitoleic acid were identified as the significant metabolites in the RA group because their levels were markedly lower in the RA group. These results indicate that the fatty acid metabolism was more activated in the non-RA group than in the RA group.

This study has some limitations in the sample size and gender ratio. Although the sample size was relatively small here, the OPLS-DA model was well validated by the permutation test (Figure S1-a), and the potential biomarkers of RA were also verified by external validation (Figure S1-b) and AUC (Table 2). The gender ratio was not controlled in each group in this study, but among the 20 biomarkers of RA found from 13 RA and 25 non-RA patients without gender ratio control, 14 metabolites reappeared as the biomarkers of RA from 13 RA and 5 non-RA patients with gender ratio control (Table S2). These results agreed with previous reports that the metabolic profiles of RA did not significantly affected by gender [16,39].

In conclusion, this is the first report on the identification of potential biomarkers for RA using human synovial fluid of RA and non-RA patients by metabolomics for the diagnosis of RA distinguished from other inflammatory arthritis such as AS, BD, and gout. We also demonstrated that metabolic profiling may be a useful tool to discover biomarkers, and envision a holistic view of metabolism for diseases.

## Supporting Information

**Figure S1 OPLS model of the metabolite profiles of RA and non-RA groups. (a) Validation of the OPLS-DA model using 100 permutation test.** Y-axis intercept of R2 and Q2 were 0.514 and −0.231, respectively. (b) Y-predicted scatter plot of the OPLS-DA model validated with RA and non-RA patients from another cohort. Red, RA patients; Blue, non-RA patients; Orange, RA and non-RA patients from another cohort.

**Figure S2 Fold changes of abundances of 20 metabolites in synovial fluid selected as potential biomarkers for RA.** Positive values indicate the increased fold changes in the RA group and negative values the increased fold changes in the non-RA group.

**Table S1** Metabolites identified from GC/TOF MS and BinBase analyses of synovial fluid.

**Table S2** The potential biomarkers of RA found from metabolite analysis of synovial fluid with and without controlling gender ratios of RA and non-RA patients.

## Author Contributions

Conceived and designed the experiments: HSC KHK. Performed the experiments: SK JH JX YHJ. Analyzed the data: SK JH HSC KHK. Contributed reagents/materials/analysis tools: SK JH HSC KHK. Wrote the paper: SK JH HSC KHK.

## References

1. Cammarata RJ, Rodnan GP, Fennell RH (1967) Serum anti-γ-globulin and antinuclear factors in the aged. JAMA-J Am Med Assoc 199: 455–458.
2. Litwin SD, Singer JM (1965) Studies of the incidence and significance of anti-gamma globulin factors in the aging. Arthritis Rheum 8: 538–550.
3. Rantapaa-Dahlqvist S, de Jong BAW, Berglin E, Hallmans G, Wadell G, et al. (2003) Antibodies against cyclic citrullinated peptide and IgA rheumatoid factor predict the development of rheumatoid arthritis. Arthritis Rheum 48: 2741–2749.
4. Humphreys JH, Symmons DP (2012) Postpublication validation of the 2010 American College of Rheumatology/European League Against Rheumatism classification criteria for rheumatoid arthritis: where do we stand? Curr Opin Rheumatol 25(2): 157–163.
5. Kallberg H, Padyukov L, Plenge RM, Ronnelid J, Gregersen PK, et al. (2007) Gene-gene and gene-environment interactions involving HLA-DRB1, PTPN22, and smoking in two subsets of rheumatoid arthritis. Am J Hum Genet 80: 867–875.
6. Teixeira VH, Olaso R, Martin-Magniette ML, Lasbleiz S, Jacq L, et al. (2009) Transcriptome analysis describing new immunity and defense genes in peripheral blood mononuclear cells of rheumatoid arthritis patients. PLOS ONE 4(8): e6803.
7. Tanino M, Matoba R, Nakamura S, Kameda H, Amano K, et al. (2009) Prediction of efficacy of anti-TNF biologic agent, infliximab, for rheumatoid arthritis patients using a comprehensive transcriptome analysis of white blood cells. Biochem Biophys Res Commun 387: 261–265.
8. Villas-Boas SG, Roessner-Tunali U, Hansen MAE, Smedsgaard J, Nielsen J (2007) Metabolome Analysis: An Introduction. Hoboken, NJ: John Wiley and Sons, Inc.
9. Bogdanov M, Matson WR, Wang L, Matson T, Saunders-Pullman R, et al. (2008) Metabolomic profiling to develop blood biomarkers for Parkinson's disease. Brain 131: 389–396.
10. Zhang J, Bowers J, Liu LY, Wei SW, Gowda GAN, et al. (2012) Esophageal cancer metabolite biomarkers detected by LC-MS and NMR methods. PLOS ONE 7(1): e30181.
11. Chen TL, Xie GX, Wang XY, Fan J, Qiu YP, et al. (2011) Serum and urine metabolite profiling reveals potential biomarkers of human hepatocellular carcinoma. Mol Cell Proteomics 10(7): M110.004945.
12. Huang ZZ, Lin L, Gao Y, Chen YJ, Yan XM, et al. (2011) Bladder cancer determination via two urinary metabolites: A biomarker pattern approach. Mol Cell Proteomics 10(10): M111.007922.
13. Bell JD, Sadler PJ, Morris VC, Levander OA (1991) Effect of aging and diet on proton NMR spectra of rat urine. Magn Reson Med 17: 414–422.
14. Connor SC, Hansen MK, Corner A, Smith RF, Ryan TE (2010) Integration of metabolomics and transcriptomics data to aid biomarker discovery in type 2 diabetes. Mol Biosyst 6: 909–921.
15. Holmes E, Wilson ID, Nicholson JK (2008) Metabolic phenotyping in health and disease. Cell 134: 714–717.
16. Lauridsen MB, Bliddal H, Christensen R, Danneskiold-Samsoe B, Bennett R, et al. (2010) ¹H NMR Spectroscopy-based interventional metabolic phenotyping: A cohort study of rheumatoid arthritis patients. J Proteome Res 9: 4545–4553.
17. Madsen RK, Lundstedt T, Gabrielsson J, Sennbro CJ, Alenius GM, et al. (2011) Diagnostic properties of metabolic perturbations in rheumatoid arthritis. Arthritis Res Ther 13.
18. Borenstein DG, Gibbs CA, Jacobs RP (1982) Gas-liquid chromatographic analysis of synovial fluid. Arthritis Rheum 25: 947–953.
19. Lee DY, Fiehn O (2008) High quality metabolomic data for Chlamydomonas reinhardtii. Plant Methods 4: 7.
20. Fiehn O, Wohlgemuth G, Scholz M, Kind T, Lee DY, et al. (2008) Quality control for plant metabolomics: reporting MSI-compliant studies. Plant J 53: 691–704.
21. Hutschenreuther A, Kiontke A, Birkenmeier G, Birkemeyer C (2012) Comparison of extraction conditions and normalization approaches for cellular metabolomics of adherent growing cells with GC-MS. Anal Methods 4: 1953–1963.
22. Lee DY, Park JJ, Barupal DK, Fiehn O (2012) System Response of Metabolic Networks in Chlamydomonas reinhardtii to Total Available Ammonium. Mol Cell Proteomics 11: 973–988.
23. Denkert C, Budczies J, Kind T, Weichert W, Tablack P, et al. (2006) Mass spectrometry-based metabolic profiling reveals different metabolite patterns in invasive ovarian carcinomas and ovarian borderline tumors. Cancer Res 66: 10795–10804.
24. Saeed AI, Bhagabati NK, Braisted JC, Liang W, Sharov V, et al. (2006) TM4 microarray software suite. Methods Enzymol 411: 134–193.
25. Umetrics AB (2005) User's Guide to SIMCA-P, SIMCA-P+ version 11.0. Umeå, Sweden: Umetrics AB.
26. Lalkhen AG, McCluskey A (2008) Clinical tests: sensitivity and specificity. Contin Educ Anaesth Crit Care Pain 8: 221–223.
27. Swets JA (1988) Measuring the accuracy of diagnostic systems. Science 240: 1285–1293.
28. Lasko TA, Bhagwat JG, Zou KH, Ohno-Machado L (2005) The use of receiver operating characteristic curves in biomedical informatics. J Biomed Inform 38: 404–415.
29. Greiner M, Pfeiffer D, Smith RD (2000) Principles and practical application of the receiver-operating characteristic analysis for diagnostic tests. Prev Vet Med 45: 23–41.
30. Mamas M, Dunn WB, Neyses L, Goodacre R (2011) The role of metabolites and metabolomics in clinically applicable biomarkers of disease. Arch Toxicol 85: 5–17.
31. Madsen R, Lundstedt T, Trygg J (2010) Chemometrics in metabolomics-A review in human disease diagnosis. Anal Chim Acta 659: 23–33.
32. Vinayavekhin N, Homan EA, Saghatelian A (2010) Exploring Disease through Metabolomics. ACS Chem Biol 5: 91–103.
33. Zhai G, Wang-Sattler R, Hart DJ, Arden NK, Hakim AJ, et al. (2010) Serum branched-chain amino acid to histidine ratio: a novel metabolomic biomarker of knee osteoarthritis. Ann Rheum Dis 69: 1227–1231.
34. Hugle T, Kovacs H, Heijnen I, Daikeler T, Baisch U, et al. (2012) Synovial fluid metabolomics in different forms of arthritis assessed by nuclear magnetic resonance spectroscopy. Clin Exp Rheumatol 30: 240–245.
35. Tarcsa E, Marekov LN, Mei G, Melino G, Lee SC, et al. (1996) Protein unfolding by peptidylarginine deiminase – Substrate specificity and structural

relationships of the natural substrates trichohyalin and filaggrin. J Biol Chem 271: 30709–30716.

36. Bas S, Perneger TV, Seitz M, Tiercy JM, Roux-Lombard P, et al. (2002) Diagnostic tests for rheumatoid arthritis: comparison of anti-cyclic citrullinated peptide antibodies, anti-keratin antibodies and IgM rheumatoid factors. Rheumatology 41: 809–814.

37. Jetten MSM, Pitoc GA, Follettie MT, Sinskey AJ (1994) Regulation of phospho(enol)-pyruvate-and oxaloacetate-converting enzymes in *Corynebacterium glutamicum*. Appl Microbiol Biotechnol 41: 47–52.

38. Kremer JM, Lawrence DA, Jubiz W, Digiacomo R, Rynes R, et al. (1990) Dietary fish oil and olive oil supplementation in patients with rheumatoid arthritis. Arthritis Rheum 33: 810–820.

39. Xie GX, Chen TL, Qiu YP, Shi P, Zheng XJ, et al. (2012) Urine metabolite profiling offers potential early diagnosis of oral cancer. Metabolomics 8: 220–231.

# 2

# Increased Frequencies of Th22 Cells as well as Th17 Cells in the Peripheral Blood of Patients with Ankylosing Spondylitis and Rheumatoid Arthritis

Lei Zhang[1][○], Yong-gang Li[1][○], Yu-hua Li[2][○], Lei Qi[1], Xin-guang Liu[3], Cun-zhong Yuan[4], Nai-wen Hu[5], Dao-xin Ma[3]*, Zhen-feng Li[1], Qiang Yang[1], Wei Li[6], Jian-min Li[1]*

1 Department of Orthopedics, Qilu Hospital, Shandong University, Jinan, China, 2 Department of Emergency, Qilu Hospital, Shandong University, Jinan, China, 3 Department of Hematology, Qilu Hospital, Shandong University, Jinan, China, 4 Department of Obstetrics and Gynecology, Qilu Hospital, Shandong University, Jinan, China, 5 Department of Rheumatology, Provincial Hospital affiliated to Shandong University, Jinan, China, 6 Department of Clinical Laboratory, Qilu Hospital, Shandong University, Jinan, China

## Abstract

*Background:* T-helper (Th) 22 is involved in the pathogenesis of inflammatory diseases. The roles of Th22 cells in the pathophysiological of ankylosing spondylitis (AS) and rheumatoid arthritis (RA) remain unsettled. So we examined the frequencies of Th22 cells, Th17 cells and Th1 cells in peripheral blood (PB) from patients with AS and patients with RA compared with both healthy controls as well as patients with osteoarthritis.

*Design and Methods:* We studied 32 AS patients, 20 RA patients, 10 OA patients and 20 healthy controls. The expression of IL-22, IL-17 and IFN-$\gamma$ were examined in AS, RA, OA patients and healthy controls by flow cytometry. Plasma IL-22 and IL-17 levels were examined by enzyme-linked immunosorbent assay.

*Results:* Th22 cells, Th17 cells and interleukin-22 were significantly elevated in AS and RA patients compared with OA patients and healthy controls. Moreover, Th22 cells showed positive correlation with Th17 cells as well as interleukin-22 in AS and RA patients. However, positive correlation between IL-22 and Th17 cells was only found in AS patients not in RA patients. In addition, the percentages of both Th22 cells and Th17 cells correlated positively with disease activity only in RA patients not in AS patients.

*Conclusions:* The frequencies of both Th22 cells and Th17 cells were elevated in PB from patients with AS and patients with RA. These findings suggest that Th22 cells and Th17 cells may be implicated in the pathogenesis of AS and RA, and Th22 cells and Th17 cells may be reasonable cellular targets for therapeutic intervention.

**Editor:** Gernot Zissel, University Medical Center Freiburg, Germany

**Funding:** This study was partially supported by research funding from the National Natural Science Foundation (30600680, 81070407 and 30973018), the Shandong Technological Development Project (2005BS03022, Q2008C07, and BS2009SW014), and Graduate Independent Innovation Foundation of Shandong University, GIIFSDU (yzc21300071613082, yzc10147). (http://www.nsfc.gov.cn/Portal0/default152.htm) (http://www.art.sdu.edu.cn/2011/0321/931.html). The funders had no role in study design, data collection and analysis, decision to publish, or preparation of the manuscript.

**Competing Interests:** The authors have declared that no competing interests exist.

* E-mail: jianminli123456@163.com (J-mL); daoxinma@hotmail.com (D-xM)

○ These authors contributed equally to this work.

## Introduction

Ankylosing spondylitis (AS) is a chronic inammatory disease that is characterized by mainly involving bilateral sacroiliitis and axial joints, but sometimes peripheral joints and extra-articular organs are also involved [1]. Rheumatoid arthritis (RA), which represents an example of autoimmunity disease, is another form of arthritis. The abnormality of T cells is implicated in the pathogenesis of many autoimmune diseases, and many autoimmune diseases, especially arthritis, were considered to be mainly driven by Th1 cells [1–3]. A new IL-17-producing T cell subset, termed Th17 cells, has been described in recent years [4–7]. It has been established that Th17 cells play critical roles in several animal models of autoimmunity, such as experimental allergic encepha-

lomyelitis (EAE) [8] and murine arthritis models [9,10]. Besides, Th17 cells are considered to be involved in many human inflammatory diseases, including multiple sclerosis, psoriasis and inflammatory arthritis [11–15]. As to AS and RA, increased Th17 cells were found in PBMC from patients with AS and RA [16]. IL-17, secreted mainly by Th17 cells, is a cytokine shown to stimulate RA synovial fibroblast (RASF) to release several mediators of joint inflammation including IL-6, IL-8, GM-CSF and PGE2 [17–19]. Moreover, elevated serum levels of IL-17 and IL-23 has been reported in AS which is one of the forms of arthritis [20].

IL-22, a member of IL-10 cytokine family, exerts its effects via a heterodimeric transmembrane receptor complex consisting of IL-10R2 and IL-22R1 [21]. IL-22 has been believed as an important player in regulating inflammatory responses associated with many inflammatory diseases. Higher expression of IL-22 mRNA was observed in psoriatic skin lesion, and elevated serum IL-22 levels were found in patients with psoriasis [22]. In addition, the involvement of IL-22 in other inflammatory diseases such as inflammatory bowel disease [23] also proves its proinflammatory roles. However, diminishing intestinal inflammatory in a mouse model of ulcerative colitis and providing protection to hepatocytes during acute liver inflammation by IL-22 demonstrate its anti-inflammatory properties [24]. The situation of IL-22 was not completely consistent in autoimmune diseases. Consistent with psoriasis, increased IL-22 has also been found in serum samples from RA and Crohn disease patients. On the contrary, decreased plasma IL-22 levels were found in patients with SLE [25]. So, diverse pathogenic mechanisms and tissue microenvironments may result in different contributions of IL-22 in autoimmune disease development. The precise pathophysiologic function of IL-22 remains unclear, and the involvement of IL-22 in AS and RA remains to be established.

Th22 subset is a more recently identified new human T helper subset, which is characterized by abundant secretion of IL-22 but not IL-17 or IFN-$\gamma$ [26–28]. Th22 cells express the chemokine receptors CCR4, CCR6 and CCR10 [26]. Moreover, this newly identified CD4$^+$ T cells clones have low or undetectable expression of Th1 and Th17 transcription factor T-bet and ROR$\gamma$t, and arylhydrocarbon receptor (AHR) has been considered to be the key transcription factor of Th22 subset [26]. In addition, naïve T cells differentiate toward the Th22 phenotype in the presence of IL-6 and TNF-$\alpha$[26]. All of above provide strong evidence that Th22 cells represent an independent and terminally differentiated T cells subtype. It has been reported that Th22 cells were detected in psoriatic skin lesions. Moreover, the increasing circulating Th22 cells [29] suggest that Th22 cells may be implicated in the pathogenesis of psoriasis which is a chronic inammatory disease. In addition, elevated Th22 cells in peripheral blood of RA patients have also been reported in our previous study. Thus, the involvement of Th22 cells in other chronic inammatory diseases needs to be further investigated.

The roles of both Th22 cells and IL-22 in the pathogenesis of ankylosing spondylitis and rheumatoid arthritis are still unclear and remain to be clarified. Therefore, to investigate their roles in the pathogenesis of AS and RA, we examined the frequencies of Th22 cells in peripheral blood as well as the levels of plasma IL-22 of both AS and RA patients, and assayed their correlations with disease activity in this study.

## Materials and Methods

### Ethics Statement

Enrollment took place between May, 2010 and April, 2011 in two centers: Qilu Hospital, Shandong University and Shandong Provincial Hospital, Shandong University, China. Our research has been approved by both the Medical Ethical Committee of Qilu Hospital, Shandong University and the Medical Ethical Committee of Shandong Provincial Hospital, Shandong University. A written informed consent document has been obtained from each participant.

### Patients and Controls

A total of 32 patients with AS according to the modified New York criteria [30] ere recruited in this study. The Bath Ankylosing Spondylitis Disease Activity Index (BASDAI) score [31] were measured for the patients with AS. All patients were HLA-B27-positive. This group consisted of 27 men and 5 women, with mean ± SD disease duration of 8.6±5.9 years. The mean age of the

patients was 36.6±10.2 years. A total of 20 patients with active RA according to the criteria of the American College of Rheumatology were included in this study [32]. The DAS28 score [33] were measured for the patients with RA. This group consisted of 16 women and 4 men, with mean ± SD disease duration of 8.9±3.9 years. The mean age of the patients was 47.5±9.2 years. The demographic and key clinical information of AS and RA patients are summarized in Table 1 and Table 2. All of the patients did not receive immunosuppressive or immunomodulatory drugs for at least 2 months when sampling. The major previous treatment of AS and RA patients were shown in Table S1 and Table S2. Ten osteoarthritis (OA) patients (3 females and 7 males; mean age 48.9±10.3 years) as disease controls and twenty healthy controls (5 females and 15 males; mean age 37.9±9.1 years) were also recruited in the study, and all of them did not have any rheumatologic conditions.

### Flow Cytometric Analysis

Intracellular cytokines were studied by flow cytometry to reflex the cytokine-producing cells. Briefly, heparinized peripheral whole blood (400 μl) with an equal volume of Roswell Park Memorial Institute 1640 medium were incubated for 4 h at 37°C, 5% CO2 in the presence of 25 ng/mL of phorbol myristate acetate (PMA), 1 μg/mL of ionomycin, and 1.7 μg/ml Golgiplug(Monensin; all from Alexis Biochemicals, San Diego, CA, USA). PMA and ionomycin are pharmacological T-cell-activating agents that mimic signals generated by the T-cell receptor (TCR) complex and have the advantage of stimulating T cells of any antigen specificity. Monensin was used to block intracellular transport mechanisms, thereby leading to an accumulation of cytokines in the cells. After incubation, the cells were stained with PE-Cy5-conjugated anti-CD4 monoclonal antibodies (clone: RPA-T4, Cat: 45-0049-42) at room temperature in the dark for 20 min. The cells were next stained with FITC-conjugated anti-interferon (IFN)-$\gamma$ monoclonal antibodies (clone: 4S-BS, Cat: 11-7319-82), PE-conjugated anti-IL-17A monoclonal antibodies (clone: eBio64DEC17, Cat: 12-7179-42) and APC-conjugated anti-IL22 monoclonal antibodies (clone: 22URTI, Cat: 50-7229-42) after fixation and permeabilization. All the antibodies were from eBioscience, San Diego, CA, USA. Isotype controls were given to enable correct compensation and confirm antibody specificity. Stained cells were analyzed by flow cytometric analysis using a FACScan cytometer equipped with CellQuest software (BD Bioscience PharMingen). Th22, Th17, Th1 and Th1/Th17 cells

**Table 1.** Characteristics of the patients with Ankylosing Spondylitis.*

| Characteristics | value |
|---|---|
| Age(y) | 36.6±10.2 |
| Sex(male/female) | 27/5 |
| Disease duration(y) | 8.6±5.9 |
| ESR(mm/h) | 38.2±20.8 |
| ESR(mm/h) of Healthy Control | 9.5±4.2 |
| CRP(mg/L) | 24.9±13.7 |
| CRP(mg/L) of Healthy Control | 3.4±1.6 |
| BASDAI score | 3.2±1.7 |
| HLA-B27,positive member | 32 |

*BASDAI = Bath Ankylosing Spondylitis Disease Activity Index (range 0–10); ESR = erythrocyte sedimentation rate; CRP = C-reactive protein.

**Table 2.** Demographic and clinical characteristics of RA patients.*

| Characteristics | value |
|---|---|
| No. of patients | 20 |
| Age(y) | 47.5±9.2 |
| Sex(male/female) | 4/16 |
| Disease duration(y) | 8.9±3.9 |
| RF | 14/20(70%) |
| ESR(mm/h) | 35.8±27.9 |
| CRP(mg/L) | 27.1±23.3 |
| No. of swollen joints | 7.3±3.7 |
| No. of tender joints | 8.1±3.8 |
| DAS28 | 5.2±1.4 |

*RF = rheumatoid factor; ESR = erythrocyte sedimentation rate; CRP = C-reactive protein; DAS28 = Disease Activity Score in 28 joints.

were defined as $CD4^+IFN\gamma^-IL17^-IL-22^+$, $CD4^+IFN\gamma^-IL17^+$, $CD4^+IFN\gamma^+$ and $CD4^+IFN\gamma^+IL17^+$T cells respectively.

## IL-22 and IL-17 Enzyme-linked Immunosorbent Assay (ELISA)

Peripheral blood was collected into heparin-anticoagulant vacetainer tubes. Plasma was obtained from all subjects by centrifugation and stored at –80°C for determination of cytokines. Plasma IL-22 (Cat: BMS2047) and IL-17 (Cat: BMS2017) levels were determined with a quantitative sandwich enzyme immunoassay technique in accordance with the manufacturer's recommendations (lower detection limit 9 pg/ml; eBioscience).

## Clinical Assessment

BASDAI score of AS patients and disease activity score in 28-joints (DAS28) of RA patients was calculated in our study. At the time of clinical assessment for disease activity, blood samples were collected for the measurement of levels of C-reactive protein (CRP) and ESR.

## Statistical Analysis

Results were expressed as mean ± SD or median (range). Statistical significance of Th22, Th17, Th1 and plasma IL-22 as well as IL-17 among patients with AS, RA, OA and HC was determined by ANOVA, and difference between two groups was determined by Newman–Keuls multiple comparison test ($q$ test) unless the data were not normally distributed, in which case Kruskal - Wallis test ($H$ test) and Nemenyi test were used. The Pearson or Spearman correlation test was used for correlation analysis depending on data distribution. All tests were performed by SPSS 17.0 system. P value less than 0.05 was considered statistically significant.

## Results

### Elevated Th22 Cells Correlated with Increased Plasma Levels of IL-22 in AS and RA Patients

We analyzed the frequency of Th22 cells based on cytokine patterns after in vitro activation by PMA/ionomycin in short-term cultures. The expression of a typical dot-plot of Th22 cells in representative AS, RA as well as OA patients and healthy controls was shown in Fig. 1a. The percentage of Th22 cells was significantly

elevated in AS (1.27±0.42%) and RA (1.37±0.49%) patients compared to OA patients (0.70±0.19%) or healthy controls (0.68±0.18%) (Fig. 1b).

In addition, we also quantified the number of Th22 cells per volume (50µL) of peripheral blood. The number of Th22 cells was significantly increased in AS (204±34) and RA (211±43) patients compared with healthy controls (123±23) after stimulation with phorbol myristate acetate, ionomycin, and monensin for 4 h (Fig. S2a).

Plasma levels of IL-22 were examined by ELISA. The levels of IL-22 were significantly increased in AS (41.03±16.00pg/ml) and RA (44.53±29.84pg/ml) patients compared to OA patients (24.53±3.45pg/ml) and healthy controls (25.33±3.75pg/ml) (Fig. 2a).

A positive correlation was found between Th22 cells and plasma levels of IL-22 in AS (r = 0.743, P<0.001; Fig. 3a) and RA (r = 0.548, P = 0.027; Fig. 3b) patients. Moreover, positive correlations were also found between IL-22 plasma levels and Th17 cells (r = 0.587, P = 0.045; Fig. 3c) in AS patients. However, no corresponding correlation was found in RA patients (P = 0.801) (Fig. S1l).

### Elevated Th17 Cells in AS and RA Patients

The expression of a typical dot-plot of Th17 cells in representative AS, RA, OA patients and healthy controls was shown in Fig. 4a. We found significantly increased percentage of Th17 cells in AS (2.58±0.86%) and RA (2.57±0.72%) patients compared with OA patients (1.15±0.31%) and healthy controls (1.07±0.26%)(Fig. 4b). Consistently, the number of Th17 cells per volume (50µL) of peripheral blood was significantly increased in AS (320±36) and RA (337±39) patients compared with healthy controls (214±26) after stimulation with phorbol myristate acetate, ionomycin, and monensin for 4 h (Fig. S2b). However, there was no significant difference regarding plasma IL-17 between each group. (AS: 16.28±4.25, P>0.05; RA: 15.02±4.60, P>0.05; OA: 14.80±2.88, P>0.05; HC: 14.39±2.72, P>0.05) (Fig. 2b).

As to Th1 cells, there was no significant difference between each group. (AS: 11.05±3.41%, P>0.05; RA: 11.13±4.09%, P>0.05; OA:10.73±2.50%, P>0.05; HC:10.37±2.00, P>0.05) (Fig. 1a, b).

### Increased Expression of IL-17 and IL-22 Double-Positive CD4 T Cells as well as IL-17 and IFN-γ Double-Positive CD4 T Cells in AS and RA Patients

For these experiments, we also examined the frequencies of $CD4^+IFN\gamma^-IL17^+IL-22^+$ T cells and $CD4^+IFN\gamma^+IL17^+$ T cells. Though most Th17 cells did not simultaneously express both IL-22 and IL-17, the percentage of $CD4^+IFN\gamma^-IL17^+IL-22^+$ T cells was significantly increased in AS (0.63±0.34%)) and RA (0.65±0.29%) patients compared with OA patients (0.20±0.04%) and healthy controls (0.19±0.05%)(Fig. 1b). In addition, ratios of Th1/Th17 cells were significantly increased in AS patients (0.63±0.35%) and RA patients (0.66±0.21%) compared to OA patients (0.22±0.07%) and healthy controls (0.22±0.06%). (Fig. 4b).

### Correlation between Th22, Th17 and Th1 Cells in AS and RA Patients

In AS patients, there was a significant positive correlation between Th22 cells and Th17 cells (r = 0.676, P<0.001) (Fig. 5a). Similarly, a positive correlation was also found between Th22 cells and Th17 cells (r = 0.46, P = 0.041) in RA patients (Fig. 5b). However, Th1 cells failed to show a significant correlation with Th22 cells and Th17 cells.

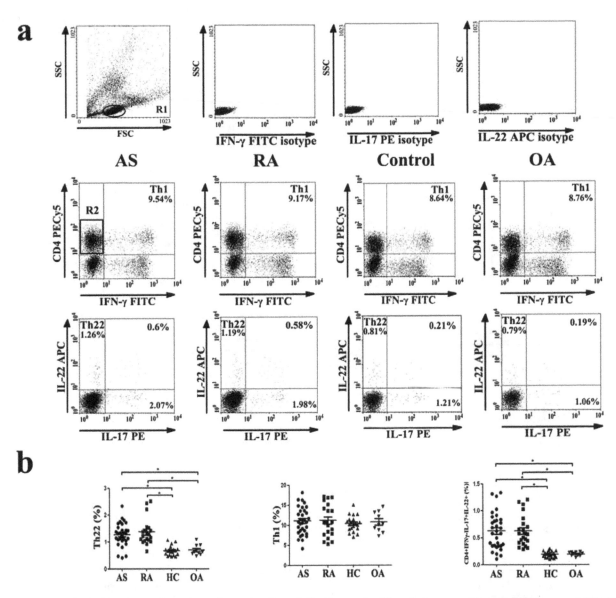

**Figure 1. Circulating Th22 cells and CD4⁺IFNγ⁻IL17⁺IL-22⁺ T cells are significantly increased in ankylosing spondylitis (AS) patients and rheumatoid arthritis (RA) patients compared with osteoarthritis (OA) patients and healthy controls. a,** Representative flow cytometry dot plots example of each group. **b,** The percentages of circulating Th22 cells (left panel), Th1 cells (middle panel) and CD4⁺IFNγ⁻IL17⁺IL-22⁺ T cells (right panel) from AS, RA, OA patients and healthy controls after stimulation with phorbol myristate acetate, ionomycin, and monensin for 4 h. (* = $P<0.05$).

## The Correlation of the Frequencies of Th22 Cells and Th17 Cells with Disease Activity or Laboratory Parameters in AS and RA Patients

In patients with RA, there were positive correlations between the percentage of Th22 cells and CRP level or DAS28 (r = 0.576, $P$ = 0.008 or r = 0.544, $P$ = 0.013 respectively) (Fig. 6 a, b). Consistently, positive correlations were also found between the percentage of Th17 cells (r = 0.709, $P<0.001$ or r = 0.706, $P<0.001$ respectively) (Fig. 6 c, d) and CRP level as well as DAS28. However, the percentage of Th1 cells was not correlated with either CRP level or DAS28 ($P$ = 0.105 or $P$ = 0.205), and plasma level of IL-22 or IL-17 failed to show a statistical correlation with CRP level or DAS28 ($P=0.622$ and $P$ = 0.357 or $P=0.317$ and $P=0.872$) in RA patients (Fig. S1j, k). In patients with AS, there was no correlation between the percentage of Th22

cells and clinical parameters, including ESR ($P=0.964$), CRP ($P=0.393$) and BASDAI score ($P=0.226$) (Fig. S1a, b, c). Consistently, no correlation was found between plasma level of IL-22 and clinical parameters in AS patients, including ESR ($P=0.918$), CRP ($P=0.862$) and BASDAI score ($P=0.320$) (Fig. S1g, h, i). Correlation analysis between the percentage of Th17 cells and clinical parameters also showed no association ($P=0.189$, $P=0.852$ and $P=0.733$ respectively) (Fig. S1d, e, f).

### Discussion

Th22 cells, a recently defined lineage of T cells distinct from Th1, Th2 and Th17 cells, have been believed to play a complicated and important role in inflammatory and autoimmune diseases. The function of Th22 cells is achieved through the signature cytokine they secreted. Th17 cells have already been

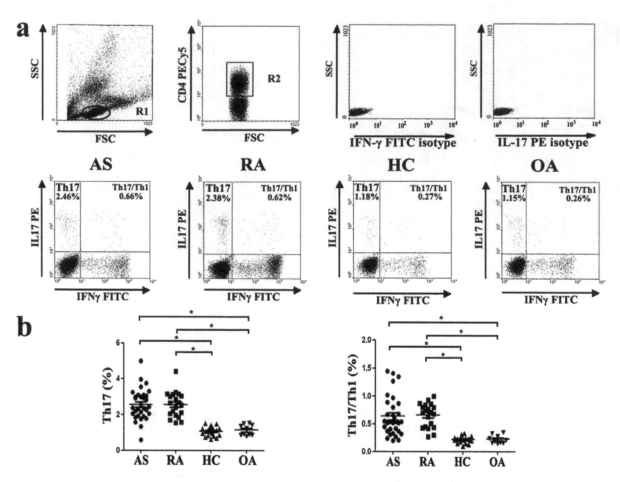

**Figure 2. Concentrations of IL-22 and IL-17 in plasma of non-stimulated peripheral blood from AS, RA, OA patients and healthy controls. a,** Concentrations of IL-22 in plasma from AS, RA, OA patients and healthy controls. The levels of IL-22 was significantly increased in AS and RA patients compared with OA patients or healthy controls. **b,** Concentrations of IL-17 in plasma from AS, RA, OA patients and healthy controls. As to IL-17, there was no significant difference between AS or RA patients and OA as well as healthy controls (* = $P < 0.05$).

proposed to be the primary driver of autoimmune diseases, including rheumatoid arthritis. However, the potential role of Th22 cells in inflammatory arthritis such as AS and RA is far from clear.

To determine whether Th22 is involved in AS and RA, the percentages of Th22 cells were examined in the peripheral blood of patients with AS, RA OA, and healthy controls in this study. This is the first study that evaluates the relative abundance of

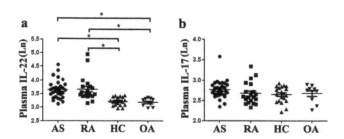

**Figure 3. Correlation between the percentages of each T cell subset and the plasma IL-22 concentrations in AS or RA patients. a and b,** Positive correlation was found between Th22 cells and IL-22 in AS (**a**) and RA (**b**) patients. **c,** Positive correlation was found between Th17 cells and IL-22 in AS patients.

Th22 cells in peripheral blood of RA and AS patients. Our results demonstrated that the percentages of Th22 cells were significantly elevated in the peripheral blood of patients with AS and also in those with RA compared with OA patients and healthy controls, which was consistent with our previous experiments on RA [34]. Moreover, we also quantified the number of Th22 cells in per volume blood. Consistent with the results of the percentage, the number of Th22 cells in per volume of blood was significantly increased in AS and RA patients compared to healthy controls. Likewise, increased Th22 cells has been observed in peripheral blood of patients with psoriasis [29], which implicating the involvement of Th22 cells in the chronic inflammatory skin disorder. These observations are compatible with the idea that Th22 cells may contribute to the pathogenesis of both RA and AS, which are two types of inflammatory arthritis. In the present study, correlation was also found between levels of Th22 cells and disease activity as assessed by DAS28 or the CRP concentration in RA. However, such correlation was not observed in AS. The possible explanation for this inconsistency between AS and RA is that many patients with AS do not have elevated CRP or ESR levels, so it is more difficult to assess disease activity in AS. It is known that Th17 cells are enriched in the joints of RA patients and co-express the chemokine receptor CCR6 and CCR4 [35]. Besides, CCL20 [36] as well as CCL22 [37], the ligand of CCR6 and CCR4 respectively, have already been observed in synovial fluid of

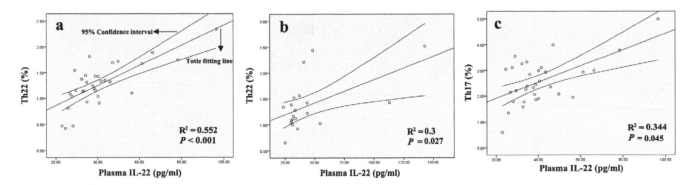

**Figure 4. Circulating Th17 cells and Th17/Th1 cells are significantly increased in ankylosing spondylitis (AS) patients and rheumatoid arthritis (RA) patients compared with osteoarthritis (OA) patients and healthy controls. a,** Representative flow cytometry dot plots example of each group. **b,** The percentages of circulating Th17 cells (left panel) and Th17/Th1 cells (right panel) from AS, RA, OA patients and healthy controls after stimulation with phorbol myristate acetate, ionomycin, and monensin for 4 h (* = *P*<0.05).

human. Thus, all signs indicate that the interaction between receptor and ligand may play an important role in attracting Th17 cells to the joints in RA. Similar to Th17 cells, Th22 cells also co-express the chemokine receptor CCR6 and CCR4. So, we can reasonable believe that Th22 cells might selectively migrate to the joints from peripheral blood in the similar way. Moreover, we also speculated that Th22 cells might be elevated in the joints of RA and AS patients, which could play a pathogenic role in the lesions. Otherwise, what the pathogenic role does the Th22 cells play in AS and RA when migrating to the lesion remain to be elucidated. Then, we would focus our further investigation on the involvement of this new subset in synovial fluid of patients' joints.

IL-22, a cytokine of IL-10 family, is the most important functional cytokine of Th22 cells. Considerable evidence suggests that IL-22 may be involved in the pathogenesis of many inflammatory diseases, but its pathophysiologic function is not well known. To investigate the potential role of IL-22 in AS and RA patients, we examined the concentrations of plasma IL-22 in our experiments. In line with our previous study, elevated levels of plasma IL-22 were also detected in AS and RA patients in the present study, implicating that IL-22 may be involved in the pathogenesis of both AS and RA. IL-22 has been demonstrated to

exert its biological effects via binding to the heterodimeric receptor complex, including IL-22R1 and IL-10R2, and IL-22 activates Jak1 and Tyk2, which further activates STAT-1, STAT-3 and STAT-5 [38]. It has already been reported that IL-22R1 mRNA was expressed in RA synovial tissue. In addition, activation of ERK-1/2 as wells as p38 MAPK by IL-22 has also been reported in RA [39]. In vitro, recombinant IL-22 promoted proliferation of synovial fibroblasts of RA patients (RASF) and increased production of monocyte chemoattractant protein 1 (MCP-1) by RASF. Thus, we speculated the similar effect of IL-22 in AS patients as in RA patients. More recently, IL-22 serum levels were demonstrated to be associated with radiographic progression in rheumatoid arthritis [40], which further improved the importance of IL-22 in chronic inflammatory arthritis. In our study, plasma IL-22 levels correlated positively with Th22 cells in both AS patients and RA patients. In addition, correlation between plasma IL-22 level and Th17 cells were observed in AS patients. By contrast, no association of plasma IL-22 levels with Th17 cells was found in RA patients. Th22 cells, Th17 cells and Th1 cells are the main T cells subsets secreting IL22 [41,26,28,42]. The correlation between Th17 cells and IL-22 in AS supported the idea that Th17 subset was an important T cells subset secreting IL-22 in

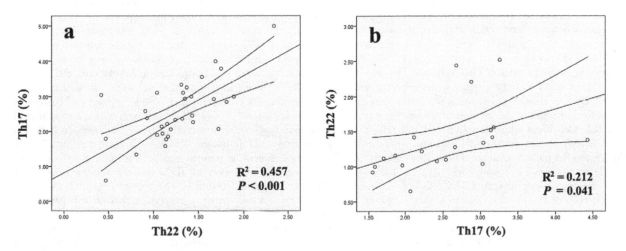

**Figure 5. Correlation between the percentages of Th22 cells and the percentages of Th17 cells in AS and RA patients. a,** Positive correlation was found between Th22 cells and Th17 cells in AS patients. **b,** Positive correlation was found between Th22 cells and Th17 cells in RA patients.

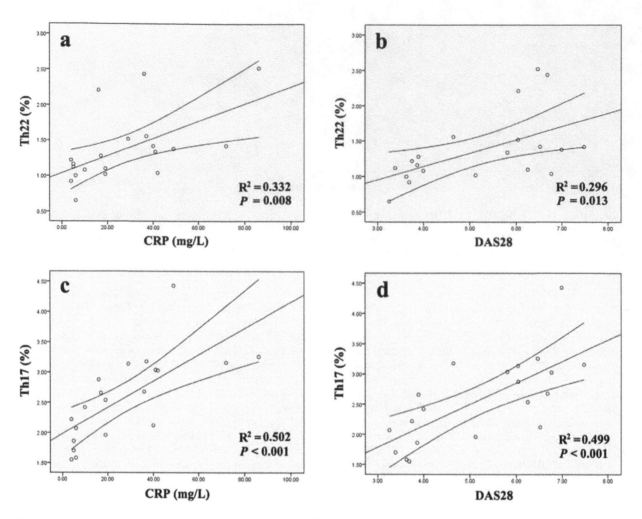

**Figure 6. Correlation between the percentages of Th22 cells as well as Th17 cells and CRP levels as well as DAS28.**

peripheral blood of AS patients. Otherwise, no correlations in RA patients suggested that Th22 cells may produced much greater portion of total IL-22, and Th17 cells may produced a relatively smaller portion of total IL-22 in peripheral blood of RA patients than AS patients. So far, the pathophysiologic role of IL-22 in both AS and RA is not fully understood and need further investigation.

Considerable evidence suggests Th17 cells and Th1 cells have been involved in the development of autoimmune diseases [43,44]. Thus, we examined the frequencies of Th17 cells and Th1 cells in each group in this experiment. In consistence with the experiment of Hui *et al* [16], the percentages of Th17 cells were demonstrated to be significantly increased in the peripheral blood of patients with AS and RA. Consistent with the results of Th22 cells, the number of Th17 cells in per volume of blood was significantly increased in AS and RA patients compared to healthy controls. In contrast to the results for Th17 and Th22 cell, no statistical difference was detected in percentages of Th1 cells between each group. Our observations supported the idea that Th17 cells contributed to the pathogenesis of AS and RA. Furthermore, we also examined the correlation between disease activity of AS or RA and the percentages Th17 cells. Like Th22 cells, there was a positive correlation between disease activity and Th17 in RA patients but not in AS patients. This inconsistent results between T cells and disease activity in AS is unclear, and needs further study. In this study, a positive correlation was found between the

frequencies Th22 cells and Th17 cells in peripheral blood of patients with both AS and RA. This co-elevated level of Th22 cells and Th17 cells suggests these two T cell subsets may play a synergistic role in AS and RA, and the specific links between Th22 cells and Th17 cells need further investigation.

IL-17, the main cytokine of Th17 cells, contributes to the pathogenesis of arthritis as has been demonstrated in many experimental arthritis models. Although elevated levels of IL-17 have been observed in synovial fluid of RA patients, the levels of this T cell cytokine in plasma of these patients is hard to detect. Furthermore, the reports on IL-17 levels in plasma of RA or AS patients are inconsistent [35,20]. The levels of IL-17 in plasma of each group were also measured in this experiment. In line with recent report [35], plasma IL-17 levels were not significantly different between the patients and healthy controls in our study. Moreover, the situation of IL-17 in autoimmune diseases is different. Increased levels of IL-17 have been shown in the serum of systemic sclerosis patients, but not in that of SLE patients or healthy controls.

In humans, it is not unusual to encounter dual +Th1/Th17 cells. It has previously been demonstrated that T cells from synovial fluid of RA can co-express IL-17 and IFN-γ [45], and both IL-17 and IFN-γ can be secreted by T cells derived from the joints [46]. In addition, IL-17 and IFN-γ cytokines have been shown to be co-expressed in human memory CD4+CD45+RO+ T cells from treatment-naïve early RA patients [47]. So we examined the percentages of Th17/Th1 cells. Consistent with a recent report in psoriasis [29], Th17/Th1 cells were increased in peripheral blood of AS and RA compared with OA and healthy controls. However, cells secreting IFN-γ alone were much more than those secreting IL-17 after stimulating with PMA and ionomycin; therefore, the contribution by Th17 cells to total IFN-γ secretion would be very low. Because Th17 cells also produced IL-22, Th17 cells that were positive for IL-22 were examined in this study. It has been shown that IL-22-positive Th17 cells were only observed in human but not in mouse [48]. In this experiment, increasing percentages of CD4+IL-22+IL-17+IFNγ- T cells were detected in peripheral blood from AS and RA patients compared to OA patients and healthy controls. Our results were in line with the study of Colin *et al* [47], which demonstrated increased percentages of IL-17+ and IL-22+CD4+ T cells in PBMCs from treatment-naïve patients with early RA. IL-22 production by Th17 cells has been demonstrated to be dependent on IL-23 [49], and elevated serum IL-23 level was detected in the patients with AS [20]. Our data suggest that the tendency to develop both CD4+IL-22+IL-17+IFNγ- T cells and Th1/Th17 cells may be a common immunologic characteristic shown in AS and RA patients.

In conclusion, our experiments showed that the frequencies of Th22 cells and Th17 cells were significantly increased in AS and RA patients compared to OA patients and healthy controls. Plasma IL-22 levels, which correlated positively with Th22 cells, were also demonstrated to be elevated in both AS and RA patients. The increasing percentages of Th22 cells and Th17 cells and the elevation of IL-22 may play important roles in the pathogenesis of AS and RA. Thus, Th22 cells and IL-22 as well as Th17 cells may prove to be a promising therapeutic targets for AS and RA. Further studies are awaited to clarify the pathophysiologic role of Th22 in AS and RA and determine the situation of Th22 cells in AS and RA patients' joints.

## References

1. Mosmann TR, Coffman RL (1989) TH1 and TH2 cells: different patterns of lymphokine secretion lead to different functional properties. Annu Rev Immunol 7: 145–173.
2. Dolhain RJ, van der Heiden AN, ter Haar NT, Breedveld FC, Miltenburg AM (1996) Shift toward T lymphocytes with a T helper 1 cytokine-secretion profile in the joints of patients with rheumatoid arthritis. Arthritis Rheum 39: 1961–1969.
3. Wedderburn LR, Robinson N, Patel A, Varsani H, Woo P (2000) Selective recruitment of polarized T cells expressing CCR5 and CXCR3 to the inflamed joints of children with juvenile idiopathic arthritis. Arthritis Rheum 43: 765–774.
4. Mangan PR, Harrington LE, O'Quinn DB, Helms WS, Bullard DC, et al. (2006) Transforming growth factor-beta induces development of the T(H)17 lineage. Nature 441: 231–234.
5. Harrington LE, Hatton RD, Mangan PR, Turner H, Murphy TL, et al. (2005) Interleukin 17-producing CD4+ effector T cells develop via a lineage distinct from the T helper type 1 and 2 lineages. Nat Immunol 6: 1123–1132.
6. Park H, Li Z, Yang XO, Chang SH, Nurieva R, et al. (2005) A distinct lineage of CD4 T cells regulates tissue inflammation by producing interleukin 17. Nat Immunol 6: 1133–1141.
7. Bettelli E, Korn T, Oukka M, Kuchroo VK (2008) Induction and effector functions of T(H)17 cells. Nature 453: 1051–1057.
8. Cua DJ, Sherlock J, Chen Y, Murphy CA, Joyce B, et al. (2003) Interleukin-23 rather than interleukin-12 is the critical cytokine for autoimmune inflammation of the brain. Nature 421: 744–748.
9. Murphy CA, Langrish CL, Chen Y, Blumenschein W, McClanahan T, et al. (2003) Divergent pro- and antiinflammatory roles for IL-23 and IL-12 in joint autoimmune inflammation. J Exp Med 198: 1951–1957.
10. Hirota K, Hashimoto M, Yoshitomi H, Tanaka S, Nomura T, et al. (2007) T cell self-reactivity forms a cytokine milieu for spontaneous development of IL-17+ Th cells that cause autoimmune arthritis. J Exp Med 204: 41–47.
11. Kebir H, Kreymborg K, Ifergan I, Dodelet-Devillers A, Cayrol R, et al. (2007) Human TH17 lymphocytes promote blood-brain barrier disruption and central nervous system inflammation. Nat Med 13: 1173–1175.
12. Fitch E, Harper E, Skorcheva I, Kurtz SE, Blauvelt A (2007) Pathophysiology of psoriasis: recent advances on IL-23 and Th17 cytokines. Curr Rheumatol Rep 9: 461–467.
13. Schmechel S, Konrad A, Diegelmann J, Glas J, Wetzke M, et al. (2008) Linking genetic susceptibility to Crohn's disease with Th17 cell function: IL-22 serum levels are increased in Crohn's disease and correlate with disease activity and IL23R genotype status. Inflamm Bowel Dis 14: 204–212.
14. Miossec P (2007) Interleukin-17 in fashion, at last: ten years after its description, its cellular source has been identified. Arthritis Rheum 56: 2111–2115.
15. Gaston JS (2008) Cytokines in arthritis--the 'big numbers' move centre stage. Rheumatology (Oxford) 47: 8–12.
16. Shen H, Goodall JC, Hill Gaston JS (2009) Frequency and phenotype of peripheral blood Th17 cells in ankylosing spondylitis and rheumatoid arthritis. Arthritis Rheum 60: 1647–1656.
17. Chabaud M, Durand JM, Buchs N, Fossiez F, Page G, et al. (1999) Human interleukin-17: A T cell-derived proinflammatory cytokine produced by the rheumatoid synovium. Arthritis Rheum 42: 963–970.
18. Miossec P (2003) Interleukin-17 in rheumatoid arthritis: if T cells were to contribute to inflammation and destruction through synergy. Arthritis Rheum 48: 594–601.
19. Parsonage G, Filer A, Bik M, Hardie D, Lax S, et al. (2008) Prolonged, granulocyte-macrophage colony-stimulating factor-dependent, neutrophil survival following rheumatoid synovial fibroblast activation by IL-17 and TNFalpha. Arthritis Res Ther 10: R47.
20. Mei Y, Pan F, Gao J, Ge R, Duan Z, et al. (2011) Increased serum IL-17 and IL-23 in the patient with ankylosing spondylitis. Clin Rheumatol 30: 269–273.
21. Renauld JC (2003) Class II cytokine receptors and their ligands: key antiviral and inflammatory modulators. Nat Rev Immunol 3: 667–676.
22. Lo YH, Torii K, Saito C, Furuhashi T, Maeda A, et al. (2010) Serum IL-22 correlates with psoriatic severity and serum IL-6 correlates with susceptibility to phototherapy. J Dermatol Sci 58: 225–227.
23. Brand S, Beigel F, Olszak T, Zitzmann K, Eichhorst ST, et al. (2006) IL-22 is increased in active Crohn's disease and promotes proinflammatory gene

## Supporting Information

**Figure S1 a, b and c,** No positive correlations were found between the percentage of Th22 cells and ESR, CRP as well as BASDAI in AS patients. d, e and f, No positive correlations were found between the percentage of Th17 cells and ESR, CRP as well as BASDAI in AS patients. **g, h and i,** No positive correlations were found between the levels of plasma IL-22 and ESR, CRP as well as BASDAI in AS patients. **j and k,** No positive correlations were found between the levels of plasma IL-22 and CRP as well as DAS28 in RA patients. **i,** No positive correlation was found between the levels of plasma IL-22 and the percentage of Th17 cells in RA patients.

**Figure S2** The number of Th22 cells and Th17 cells in per volume of peripheral blood in AS patients, RA patients and healthy controls. **a,** The number of Th22 cells was significantly increased in AS and RA patients compared with healthy controls after stimulation with phorbol myristate acetate, ionomycin, and monensin for 4 h. **b,** The number of Th17 cells was significantly increased in AS and RA patients compared with healthy controls after stimulation with phorbol myristate acetate, ionomycin, and monensin for 4 h. (* = $P<0.05$)

**Table S1**   Major previous treatment of each patient of AS*

**Table S2**   Major previous treatment of each patient of RA*

## Author Contributions

Conceived and designed the experiments: JL LZ DM YgL YhL. Performed the experiments: NH QY ZL WL LQ. Analyzed the data: CY LZ XL. Contributed reagents/materials/analysis tools: XL LZ WL. Wrote the paper: JL LZ YgL.

expression and intestinal epithelial cell migration. Am J Physiol Gastrointest Liver Physiol 290: G827–838.

24. Zenewicz LA, Yancopoulos GD, Valenzuela DM, Murphy AJ, Karow M, et al. (2007) Interleukin-22 but not interleukin-17 provides protection to hepatocytes during acute liver inflammation. Immunity 27: 647–659.

25. Cheng F, Guo Z, Xu H, Yan D, Li Q (2009) Decreased plasma IL22 levels, but not increased IL17 and IL23 levels, correlate with disease activity in patients with systemic lupus erythematosus. Ann Rheum Dis 68: 604–606.

26. Duhen T, Geiger R, Jarrossay D, Lanzavecchia A, Sallusto F (2009) Production of interleukin 22 but not interleukin 17 by a subset of human skin-homing memory T cells. Nat Immunol 10: 857–863.

27. Eyerich S, Eyerich K, Pennino D, Carbone T, Nasorri F, et al. (2009) Th22 cells represent a distinct human T cell subset involved in epidermal immunity and remodeling. J Clin Invest 119: 3573–3585.

28. Trifari S, Kaplan CD, Tran EH, Crellin NK, Spits H (2009) Identification of a human helper T cell population that has abundant production of interleukin 22 and is distinct from T(H)-17, T(H)1 and T(H)2 cells. Nat Immunol 10: 864–871.

29. Kagami S, Rizzo HL, Lee JJ, Koguchi Y, Blauvelt A (2010) Circulating Th17, Th22, and Th1 cells are increased in psoriasis. J Invest Dermatol 130: 1373–1383.

30. van der Linden S, Valkenburg HA, Cats A (1984) Evaluation of diagnostic criteria for ankylosing spondylitis. A proposal for modification of the New York criteria. Arthritis Rheum 27: 361–368.

31. Garrett S, Jenkinson T, Kennedy LG, Whitelock H, Gaisford P, et al. (1994) A new approach to defining disease status in ankylosing spondylitis: the Bath Ankylosing Spondylitis Disease Activity Index. J Rheumatol 21: 2286–2291.

32. Arnett FC, Edworthy SM, Bloch DA, McShane DJ, Fries JF, et al. (1988) The American Rheumatism Association 1987 revised criteria for the classification of rheumatoid arthritis. Arthritis Rheum 31: 315–324.

33. Prevoo ML, van't Hof MA, Kuper HH, van Leeuwen MA, van de Putte LB, et al. (1995) Modified disease activity scores that include twenty-eight-joint counts. Development and validation in a prospective longitudinal study of patients with rheumatoid arthritis. Arthritis Rheum 38: 44–48.

34. Zhang L, Li JM, Liu XG, Ma DX, Hu NW, et al. (2011) Elevated Th22 cells correlated with Th17 cells in patients with rheumatoid arthritis. J Clin Immunol 31: 606–614.

35. Leipe J, Grunke M, Dechant C, Reindl C, Kerzendorf U, et al. (2010) Role of Th17 cells in human autoimmune arthritis. Arthritis Rheum 62: 2876–2885.

36. Hirota K, Yoshitomi H, Hashimoto M, Maeda S, Teradaira S, et al. (2007) Preferential recruitment of CCR6-expressing Th17 cells to inflamed joints via CCL20 in rheumatoid arthritis and its animal model. J Exp Med 204: 2803–2812.

37. Flytlie HA, Hvid M, Lindgreen E, Kofod-Olsen E, Petersen EL, et al. (2010) Expression of MDC/CCL22 and its receptor CCR4 in rheumatoid arthritis, psoriatic arthritis and osteoarthritis. Cytokine 49: 24–29.

38. Lejeune D, Dumoutier L, Constantinescu S, Kruijer W, Schuringa JJ, et al. (2002) Interleukin-22 (IL-22) activates the JAK/STAT, ERK, JNK, and p38 MAP kinase pathways in a rat hepatoma cell line. Pathways that are shared with and distinct from IL-10. J Biol Chem 277: 33676–33682.

39. Ikeuchi H, Kuroiwa T, Hiramatsu N, Kaneko Y, Hiromura K, et al. (2005) Expression of interleukin-22 in rheumatoid arthritis: potential role as a proinflammatory cytokine. Arthritis Rheum 52: 1037–1046.

40. Leipe J, Schramm MA, Grunke M, Baeuerle M, Dechant C, et al. (2011) Interleukin 22 serum levels are associated with radiographic progression in rheumatoid arthritis. Ann Rheum Dis 70: 1453–1457.

41. Wolk K, Kunz S, Asadullah K, Sabat R (2002) Cutting edge: immune cells as sources and targets of the IL-10 family members? J Immunol 168: 5397–5402.

42. Volpe E, Servant N, Zollinger R, Bogiatzi SI, Hupe P, et al. (2008) A critical function for transforming growth factor-beta, interleukin 23 and proinflammatory cytokines in driving and modulating human T(H)-17 responses. Nat Immunol 9: 650–657.

43. Shahrara S, Huang Q, Mandelin AM, 2nd, Pope RM (2008) TH-17 cells in rheumatoid arthritis. Arthritis Res Ther 10: R93.

44. Bettelli E, Oukka M, Kuchroo VK (2007) T(H)-17 cells in the circle of immunity and autoimmunity. Nat Immunol 8: 345–350.

45. Lubberts E, Joosten LA, Oppers B, van den Bersselaar L, Coenen-de Roo CJ, et al. (2001) IL-1-independent role of IL-17 in synovial inflammation and joint destruction during collagen-induced arthritis. J Immunol 167: 1004–1013.

46. Lubberts E, Koenders MI, Oppers-Walgreen B, van den Bersselaar L, Coenen-de Roo CJ, et al. (2004) Treatment with a neutralizing anti-murine interleukin-17 antibody after the onset of collagen-induced arthritis reduces joint inflammation, cartilage destruction, and bone erosion. Arthritis Rheum 50: 650–659.

47. Colin EM, Asmawidjaja PS, van Hamburg JP, Mus AM, van Driel M, et al. (2010) 1,25-dihydroxyvitamin D3 modulates Th17 polarization and interleukin-22 expression by memory T cells from patients with early rheumatoid arthritis. Arthritis Rheum 62: 132–142.

48. Okey AB, Franc MA, Moffat ID, Tijet N, Boutros PC, et al. (2005) Toxicological implications of polymorphisms in receptors for xenobiotic chemicals: the case of the aryl hydrocarbon receptor. Toxicol Appl Pharmacol 207: 43–51.

49. Zheng Y, Danilenko DM, Valdez P, Kasman I, Eastham-Anderson J, et al. (2007) Interleukin-22, a T(H)17 cytokine, mediates IL-23-induced dermal inflammation and acanthosis. Nature 445: 648–651.

# 3

# Both Baseline Clinical Factors and Genetic Polymorphisms Influence the Development of Severe Functional Status in Ankylosing Spondylitis

**Ruxandra Schiotis[1,2]\*, Nerea Bartolomé[3], Alejandra Sánchez[4], Magdalena Szczypiorska[3], Jesús Sanz[4], Eduardo Cuende[5], Eduardo Collantes Estevez[2], Antonio Martínez[3], Diego Tejedor[3], Marta Artieda[3], Anca Buzoianu[6], Juan Mulero[4]**

1 Department of Pharmacology, "Iuliu Hatieganu" University of Medicine and Pharmacy and SCBI- Rheumatology Department, Cluj-Napoca, Romania, 2 Department of Rheumatology, University Hospital "Reina Sofía"/IMIBIC, Córdoba, Spain, 3 Department of R+D, Progenika Biopharma SA, Derio-Vizcaya, Spain, 4 Department of Rheumatology, "Puerta de Hierro Majadahonda", University Hospital, Madrid, Spain, 5 Department of Rheumatology, University Hospital "Príncipe de Asturias", Alcalá de Henares, Madrid, Spain, 6 Department of Pharmacology, "Iuliu Hatieganu" University of Medicine and Pharmacy, Cluj-Napoca, Romania

## Abstract

Functional severity in ankylosing spondylitis (AS) patients is variable and difficult to predict early. The aim of our study was to assess whether a combination of baseline clinical factors and genetic markers may predict the development of severe functional status in AS. We performed a cross-sectional association study on AS patients included in the Spanish National Registry of Spondyloarthropathies—REGISPONSER. Bath Ankylosing Spondylitis Functional Index (BASFI) was standardized by adjusting for disease duration since the first symptoms (BASFI/t). We considered as severe functional status the values of BASFI/t in the top of the 60th (p60), 65th (p65), 70th (p70), and 75th (p75) percentile. We selected 384 single nucleotide polymorphisms (SNPs) distributed in 190 genes to be analyzed. The study cohort included 456 patients with mean age 50.8($\pm$10.5) years and with mean disease duration since first symptoms 24.7 ($\pm$10.1) years. Older age at disease onset and neck pain at baseline showed statistical significant association with severe BASFI/t. Polymorphisms associated in the allele frequencies test with severe BASFI/t in all classifications were: *rs2542151* (p60 [$P=.04$], p65 [$P=.04$], p70 [$P=.001$] and p75 [$P=.001$]) and *rs2254441* (p60 [$P=.004$], p65 [$P=.02$], p70 [$P=.01$] and p75 [$P<.001$]).. Genotype association, after adjustment for covariates, found an association in three of the four patients' classifications for rs2542151 and in two of the classifications for rs2254441.Forward logistic regression did not identify any model with a good predictive power for severe functional development.  In our study we identified clinical factors and 24 polymorphisms associated with development of severe functional status in AS patients. Validation of these results in other cohorts is required.

**Editor:** Amr H. Sawalha, University of Michigan, United States of America

**Funding:** This work was supported by the Ministerio de Ciencia e Innovación of Spain [Proyect PSE-01000-2006-1] and by Progenika Biopharma S.A. The funders had no role in study design, data collection and analysis, decision to publish, or preparation of the manuscript.

**Competing Interests:** The authors declare the following interests: M.S., N.B., M.A., A.M. and D.T. are currently employees of Progenika Biopharma, SA. A.S. is supported by an unrestricted grant from Pfizer. All other authors have declared no conflicts of interest.

\* E-mail: Elena.Schiotis@umfcluj.ro

## Introduction

Ankylosing spondylitis (AS) is a chronic progressive inflammatory disease affecting the spine and peripheral joints. It is largely confirmed that susceptibility to AS is genetically determined with *HLA-B27* as a major genetic contributor to the disease [1–3] and that environmental factors also play a role in susceptibility to the disease. In the last few years, several other genes have been reported to be involved in AS susceptibility [4–9].

Although the assessment of physical function is only one of several aspects of assessing disease severity, it is one of the most important measures of structural damage outcome in AS, as it directly influences the quality of life of patients and the economic costs of the disease [10–11]. Impairment of physical function can be subdivided into a reversible and an irreversible component. In this concept the reversible component is due to disease activity (signs and symptoms of the disease) and the irreversible component

is due to structural damage that has occurred as a consequence of the disease, such as syndesmophytes and vertebral bridging. Functional severity was found to be independently determined by both the reversible factors such as disease activity and the irreversible factors such as structural damage [12] but the loss of functional capacity in each patient was not predictable from early disease stages [13].

There is evidence that several clinical parameters such as hip involvement, disease duration, erythrocyte sedimentation rate (ESR), C-reactive protein (CRP) levels, smoking, and lower socioeconomic status are associated with worse function [13–14]. Nevertheless, much of the variability in disease functional severity in AS remains unexplained, suggesting that genetic factors could have a greater influence than environmental factors on AS progression [13].

A genetic component has been demonstrated for AS functional severity [15]. However, very little is known about the specific genes or genetic markers inside and outside the major histocompatibility gene complex (MHC) involved in the functional component of the disease [16–20].

Understanding the genetic basis of functional severity in AS would be of major value to differentiate at early stages patients at high risk of severe functional impairment and patients with a lower risk. Thus, clinicians could better select and optimize the preventive and therapeutic approach for each patient as of the time of diagnosis of the disease by objectively distributing high cost treatments.

Taking into consideration the fact that impairment of physical function may be partially controlled by the appropriate treatment, the aim of our study was to identify the baseline clinical and genetic factors that determine individual development of functional severity in AS.

## Materials and Methods

### Patients with AS

We performed a cross-sectional association study on Spanish AS patients which were recruited from 25 hospitals which participated in the Spanish National Spondyloarthropathies Registry (REGIS-PONSER) [21]. Patients fulfilled the modified New York Criteria for AS [22] and had at least 10 years of follow-up from the first symptoms of the disease. Baseline characteristics of the patients at the beginning of the disease were recorded as potential prognostic predictors. Specifically, clinical and demographic data, sex, age at disease onset, family history of spondyloarthropathies (SpA), initial symptoms of SpA (inflammatory low back pain, neck pain, enthesitis, dactylitis, tarsitis, sacroiliac syndrome, coxitis, lower limb arthritis, and upper limb arthritis), and the number of initial SpA symptoms.

### Demographic and clinical characteristics of the AS population

The studied cohort included 456 AS patients (348 males and 108 females) with a mean age of 50.8±10.5 years, 26.1±9.1 years at disease onset and 34.6±11.4 years at diagnosis. The average time of evolution, from disease onset, was 24.7±10.1 years. *HLA-B27* was positive in 84.9% of the patients and 19.3% had a family history of spondyloarthropathies (SpA). Patients had mean BASFI at baseline 4.0±2.8, with mean BASFI/t (years) of 0.17±0.13.

### Functional phenotype

To measure functional impairment we used the BASFI score, standardized by adjusting for disease duration since first symptoms, denominated here BASFI/t. BASFI is a validated index that focuses on 10 questions pertaining to function, measured on a visual analog scale (VAS). The mean of the 10 questions generates the score, with 10 denoting worst possible functional status [23].

There are no validated threshold values for classifying AS patients into mild or severe categories according to their BASFI score standardized by disease duration (BASFI/t). Therefore, to define functional severity we performed four association analyses using the $\chi$2-test with different criteria. Based on the opinion of the clinicians who participated in this study, who estimated that approximately 25% to 40% of AS patients had severe functional damage, we defined as severe functional status the values of BASFI/t in the top 60th (p60), 65th (p65), 70th (p70) or 75th (p75) percentiles. The cut-off values for BASFI/t severe phenotype for each percentile were: 0.19 for p60, 0.21 for p65, 0.22 for p70, and 0.25 for p75 respectively.

### HLA-B27 typing and SNP genotyping

Genomic DNA was isolated from saliva samples using the Oragene™ DNA Self-Collection kit (DNA Genotek Inc., Ottawa, Canada), according to the manufacturer's extraction protocol. All samples were tested for the presence of the HLA-B27 allele by conventional PCR using the primers reported by Olerup et al [24]. A region of 236 bp on exon 8 from the p53 gene was used as an internal control for the performance of the PCR [25].

After an extensive bibliographic search we selected 384 SNPs distributed in 190 genes to be analyzed in this study. We selected all the SNPs previously reported in Caucasians as associated with AS or with other SpA (psoriatic arthritis, juvenile idiopathic arthritis, reactive arthritis, undifferentiated arthritis, and inflammatory bowel disease–associated spondyloarthropathy). Besides those SNPs, we included some SNPs in genes described in the literature as associated to other autoimmune diseases and to bone-related disorders, since we considered them as potential candidates to be implicated in AS severity. Finally, we included tag SNPs in genes from the metabolic pathways of the two most important genes considered to be involved in AS: ERAP1 and IL-23R. The tag SNPs were selected from the HapMap CEU panel (the minor allele frequency at each locus was required to be >0.05 in Caucasian population, with an r2-value of <0.8 between adjacent markers). SNP genotyping was performed using the Illumina Golden gate genotyping platform (Illumina, Inc., San Diego, CA, USA) [26].

### Statistical analysis

Statistical analysis was performed with SPSS v 15.0 (SPSS, Chicago, IL, USA) and SVS v 7.3.1 (Golden Helix Inc., Bozeman, Montana, USA) softwares.

All quantitative data are presented as mean and standard deviation (± SD) and all qualitative data as absolute frequencies and percentages. To assess the association between clinical variables and BASFI/t severe phenotype an unvaried analysis was performed using the chi-square ($\chi$2) test for categorical variables and the unpaired $t$ test for continuous variables.

A test for deviation from Hardy-Weinberg equilibrium (HWE) was performed for each SNP. Pruning of the initial genotype dataset with default parameters (exclusion of SNPs with poor genotype cloud clustering, of SNPs with call-rate <85%, of SNPs with severe deviation from HWE (P<.0001) and of samples with call rate <85%) led to 456 samples and 344 SNPs [27–30]. Association test between allele and genotype frequencies and BASFI/t severe phenotype was performed by the chi-square ($\chi$2) test. P-values were calculated using a single-value permutation test (1000 permutations). The minor allele frequency at all loci was above 10%…Logistic regression analysis was used to discard weather the baseline clinical factors associated with severe function could be confounding for the association between BASFI/t severe phenotype and the SNPs genotypes. P values of <.05 were considered statistically significant and p values of (.05≥p<.1) borderline.

Clinical factors and SNPs were then studied by means of multivariate logistic regression. Individual *P* values of the SNPs and of the clinical variables were ranked and only those most significantly associated with the severe functional phenotype were included in the multivariate analysis as potential predictors (P<.1 in the allele frequencies association test).. The multivariate analysis was performed for all four defined classifications of functional severity (p60, p65, p70, and p75). BASFI/t was considered as dependent variable and baseline clinical variables and SNPs were included as predictors. The predictive discrimination of the models was tested both by Hosmer-Lemeshow statistic and the receiver operating characteristic curve (ROC) with 95% confidence interval (CI). An area under the ROC curve (AUC) above 0.75 was considered as an indicator of a good predictive precision of the model.

### Ethical approval

This study was approved by the Ethics Committee of "Reina Sofia" University Hospital, Córdoba and "Puerta de Hierro Majadahonda" University Hospital, Madrid, Spain. Each patient signed an informed consent form upon inclusion in REGISPON-SER-AS, in accordance with the fundamental principles set out in the Declaration of Human Rights in Helsinki.

## Results

### Baseline clinical variables and SNPs associated with functional severity in AS patients

Of the baseline clinical variables analyzed, the association with BASFI/t severe phenotype for neck pain and older age at disease onset was found to be statistically significant. A slight association was also found for low back pain (p60) and HLA-B27 (p65 and p70) (Table 1).

In the allele frequencies test, from the SNPs analyzed, we identified 24 polymorphisms associated with functional severe phenotype in at least one of the patient classifications. Two SNPs showed consistent association with BASFI/t and were significantly associated in all four patient classifications: rs2542151 in the protein tyrosine phosphatase non-receptor type 2 (*PTPN2*) gene [p60 (*P* = .046), p65 (*P* = .006), p70 (*P* = .002) and p75 (*P* = .001)] and rs2254441 in the proline-serine-threonine phosphatase-interacting protein 1 (*PSTPIP1*) gene [p60 (*P* = .036), p65 (*P* = .017), p70 (*P* = .010) and p75 (*P* = .001)]. Five SNPs (*rs10065172. rs2268624, rs4986790, rs4986791, rs3736228*) were associated with BASFI/t in three of the four patient classifications and eight polymorphisms (*rs6887695, rs17481856, rs2280153, rs1217414, rs4958847, rs2227982, rs17551710, rs1248634*) in two classifications. The other nine polymorphisms (*rs6822844, rs11959820, rs3117222, rs660895, rs1061622 rs13151961, rs27044, rs6254, rs743572*) were found significantly associated with BASFI/t for only one of the patient classifications (Table 2).

As we found that age at disease onset and neck pain at onset were the clinical factors associated with BASFI/t severe phenotype, they were entered in the logistic regression modeling as covariates. The results of the genotype frequencies test showed that the SNP *rs2542151* in the *PTPN2* gene was significantly associated to BASFI/t in three of the four patients' classifications

after adjustment for age at disease onset and neck pain (Table 2). There were other four SNPs with significant or borderline genotype associations in two of the patients' classifications after adjustment for age at disease onset and neck pain, *rs2254441* in the *PSTPIP1* gene, *rs2268624* in the *TGFB3* gene, and *rs4986790* and *rs4986791* in the TLR4 gene. The rest of SNPs were not associated to BASFI/t in the genotype test after correction for age at disease onset and neck pain at onset.

For further investigate the association between clinical-genetic variables and functional severe phenotype in AS, we performed a multivariate analysis using BASFI/t (severe/mild) as dependent variable and as covariates the clinical and genetic variables most significantly associated with BASFI/t ((p<0,1 in the allele frequencies association test). We did not find any model with a good predictive accuracy for BASFI/t for any of the patient classifications, p60, p65, p70, and p75 as none of the ROC curves of the predictive models attained an area under the curve (AUC) above 0.75.

## Discussion

This is a pioneering study performed on daily clinical patients which sought the clinical and genetic factors of influence in the development of functional severity in AS. Maintaining a good functional status is the main aim of pharmacologic treatment in current clinical practice. Reliable markers that could be applied early in the disease course to identify patients with potential severe functional outcome would be of major value for clinicians to consequently select the most suitable treatment strategy. The results of our study found that older age and neck pain at disease onset and several new SNPs, particularly *rs2542151 (PTPN2)* and *rs2254441 (PSTPIP1)*, are predictors of severe functional impairment in AS. However, the combination of the genetic and clinical factors identified in our study was not sufficient to develop a predictive model with a good accuracy for AS functional outcome; therefore, additional predictors are required.

We found neck pain and older age at disease onset as the main clinical variables associated with severe AS functional status. Neck pain at onset, which in AS may arise from either mechanical or inflammatory lesions, presented a consistent association in all four patient classifications studied [p75 (*P* = .040), p70 (*P* = .002), p65 (*P* = .004), p60 (*P* = .011)]. To the best of our knowledge, this is the first study which has found neck pain as a predictor for AS functionality. There is conflicting evidence about the role of age at disease onset as a predictor of disease severity, with some studies finding an association and others failing to support this [31–35]. Patients included in our study were young adults at disease onset, with mean age of 26.1±9.1 years. Interestingly, we found a statistically significant association between older age at disease onset and BASFI/t severe phenotype (p75, p70, p65, p60; *P*<.001). This result is in accordance with a recent study which found that the likelihood of developing more severe radiographic damage was greater among patients with an older age at disease onset [36]. The authors suggested that this association could result if patients with an older age at disease onset are asymptomatic early in their illness or if they have occasional or milder symptoms, which might cause them to underestimate the duration of their disease. Supporting previous studies [36–38], we found that *HLA-B27* was poorly associated with functional severity; thus, we only identified statistically significant association in two of the percentiles studied [p65 (*P* = .050), p70 (*P* = .049)]. Surprisingly, we did not find coxitis at baseline to be associated with development of severe physical function as found in several

**Table 1.** Baseline clinical variables associated with functional severity in AS patients.

| Clinical Variable | p value | | | |
|---|---|---|---|---|
| | BASFI/t p75 | BASFI/t p70 | BASFI/t p65 | BASFI/t p60 |
| Age at disease onset | <.001 | <.001 | <.001 | <.001 |
| Neck pain | .040 | .002 | .004 | .011 |
| Low back pain | NS | NS | NS | .030 |
| HLA-B27 | NS | .050 | .049 | NS |

NS- no statistically significant.

**Table 2.** SNPs associated with functional severity in AS patients.

| SNP Name | Gene Symbol | Risk Allele | Allele frequencies test, p value[§] | | | |
|---|---|---|---|---|---|---|
| | | | BASFI/t p75 | BASFI/t p70 | BASFI/t p65 | BASFI/t p60 |
| rs2542151 | PTPN2 | C | 0.001* | 0.002* | 0.006* | 0.046# |
| rs2254441 | PSTPIP1 | A | 0.001* | 0.010† | 0.017# | 0.036# |
| rs2268624 | TGFB3 | G | 0.002* | 0.017* | 0,032# | NS |
| rs4986790 | TLR4 | G | 0.008† | 0.009† | 0.037# | NS |
| rs4986791 | TLR4 | A | 0.011* | 0.006* | 0.031# | NS |
| rs10065172 | IRGM | G | NS | 0,014# | 0,012# | 0.006* |
| rs3736228 | LRP5 | A | 0.049# | 0,051# | 0,056# | NS |
| rs6887695 | IL12B | C | NS | 0.038# | 0.037# | NS |
| rs17481856 | ERAP1 | G | NS | 0.035# | NS | 0.038# |
| rs2280153 | WISP3 | G | NS | NS | 0.032# | 0.014* |
| rs1217414 | PTPN22 | G | NS | 0.049# | NS | 0.034† |
| rs4958847 | IRGM | G | NS | NS | 0.042# | 0.027# |
| rs2227982 | PDCD1 | A | NS | 0.019† | 0,044# | NS |
| rs17551710 | COL6A1 | A | 0.043# | NS | NS | 0.048# |
| rs1248634 | DLG5 | A | NS | 0.047# | 0.043# | NS |
| rs6822844 | IL21 | A | NS | NS | NS | 0.031# |
| rs11959820 | PPARBC1B | C | NS | NS | NS | 0.017* |
| rs3117222 | LOC646702 | G | NS | NS | NS | 0.018* |
| rs660895 | HLA-DRB1 | G | NS | NS | 0.044† | NS |
| rs1061622 | TNFRSF1B | A | NS | NS | NS | 0.050# |
| rs13151961 | KIAA1109 | G | NS | NS | NS | 0.042# |
| rs27044 | ERAP1 | C | NS | NS | NS | 0.020* |
| rs6254 | PTH | A | 0,025# | NS | NS | NS |
| rs743572 | CYP17A1 | A | 0.032# | NS | NS | NS |

[§]- The p-values shown correspond to the allele frequencies test corrected by a single-value permutation test.
The symbols represent the results of the genotype frequencies association test before and after a logistic regression analysis using the age at disease onset and neck pain as covariates:
*Significant genotype association (p<0.05) after logistic regression analysis with adjustment for age at disease onset and neck pain;
†Borderline genotype association (0.05≥p<0.1) after logistic regression analysis with adjustment for age at disease onset and neck pain;
#Significant genotype association (p<0.05) was lost after logistic regression analysis with adjustment for age at disease onset and neck pain.

previous studies that sought clinical predictors of functional disability in AS [39–41].

Recent genome-wide association studies have provided valuable evidence supporting the involvement of genetic factors in the pathogenesis and prognosis of autoimmune diseases. The two major SNPs found in this study to be associated with development of severe physical function are located in the autoinflammatory genes PTPN2 and PSTPIP1. Our study found a consistent association between AS functional severity and the C allele of the SNP rs2542151 in the PTPN2 gene. PTPN2 is a remarkable gene, since it appears to influence most cells involved in the development of the immune system [42]. PTPN2 encodes the T cell protein tyrosine phosphatase TCPTP, a key negative regulator of inflammatory responses. Abnormalities in tyrosine phosphorylation have been found to be involved in the pathogenesis of numerous human diseases, such as developmental defects, neoplastic disorders, immunodeficiency, and autoimmunity [43]. The C allele of the SNP rs2542151 at PTPN2 gene, which we found to influence AS functional severity, was previously found to be associated with other autoimmune diseases, such as Crohn's disease, type 1 diabetes, and rheumatoid arthritis [44–45]. The fact that the SNP rs2542151 in PTPN2 is associated with different

aspects of autoimmune diseases suggests that these diseases, including AS, could share common pathogenic mechanisms.

Another consistent association between poor physical function of AS patients and SNPs was found for the A allele of the polymorphism rs2254441 in the PSTPIP1 gene. PSTPIP1 is a cytoskeleton-associated adaptor protein that regulates innate and adaptive immune responses. Although this pathway has been traditionally related to diseases associated with pyoderma gangraenosum, such as aseptic abscesses syndrome and chronic inflammatory bowel disease (IBD) [46], the SNP rs2254441 has been recently reported as associated with psoriatic juvenile idiopathic arthritis, a disease included in the spondyloarthropathies group together with AS and IBD [47].

In addition to SNPs in PTPN2 and PSTPIP1 genes, a milder association with BASFI/t severe phenotype was observed for SNPs in the immunity-related GTPase family M protein (IRGM), transforming growth factor beta 3 (TGFB3), Toll-like receptor 4 (TLR4), and LDL receptor related protein 5 (LRP5) genes. IRGM is a human immunity-related GTPase which confers autophagic defense against intracellular pathogens such as Mycobacterium tuberculosis (BCG) and Salmonella typhimurium. This gene's polymorphism rs10065172, which we found associated with AS functional severity, has been associated with increased tuberculosis risk in some populations [42] and is a well-established risk factor for IBD [43].

In addition to SNPs in *PTPN2* and *PSTPIP1* genes, a milder association with BASFI/t severe phenotype was seen for SNPs in the transforming growth factor beta 3 (*TGFB3*) and Toll-like receptor 4 (*TLR4*) genes. Regarding TGFß3, high serum levels of this protein have been linked to osteoporosis risk [48] and polymorphisms in *TGFß* have been found to be associated with ossification of the posterior longitudinal ligament of the spine (OPLL) in the Japanese population [49]. To the best of our knowledge this is the first report which linked risk from allele G of *rs2268624* in *TGFß3* with development of functional severity in AS.

The association of the SNPs *rs4986790* and *rs4986791* in the *TLR4* gene could represent the involvement of the innate immune system in the progression of AS. Dysregulation of Toll-like receptor (TLR)-related pathways, specifically upregulation of TLR4 and TLR5, has been reported in AS [50].

Of particular interest was to find an association between severe functional impairment and *rs3736228* in *LRP5* gene, since a recently published study in the Chinese population has found several other SNPs in *LRP5* to be associated with AS susceptibility [47]. The SNP *rs3736228* was also identified to be associated with gender dependent bone mass formation and may be implicated in the adaptation of bone to mechanical load in humans [48]. As far as we are concerned, this is the first report in which a link between polymorphisms involved in bone formation and AS functional severity is identified.

The strength of this study lies in the large number of clinically well characterized AS patients. However, our study has some limitations. First, we performed a cross-sectional study in which we did not analyze the treatment administered to patients as a possible factor that influences physical outcome, since we did not have reliable data about which patients were on a specific therapy prior to their inclusion in the study. The lack of information about the treatment could have introduced some bias. Secondly, in spite of the clinical and genetic factors found to influence AS functional prognosis, we could not achieve a good predictive model for development of severe functional status by combining these factors. Thus, further research in this area in other cohorts or in prospective studies is needed to confirm which of these genetic markers in combination with clinical factors could identify an accurate predictive model for AS functional severity.

In conclusion, our results confirm that severe functional status in AS is associated with both clinical and genetic factors. We found that older age and neck pain at disease onset, lymphoid tyrosine phosphatase (*PTPN2*)-*rs2542151*, proline-serine-threonine phosphatase interacting protein1 (*PSTPIP1*)-*rs2254441* polymorphisms, are potential predictors of the development of severe functional status in AS patients. Validation of these results in other cohorts is required.

## Author Contributions

Conceived and designed the experiments: RS AS JS ECE AB JM. Performed the experiments: NB MS AM DT MA. Analyzed the data: RS NB AS MS DT MA ECE JM. Contributed reagents/materials/analysis tools: AS ECE JM JS EC AB. Wrote the paper: RS AS NB ECE JM.

## References

1. Schlosstein L, Terasaki PI, Bluestone R, Pearson CM (1973) High association of an HL-A antigen, B27, with ankylosing spondylitis. N Engl J Med 288:704–6.

2. Brown MA, Pile KD, Kennedy LG, Campbell D, Andrew L, et al. (1998) A genome-wide screen for susceptibility loci in ankylosing spondylitis. Arthritis Rheum 41:588–95.

3. Carter N, Williamson L, Kennedy LG, Brown MA, Wordsworth BP (2000) Susceptibility to ankylosing spondylitis [letter]. Rheumatology (Oxford) 39: 445.

4. Burton PR, Clayton DG, Cardon LR, Craddock N, Deloukas P, et al. (2007) Association scan of 14,500 nonsynonymous SNPs in four diseases identifies autoimmunity variants. Nat Genet 39:1329–37.

5. Rueda B, Orozco G, Raya E, Fernandez-Sueiro JL, Mulero J, et al. (2008) The IL23R Arg381Gln non-synonymous polymorphism confers susceptibility to ankylosing spondylitis. Ann Rheum Dis 67:1451–4.

6. Harvey D, Pointon JJ, Evans DM, Karaderi T, Farrar C, et al. (2009) Investigating the genetic association between ERAP1 and ankylosing spondylitis. Hum Mol Genet 18:4204–12.

7. Evans DM, Spencer CC, Pointon J, Su Z, Harvey D, et al. (2011) Interaction between ERAP1 and HLA-B27 in ankylosing spondylitis implicates peptide handling in the mechanism for HLA-B27 in disease susceptibility. Nat Genet 43: 761–767.

8. Guo C, Xia Y, Yang Q, Qiu R, Zhao H, et al. (2012) Association of the ANTXR2 gene polymorphism and ankylosing spondylitis in Chinese Han. Scand J Rheumatol 41: 29–32.

9. Lin Z, Bei JX, Shen M, Li Q, Liao Z, et al. (2011) A genome-wide association study in Han Chinese identifies new susceptibility loci for ankylosing spondylitis. Nat Genet 44:73–7.

10. Cakar E, Taskaynatan MA, Dincer U, Kiralp MZ, Durmus O, et al. (2009) Work disability in ankylosing spondylitis: differences among working and work disabled patients. Clin Rheumatol 28:1309–14.

11. Ariza-Ariza R, Hernández-Cruz B, Collantes E, Batle E, Fernández-Sueiro JL, et al. (2009) Work disability in patients with ankylosing spondylitis. J Rheumatol 36:2512–6.

12. Landewé R, Dougados M, Mielants H, van der Tempel H, van der Heijde D (2009) Physical function in ankylosing spondylitis is independently determined by both disease activity and radiographic damage of the spine. Ann Rheum Dis 68:863–7.

13. Doran MF, Brophy S, MacKay K, Taylor G, Calin A (2003) Predictors of longterm outcome in ankylosing spondylitis. J Rheumatol 30:316–20.

14. Cansu DU, Calışır C, Savaş Yavaş U, Kaşifoğlu T, Korkmaz C, et al. (2011) Predictors of radiographic severity and functional disability in Turkish patients with ankylosing spondylitis. Clin Rheumatol 30:557–62.

15. Hamersma J, Cardon LR, Bradbury L, Brophy S, van der Horst-Bruinsma I, et al. (2001) Is disease severity in ankylosing spondylitis genetically determined? Arthritis Rheum 44:1396–400.

16. Brophy S, Hickey S, Menon A, Taylor G, Bradbury L, et al. (2004) Concordance of disease severity among family members with ankylosing spondylitis?. J Rheumatol 31:1775–78.

17. Brown MA, Brophy S, Bradbury L, Hamersma J, Timms A, et al. (2003) Identification of major loci controlling clinical manifestations of ankylosing spondylitis. Arthritis Rheum 48:2234–39.

18. Brown MA (2009) Progress in studies of the genetics of ankylosing spondylitis. Arthr Res & Ther 11:254–60.

19. Goedecke V, Crane AM, Jaakkola E, Kaluza W, Laiho K, et al. (2003) Interleukin 10 polymorphisms in ankylosing spondylitis. Genes Immun 4:74–6.

20. Szczypiorska M, Sánchez A, Bartolomé N, Arteta D, Sanz J, et al. (2011). ERAP1 polymorphisms and haplotypes are associated with ankylosing spondylitis susceptibility and functional severity in a Spanish population. Rheumatology (Oxford) 50:1969–75.

21. Collantes E, Zarco P, Munoz E, Juanola X, Mulero J, et al. (2007) Disease pattern of spondyloarthropathies in Spain: description of the first national registry (REGISPONSER) extended report. Rheumatology (Oxford) 46:1309–15.

22. Van der Linden S, Valkenburg HA, Cats A (1984) Evaluation of diagnostic criteria for ankylosing spondylitis. A proposal for modification of the New York criteria. Arthritis Rheum 27:361–8.

23. Calin A, Garrett S, Whitelock H, Kennedy LG, O'Hea J, et al. (1994) A new approach to defining functional ability in ankylosing spondylitis: the development of the Bath Ankylosing Spondylitis Functional Index. J Rheumatol 21:2281–5.

24. Olerup O (1994) HLA-B27 typing by a group-specific PCR amplification. Tissue Antigens 43:253–6.

25. Cho SY, Lee KG, Park SY, Lee HJ (2008) Utility of in-house PCR for HLA-B27 typing: comparison of concordance rate between PCR kit and in-house PCR. Korean J Lab Med 28:239–43.

26. Fan JB, Oliphant A, Shen R, Kermani BG, Garcia F, et al. (2003) Highly parallel SNP genotyping. Cold Spring Harb Symp Quant Biol 68:69–78.

27. Paynter RA, Skibola DR, Skibola CF, Buffler PA, Wiemels JL, et al. (2006) Accuracy of multiplexed Illumina platform-based single-nucleotide polymorphism genotyping compared between genomic and whole genome amplified DNA collected from multiple sources. Cancer Epidemiol Biomarkers Prev 15:2533–6.

28. Reich D, Patterson N, De Jager PL, McDonald GJ, Waliszewska A, et al. (2005) A whole-genome admixture scan finds a candidate locus for multiple sclerosis susceptibility. Nat Genet 37:1113–8.

29. Bartolomé N, Szczypiorska M, Sánchez A, Sanz J, Juanola-Roura X, et al. (2012). Genetic polymorphisms, inside and outside the MHC, improve prediction of AS radiographic severity in addition to clinical variables. Rheumatology (Oxford) 51:1471–8.

30. Low YL, Li Y, Humphreys K, Thalamuthu A, Li Y, et al. (2010). Multi-variant pathway association analysis reveals the importance of genetic determinants of estrogen metabolism in breast and endometrial cancer susceptibility. PLoS Genet 6:e1001012.

31. Amor B, Santos R, Nahal R, Listrat V, Dougados M (1994) Predictive factors for the long-term outcome of spondyloarthropathies. J Rheumatol 21:1883–7.

32. Boonen A, vander Cruyssen B, de Vlam K, Steinfeld S, Ribbens C, et al. (2009) Spinal radiographic changes in ankylosing spondylitis: association with clinical characteristics and functional outcome. J Rheumatol 36:1249–55.

33. Brophy S, Calin A. (2001) Ankylosing spondylitis: Interaction between genes, joints, age at onset, and disease expression. J Rheumatol 28:2283–8.

34. Gensler LS, Ward MM, Reveille JD, Learch TJ, Weisman MH, et al. (2008) Clinical, radiographic and functional differences between juvenile-onset and adult-onset ankylosing spondylitis: results from the PSOAS cohort. Ann Rheum Dis 67:233–7.

35. Robertson LP, Davis MJ (2004) A longitudinal study of disease activity and functional status in a hospital cohort of patients with ankylosing spondylitis. Rheumatology (Oxford) 43:1565–8.

36. Ward MM, Hendrey MR, Malley JD, Learch TJ, Davis JC Jr, et al. (2009) Clinical and immunogenetic prognostic factors for radiographic severity in ankylosing spondylitis. Arthritis Rheum 61:859–66.

37. Rudwaleit M, Listing J, Brandt J, Braun J, Sieper J (2004) Prediction of a major clinical response (BASDAI 50) to tumour necrosis factor a blockers in ankylosing Spondylitis. Ann Rheum Dis 63:665–70.

38. Khan MA, Kushner I, Braun WE, Zachary AA, Steinberg AG (1978) *HLA-B27* homozygosity in ankylosing spondylitis: relationship to risk and severity. Tissue Antigens 11:434–8.

39. Carette S, Graham D, Little H, Rubenstein J, Rosen P (1983) The natural disease course of ankylosing spondylitis. Arthritis Rheum 26:186–90.

40. Falkenbach A, Franke A, van der Linden S (2003) Factors associated with body function and disability in patients with ankylosing spondylitis: a cross-sectional study. J Rheumatol 30:2186–92.

41. Vander Cruyssen B, Muñoz-Gomariz E, Font P, Mulero J, de Vlam K, al. ASPECT-REGISPONSER-RESPONDIA working group (2010) Hip involvement in ankylosing spondylitis: epidemiology and risk factors associated with hip replacement surgery. Rheumatology (Oxford) 49:73–81.

42. Moore F, Colli ML, Cnop M, Esteve MI, Cardozo AK, et al. (2009) PTPN2, a candidate gene for type 1 diabetes, modulates interferon-gamma-induced pancreatic beta-cell apoptosis. Diabetes 58:1283–91.

43. Vang T, Miletic AV, Arimura Y, Tautz L, Rickert RC, et al. (2008) Protein tyrosine phosphatases in autoimmunity. Annu Rev Immunol 26:29–55.

44. Burton PR, Clayton DG, Cardon LR, Craddock N, Deloukas P, et al. (2007) Genome-wide association study of 14,000 cases of seven common diseases and 3,000 shared controls. Nature 447:661–78.

45. Morgan AR, Han DY, Huebner C, Lam WJ, Fraser AG, et al. (2010) *PTPN2* but not *PTPN22* is associated with Crohn's disease in a New Zealand population. Tissue Antigens 76:119–25.

46. Wollina U, Haroske G (2011) Pyoderma gangraenosum. Curr Opin Rheumatol 23:50–6.

47. Day TG, Ramanan AV, Hinks A, Lamb R, Packham J, et al. (2008) Autoinflammatory Genes and Susceptibility to Psoriatic Juvenile Idiopathic Arthritis. Arthritis Rheum 58:2142–6.

48. Grainger DJ, Percival J, Chiano M, Spector TD (1999) The role of serum TGF-beta isoforms as potential markers of osteoporosis. Osteoporos Int 9:398–404.

49. Kamiya M, Harada A, Mizuno M, Iwata H, Yamada Y (2001) Association between a polymorphism of the transforming growth factor-beta1 gene and genetic susceptibility to ossification of the posterior longitudinal ligament in Japanese patients. Spine 26:1264–1267.

50. Assassi S, Reveille JD, Arnett FC, Weisman MH, Ward MM, et al. (2010) Whole-blood gene expression profiling in Ankylosing Spondylitis shows upregulation of Toll-like receptor 4 and 5. J Rheumatol 38:87–98.

# 4

# Association of *ORAI1* Haplotypes with the Risk of HLA-B27 Positive Ankylosing Spondylitis

James Cheng-Chung Wei[1], Jeng-Hsien Yen[4,6], Suh-Hang Hank Juo[2,3], Wei-Chiao Chen[2], Yu-Shiuan Wang[2], Yi-Ching Chiu[2], Tusty-Jiuan Hsieh[2], Yuh-Cherng Guo[8], Chun-Huang Huang[1], Ruey-Hong Wong[1], Hui-Po Wang[10], Ke-Li Tsai[9], Yang-Chang Wu[11], Hsueh-Wei Chang[5], Edward Hsi[2], Wei-Pin Chang[7], Wei-Chiao Chang[2,3]*

**1** Division of Allergy, Immunology and Rheumatology, Department of Medicine, Chung Shan Medical University Hospital, Institute of Medicine, Chung Shan Medical University, Graduate Institute of Integrated Medicine, China Medical University, Taichung, Taiwan, **2** Department of Medical Genetics, College of Medicine, Kaohsiung Medical University, Kaohsiung, Taiwan, **3** Cancer Center, Kaohsiung Medical University Hospital, Kaohsiung, Taiwan, **4** Division of Rheumatology, Department of Internal Medicine, Kaohsiung Medical University Hospital, Kaohsiung, Taiwan, **5** Department of Biomedical Science and Environmental Biology, Kaohsiung, Taiwan, **6** Graduate Institute of Medicine, Kaohsiung Medical University, Kaohsiung, Taiwan, **7** Department of Healthcare Management, Yuanpei University, HsinChu, Taiwan, **8** Department of Neurology, Kaohsiung Municipal Hsiao-Kang Hospital, Kaohsiung Medical University, Kaohsiung, Taiwan, **9** Department of Physiology, College of Medicine, Kaohsiung Medical University, Kaohsiung, Taiwan, **10** Department of Pharmacy, Taipei Medical University, Taipei, Taiwan, **11** Graduate Institute of Integrated Medicine, China Medical University, Taichung, Taiwan

## Abstract

Ankylosing spondylitis (AS) is a chronic inflammation of the sacroiliac joints, spine and peripheral joints. The aetiology of ankylosing spondylitis is still unclear. Previous studies have indicated that genetics factors such as human leukocyte antigen *HLA-B27* associates to AS susceptibility. We carried out a case-control study to determine whether the genetic polymorphisms of *ORAI1* gene, a major component of store-operated calcium channels that involved the regulation of immune system, is a susceptibility factor to AS in a Taiwanese population. We enrolled 361 AS patients fulfilled the modified New York criteria and 379 controls from community. Five tagging single nucleotides polymorphisms (tSNPs) at *ORAI1* were selected from the data of Han Chinese population in HapMap project. Clinical statuses of AS were assessed by the Bath Ankylosing Spondylitis Disease Activity Index (BASDAI), Bath Ankylosing Spondylitis Functional Index (BASFI), and Bath Ankylosing Spondylitis Global Index (BAS-G). Our results indicated that subjects carrying the minor allele homozygote (CC) of the promoter SNP rs12313273 or TT homozygote of the SNP rs7135617 had an increased risk of HLA-B27 positive AS. The minor allele C of 3'UTR SNP rs712853 exerted a protective effect to HLA-B27 positive AS. Furthermore, the rs12313273/rs7135617 pairwise allele analysis found that C-G (OR 1.69, 95% CI 1.27, 2.25; p = 0.0003) and T-T (OR 1.75, 95% CI 1.36, 2.27; p<0.0001) haplotypes had a significantly association with the risk of HLA-B27-positive AS in comparison with the T-G carriers. This is the first study that indicate haplotypes of *ORAI1* (rs12313273 and rs7135617) are associated with the risk of HLA-B27 positive AS.

**Editor:** Proost Paul, University of Leuven, Rega Institute, Belgium

**Funding:** This study was supported by National Science Council of Taiwan (NSC 98-2320-B-037 -028 -MY2); excellence for cancer research center grant (NO.DOH99-TD-C-111-002), Department of Health, Executive Yuan, Taiwan, ROC to W.C. Chang. The funders had no role in study design, data collection and analysis, decision to publish, or preparation of the manuscript.

**Competing Interests:** The authors have declared that no competing interests exist.

\* E-mail: wcc@kmu.edu.tw

## Introduction

Ankylosing spondylitis (AS) is a systemic autoimmune disease affecting axial skeletons and peripheral joints[1]. AS ultimately limits the mobility of the spine and other joints, contributing to functional impairment[2]. Genetic factors have been strongly implicated in its pathogenesis. A twin study suggested that up to 97% of AS susceptibility was attributable to genetic factors[3]. AS was strongly associated with the human leukocyte antigen *HLA-B27* gene[4], but *HLA-B27* accounted for only 16% of the genetic load in AS[5]. HLA-B60, B61 and IL-1, IL-3R, and IL-23R complexes also have been proven to be important in the pathogenesis of AS[6–8]. A recent genome wide association study (GWAS) demonstrated immune related genes such as *ERAP1*, and

*IL-23* as strong susceptibility genes to AS[9]. Consistently, immune related genes such as Toll-like receptor 4 and Toll-like receptor 5 are overexpressed in AS patients[10]. In addition, intergenic SNP rs10865331 was found to be susceptible to AS in the Spanish population[11]. *MSX2* genetic polymorphisms were associated with AS in Japanese but not Taiwanese[12]. In the Chinese Han population, Janus kinase 2 (JAK2) polymorphisms have been implicated to be involved in the susceptibility of AS[13]. Although several genes have been proposed to explain the susceptibility of AS, most genetic associations study cannot be replicated with other populations.

Ankylosing spondylitis (AS), an inflammatory disease, affects predominantly axial skeleton and sacroiliac joints. Therefore, molecules involved in the regulation of calcification, autoimmune and/or inflammation are good candidates for the AS susceptibility genes. Calcium-dependent pathways control diverse physiological functions including enzyme metabolism, immune responses and inflammatory activation[14]. In non-excitable cells such as T cells and B cells, $Ca^{2+}$ entry was mainly through store-operated calcium channels to control immunological reactions[15]. Orai1 (also called CRACM1) consisted four transmembrane domains and functioned as a pore forming subunit of store-operated calcium channels[16]. Orai1 protein was highly expressed in bone tissues. Functional studies in *CRACM1* deficient mice indicated the dysfunction of mast cells, and attenuation of cytokine release (TNF-α and IL-6)[17]. *ORAI1*-R91W mutations disrupt the function of store-operated calcium channels resulting in the lack of $Ca^{2+}$ influx, defective T cell activation, and immunodeficiency[18]. Additionally, there were lines of evidence for a role of store-operated calcium channel in the modulation of transcription factors including NFκB and NFAT. A great number of NFκB- and/or NFAT-mediated genes were critical for maintaining the immune system[19].

In this study, we examined the association between the *ORAI1* polymorphisms and the risk for AS using a case-control study. The relationship between AS activity index (BASDAI, BASFI, BAS-G), and genetic polymorphisms of *ORAI1* was also evaluated.

## Materials and Methods

### Study Subjects

Patients were solicited sequentially at Chung Shan Medical University Hospital in Taichung, Taiwan. AS patients who met selection criteria were asked to participate in the study. Informed consent was obtained before any data was collected from the respondents. Three selection criteria were used to recruit subjects: (1) AS diagnosis by the modified New York criteria[20]; (2) fluent Chinese language speakers; and (3) no obvious cognitive impairment. Sacroiliitis was confirmed by a qualified radiologist or rheumatologists, and AS diagnosis was confirmed by a qualified rheumatologist. A total of 361 unrelated AS patients were included in the study as cases. A detailed clinical history was recorded by the physician at enrollment. 29 (8%) AS patients whose age are less than 18. The mean duration of the symptoms was 7.5 years. 100% of AS patients in this study have sacroiliitis. A total of 379 control subjects were recruited from the general population who volunteered to participate in our study while receiving a health screening examination at the Kaohsiung Medical University Hospital. All the subjects gave the consent form. The study protocol conformed to the Declaration of Helsinki and study was approved by the Institute Review Board of each Hospital.

### Clinical Evaluations

Disease activity and functional status were assessed by the Chinese versions of the BASDAI, the BASFI, and the Bath Ankylosing Spondylitis Global (BAS-G) Score. Good reliability (0.87 to 0.94) and validity (0.92 to 0.94) of these Chinese methods have been documented[21].

### Laboratory Analyses

Venous blood was collected during medical surveillance, stored at 4°C, and processed on the same day. The blood was centrifuged to separate the serum and the cells. All specimens were stored under −70°C until analysis. HLA-B27 carriage had previously been assessed by flow cytometry[22]. Genotyping is performed using TaqMan PCR. Briefly, Taqman probes are labeled with different fluorescent markers. PCR primers and TaqMan probes are designed with SNP sites. Reactions are performed in 96 well microplates with ABI 7500 thermal cycles (Applied Biosystems, Foster City, USA). Fluorescence is measured by the ABI Real Time PCR system. By reading the fluorescence from PCR product, possible genotypes can be identified. Results are analyzed with the ABI SDS software version 1.2.3.

### Statistical Analysis

Genotype distributions of the five tagging single nucleotide polymorphisms (tSNPs) were tested for Hardy-Weinberg equilibrium (HWE), which means the allelic distribution between all populations and our study was not different ($P>0.05$). Chi-squared test was used to compare the genotypes distribution or allele frequencies between AS patients and controls. Analysis of variance (ANOVA) was used to compare the mean of continuous variables (BASDAI, BASFI, and BAS-G) among different genotypes in AS patients. Multiple regression analysis was used to adjust for age and sex. A $p$ value after the Bonferroni correction less than 0.01 is considered significant. The analyses were performed by using SAS 9.1 statistical software. Linkage disequilibrium (LD) was assessed for any pair of SNPs and haplotype blocks were defined using the default setting of the Haploview software[23].

## Results

### Basic and Clinical Characteristics of the Subjects

In this study, we selected five tSNPs of *ORAI1* (rs12313273, rs6486795, rs7135617, rs12320939, and rs712853) with minor allele frequency >5% from the Han Chinese in Beijing (CHB) population in the HapMap database (http://www.hapmap.org). A graphical overview of genotyped polymorphisms was shown in Figure 1. Two polymorphisms (rs12313273, rs12320939) of *ORAI1* located in the promoter area, while two polymorphisms (rs6486795, rs7135617) in the intron and one (rs712853) in the 3′ untranslated region (UTR). A total of 361 AS patients and 379 controls were recruited in this study. Table 1 showed the characteristics of the subjects. The mean age (years) and standard deviation (S.D.) were 33.5±12.8 for cases and 28.3±15.2 for

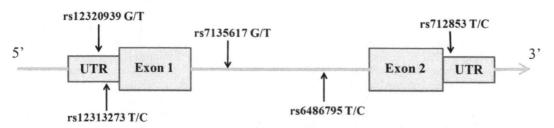

**Figure 1. A graphical overview of genotyped polymorphisms identified in relation to the exon/intron structure of the human *ORAI1* gene.**

**Table 1.** Basal characteristics and clinical features of patients with ankylosing spondylitis (AS) and of normal controls.

| Characteristics | Patients with AS | Normal Controls |
|---|---|---|
| Number of subjects | 361 | 379 |
| Gender:male, No (%) | 245 (67.9%) | 265 (69.9%)[a] |
| Age (years)[b] | 33.5±12.8 | 28.3±15.2[c] |
| Range | 6–69 | 18–80 |
| HLA-B27(+) | 315 (87.3%) | |
| BASDAI (0–10) | 4.1±2.3 | |
| BASFI (0–10) | 1.9±2.2 | |
| BAS-G (0–10) | 4.3±2.8 | |

[a]$P = 0.546$ о.
[b]means ± S.D.
[c]$P < 0.0001$.

controls. More than 67.9% of cases and 69.9% of controls were male. 87.3% (315/361) AS subjects were HLA-B27 positive and their mean BASDAI, mean BASFI, and mean BAS-G scores were 4.1±2.3, 1.9±2.2, and 4.3±2.8, respectively.

## Association of ORAI1 genetic polymorphisms for the susceptibility of HLA-B27-positive or negative patients with AS

The genotypic frequencies of SNPs among the study subjects were shown in Table 2, and the distribution of genotypes was in HWE in controls. Two SNPs, rs7135617 and rs712853, showed significant associations with HLA-B27-positive AS patients in the recessive model. The C allele of rs712853 was associated with a lower AS risk (OR: 0.46, $P = 0.002$) than the rs712853 T allele. The adjustment for age and sex did not change the association for

rs12313273 or rs712853 in the recessive model or genotype model. The association for rs7135617 or rs712853 was still significant even after the Bonferroni correction ($P < 0.01$). In addition, a borderline significant association between the genotypes and allele frequency of rs12313273 in control subjects and HLA-B27 positive patients was obtained with a $P$ value = 0.012 under the recessive model. Individuals with the rs12313273 homozygous C/C genotype had a 2.11-fold increased risk of AS compared with those with the C/T and T/T genotypes.

## No Association of ORAI1 genetic polymorphisms with the disease activity of AS

We further analyzed the relationship between disease activity (BASDAI, BASFI and BAS-G) and the five polymorphisms of ORAI1 among AS patients. BASFI is strongly affected by disease duration, therefore, adjustment for disease duration and BASFI was performed. However, none of SNPs reached a nominal significant level of 0.05 (Table 3). After adjustment for the effects of age and sex, the polymorphisms of ORAI1 still failed to show any significant association with the severity of AS (Table 3). Subset analysis on cases with HLA-B27 positive or negative did not yield any significant results (data not shown).

## Haplotype Analysis of ORAI1 genetic polymorphisms in the susceptibility of HLA-B27-positive or negative patients with AS

We calculated pairwise linkage disequilibrium (LD) (Figure 2) and analyzed three common haplotypes using the Haploview 4.2 program and PHASE version 2.1, respectively. The haplotype frequency of rs12313273/rs7135617 among the study subjects was shown in Table 4. rs12313273/rs7135617 pairwise allele analysis indicated that C–G (AOR = 1.69; 95% CI, 1.27–2.25; $P = 0.0003$), and T-T (AOR = 1.75; 95% CI, 1.36–2.27; $P < 0.0001$) had a significant association with the risk of HLA-B27-positive AS in comparison with the T-G haplotype under a recessive model.

**Table 2.** Genotyping and allele frequency of ORAI1 tSNP in HLA-B27(+) or HLA-B27(-) with ankylosing spondylitis (AS) and controls.

| | Genotype | HLA-B27(+) (n = 315) (%) | HLA-B27(-) (n = 46) (%) | Control Subjects (n = 379) (%) | Recessive Odds ratio[†] | Recessive P Value[†] | Recessive Odds ratio[‡] | Recessive P Value[‡] |
|---|---|---|---|---|---|---|---|---|
| rs12320939 | TT | 68 (22.2) | 15 (32.6) | 90 (26.1) | 0.89 | 0.511 | 1.68 | 0.138 |
| | GT | 142 (46.4) | 22 (47.8) | 165 (47.8) | | | | |
| | GG | 96 (31.4) | 9 (19.6) | 90 (26.1) | | | | |
| rs12313273 | CC | 34 (10.9) | 7 (15.6) | 20 (5.7) | 2.11 | 0.012 | 3.32 | 0.015 |
| | CT | 116 (37.3) | 18 (40.0) | 148 (41.8) | | | | |
| | TT | 161 (51.8) | 20 (44.4) | 186 (52.5) | | | | |
| rs7135617 | TT | 72 (23.2) | 6 (13.7) | 60 (17.0) | 1.70 | **0.008*** | 0.90 | 0.817 |
| | GT | 139 (44.9) | 21 (47.7) | 164 (46.6) | | | | |
| | GG | 99 (31.9) | 17 (38.6) | 128 (36.4) | | | | |
| rs6486795 | CC | 50 (16.1) | 10 (22.2) | 54 (15.6) | 1.13 | 0.581 | 1.91 | 0.108 |
| | CT | 126 (40.7) | 21 (46.7) | 159 (45.8) | | | | |
| | TT | 134 (43.2) | 14 (31.1) | 134 (38.6) | | | | |
| rs712853 | CC | 25 (8.1) | 1 (2.2) | 59 (16.2) | 0.46 | **0.002*** | 0.13 | 0.045 |
| | CT | 109 (35.3) | 24 (52.2) | 153 (42.0) | | | | |
| | TT | 175 (56.6) | 21 (45.6) | 152 (41.8) | | | | |

*Significant ($P < 0.01$) values are in bold.
†Adjusted the effects of age and sex for HLA-B27 positive patients compared with controls.
‡Adjusted the effects of age and sex for HLA-B27 negative patients compared with controls.

**Table 3.** Difference in the scores of BASDAI, BASFI, and BAS-G among AS patients stratified by different *ORAI1* alleles.

| SNP | Alleles | BASDAI | BASFI | BAS-G |
|---|---|---|---|---|
| rs12320939 | T/T | 4.1±2.4[a] | 1.7±2.1 | 4.1±2.9 |
| | G/T | 4.1±2.3 | 1.9±2.1 | 4.2±2.8 |
| | G/G | 4.3±2.3 | 2.1±2.4 | 4.5±2.8 |
| Unadjusted *P*-value | | 0.86 | 0.52 | 0.57 |
| Adjusted *P*-value | | 0.86[†] | 0.51[§] | 0.57[†] |
| rs12313273 | C/C | 3.2±2.3 | 1.3±2.1 | 3.3±2.8 |
| | C/T | 4.4±2.4 | 1.9±2.1 | 4.4±2.8 |
| | T/T | 4.2±2.2 | 2.1±2.3 | 4.4±2.9 |
| Unadjusted *P*-value | | 0.02 | 0.14 | 0.10 |
| Adjusted *P*-value | | 0.02[†] | 0.12[§] | 0.09[†] |
| rs7135617 | T/T | 4.3±2.3 | 2.3±2.5 | 4.7±2.9 |
| | G/T | 4.1±2.3 | 2.0±2.2 | 4.1±2.8 |
| | G/G | 4.1±2.4 | 1.6±1.9 | 4.2±2.8 |
| Unadjusted *P*-value | | 0.72 | 0.12 | 0.46 |
| Adjusted *P*-value | | 0.72[†] | 0.09[§] | 0.46[†] |
| rs6486795 | C/C | 3.7±2.3 | 1.5±2.0 | 3.5±2.7 |
| | C/T | 4.2±2.3 | 1.9±2.1 | 4.2±2.7 |
| | T/T | 4.2±2.2 | 2.2±2.4 | 4.6±2.9 |
| Unadjusted *P*-value | | 0.40 | 0.19 | 0.10 |
| Adjusted *P*-value | | 0.40[†] | 0.17[§] | 0.10[†] |
| rs712853 | C/C | 3.9±1.9 | 2.3±2.0 | 4.3±2.7 |
| | C/T | 4.2±2.1 | 1.8±2.1 | 4.2±2.8 |
| | T/T | 4.1±2.5 | 2.0±2.3 | 4.3±2.9 |
| Unadjusted *P*-value | | 0.88 | 0.64 | 0.95 |
| Adjusted *P*-value | | 0.88[†] | 0.61[§] | 0.95[†] |

[a]Data represent means ± S.D.
[†]Adjusted the effects of age and sex.
[§]Adjusted the effects of age, sex and disease duration.

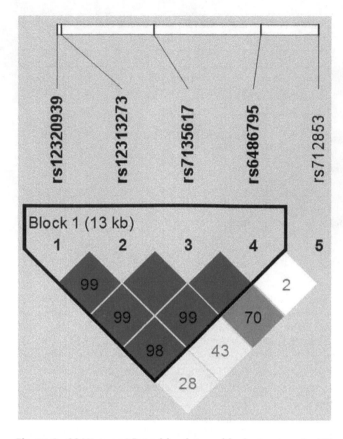

**Figure 2. *ORAI1* gene LD and haplotype block structure in AS.** The number on the cell is the LOD score of D′.

However, none of haplotypes was significantly associated with HLA-B27-negative AS patients (Table 4).

## No Association between *ORAI1* Haplotypes and the disease activity of AS

We further analyzed the relationship between disease activity and rs12313273/rs7135617 haplotypes among AS patients. As shown in table 5, none of the rs12313273/rs7135617 pairwise allele analysis tested in this study showed a significant association between AS and BASDAI, BASFI, and BAS-G. After adjustment for the effects of age, gender and disease duration, the haplotype analysis of rs12313273/rs7135617 still failed to show any significant results with the disease activity of AS.

## Discussion

Our results first revealed that genetic polymorphisms of *ORAI1* rs12313273 (located in the promoter), rs7135617 (located in the intron) and rs712853 (located in the 3′UTR) were associated with susceptibility to AS in a Taiwanese population. Results from pairwise allele analysis for rs12313273/rs7135617 indicated that C-G and T-T haplotypes associated with a significantly higher risk of HLA-B27 positive AS in comparison with the T-G haplotypes. Several lines of evidence indicated the importance of SNPs at the promoter and 3′UTR in gene expression. Studies showed that a promoter SNP of

**Table 4.** Haplotype frequency of the *ORAI1* gene in HLA-B27(+) or HLA-B27(-) patients with ankylosing spondylitis and controls.

| rs12313273/rs7135617 | HLA-B27(+) (n = 315) (%) | HLA-B27(-) (n = 46) (%) | Control Subjects (n = 379) (%) | AOR (95% CI)[†] | *P* Value[†] | AOR (95% CI)[‡] | *P* Value[‡] |
|---|---|---|---|---|---|---|---|
| C/G | 184 (30.0) | 30 (33.3) | 186 (26.8) | 1.69 (1.27–2.25) | **0.0003*** | 1.65 (0.95–2.87) | 0.078 |
| T/T | 280 (45.6) | 34 (37.8) | 282 (40.6) | 1.75 (1.36–2.27) | **<0.0001*** | 1.25 (0.73–2.13) | 0.413 |
| T/G | 150 (24.4) | 26 (28.9) | 226 (32.6) | Reference | | Reference | |

*Significant (*P<0.05*) values are in bold.
[†]Adjusted the effects of age and sex for HLA-B27 positive patients compared with controls.
[‡]Adjusted the effects of age and sex for HLA-B27 negative patients compared with controls.

**Table 5.** Difference in the scores of BASDAI, BASFI, and BAS-G among AS patients stratified by different *ORAI1* haplotypes.

| rs12313273/rs7135617 | BASDAI | BASFI | BAS-G |
|---|---|---|---|
| C/G | 4.0±2.4[a] | 1.7±2.1 | 4.0±2.8 |
| T/T | 4.2±2.3 | 2.1±2.3 | 4.4±2.8 |
| T/G | 4.2±2.2 | 1.9±2.0 | 4.4±2.8 |
| Unadjusted P-value | 0.46 | 0.07 | 0.27 |
| Adjusted P-value | 0.46[†] | 0.03[§] | 0.26[†] |

[a]Data represent mean ± S.D.
[†]Adjusted the effects of age and sex.
[§]Adjusted the effects of age, sex and disease duration.

the tumor-necrosis factor α (*TNF-α*) was associated with the development of AS via attenuation of *TNF-α* gene expression [24]. Furthermore, SNPs at the 3′UTR may interfere with mRNA stability or protein translation by interacting with microRNAs[25]. MicroRNAs have been shown to play a critical role in the regulation of gene expression in immune diseases, including psoriatic arthritis susceptibility[26]. A recent study demonstrated that a 3′UTR polymorphisms of IL-1R associated kinase (*IRAK1*) gene was associated with rheumatoid arthritis (RA) susceptibility[26]. The RA-associated SNP of *IRAK1* was in the binding site of microRNA-146a[26]. Results obtained in *IRAK1* implied that 3′UTR polymorphism at *ORAI1* might affect susceptibility to AS via similar mechanisms (microRNA-relevant expression alteration).

Despite the strong association of *HLA-B27* gene with AS, other genes within and/or outside the MHC were reported to involve in the susceptibility of AS[6,8,9]. Wei et al[8]. found that *HLA-B60* and *HLA-B61* genes were associated with AS development among *HLA-B27* negative patients which might be due to the similar T-cell epitopes of HLA-B60 and HLA-B27 [27]. In vivo, the inflammation in the joint destruction was regulated by IL-1α and IL-1β, and IL-1 receptor antagonist (IL-1Ra) combined with IL-1 receptor to inhibit the IL-1[28]. In addition, the genetic variants in the IL-1F10.3, IL-1RN.4, IL-1RN.VNTR, IL-1RN6/1 and IL-1RN6/2 were significantly associated with occurrence of AS [29]. Shiau et al., observed that the distribution of TNF-α G-238A genotypes and alleles, as well as that of G-308A genotypes and alleles, between AS patients and controls were significantly different[30]. Both IL-1β and TNF-α pathways coordinated multiple signaling events leading to the increase of intracellular calcium concentration [31]. Association study in Chinese Han population revealed that JAK2 played an important role in the susceptibility to AS [13]. The increase of cytosolic calcium resulted in the activation of JAK-STAT pathways, which, in turn, involved in the regulation of proinflammatory genes [32]. Our association studies in AS provided some indirect evidence that supported a role of calcium signaling in the susceptibility to AS. Therefore, to understand the functional role

of *ORAI1* polymorphisms in the regulation of JAK2/STAT pathways may gain more insight to the disease pathogenesis.

Calcium influx through store-operated calcium channels has been shown its importance in a variety of diseases such as hypertension, arterial injury and severe combined immunodeficiency disease (SCID)[33]. A point mutation of *ORAI1* that resulted in the reduction of store-operated $Ca^{2+}$ influx and cytokine release was found in the SCID patients[18]. The biophysical characteristics of store-operated calcium channel can be altered by the changed composition of heteromeric *ORAI* channels. The $Ca^{2+}$ selectivity of homomeric *ORAI1* or *ORAI3* was higher than that of heteromeric *ORAI1* and *ORAI3*[34]. Additionally, knockdown of *ORAI1* can inhibit cell proliferation via attenuation of store-operated $Ca^{2+}$ influx [35,36]. Importantly, overexpression of *ORAI1* may influence the successful coupling between *ORAI* subunits or lose sensitivity to the store-depletion signals that lead to the dysfunction of store-operated calcium channel [37,38]. The expression level of *ORAI* subunits hence could significantly contribute to the intracellular $Ca^{2+}$ mobilization and physiological functions. The mechanism of how *ORAI1* gene being regulated is still unclear. Our results indicated that genetic polymorphisms of *ORAI1* (rs12313273 and rs712853) were associated with the risk of AS. With these findings, our study may offer a clue to better understand the regulation mechanism of *ORAI1*.

In conclusion, our research was the first study to pinpoint the association between genetic polymorphisms of *ORAI1* and the risk of AS. Our study indicated that haplotypes of rs12313273/rs7135617 had a significantly association with the risk of HLA-B27-positive AS but none of them was associated with theHLA-B27-negatve AS. We attribute this to the case number (46 HLA-B27negative AS patients), due to a small statistical power. Another possible explanation, that should be mentioned, is that these haplotypes are associated with the HLA- B27 per se and not exactly to AS.

We also analyzed the relationship between age of onset, hip involvement, erythrocyte sedimentation rate (ESR), C reactive protein (CRP) and *ORAI1* genotypes. However, no statistically significant association between genotypes and phenotypes were found (data not shown).We acknowledged that the sample size in the study was under-powered to detect the small genetic effect of *ORAI1* in the disease activity such as BASDAI/ BASFI, BAS-G., ESR or CRP. These findings need to be replicated in another population with a larger sample size.

## Author Contributions

Conceived and designed the experiments: JC-CW J-HY S-HHJ Y-CC T-JH C-HH R-HW Y-CW W-PC W.-C. Chang. Performed the experiments: JC-CW W.-C. Chen Y-SW Y-CC T-JH C-HH R-HW W-PC. Analyzed the data: W.-C. Chen J-HY Y-CC JC-CW H-PW K-LT H-WC Y-CG W.-C.Chang EH. Contributed reagents/materials/analysis tools: W.-C. Chang. Wrote the manuscript: JC-CW Y-CC W.-C. Chang.

## References

1. Braun J, Sieper J (2007) Ankylosing spondylitis. Lancet 369: 1379–1390.
2. van der Heijde D, Calin A, Dougados M, Khan MA, van der Linden S, et al. (1999) Selection of instruments in the core set for DC-ART, SMARD, physical therapy, and clinical record keeping in ankylosing spondylitis. Progress report of the ASAS Working Group. Assessments in Ankylosing Spondylitis. J Rheumatol 26: 951–954.
3. Brown MA, Kennedy LG, MacGregor AJ, Darke C, Duncan E, et al. (1997) Susceptibility to ankylosing spondylitis in twins: the role of genes, HLA, and the environment. Arthritis Rheum 40: 1823–1828.
4. Brewerton DA, Hart FD, Nicholls A, Caffrey M, James DC, et al. (1973) Ankylosing spondylitis and HL-A 27. Lancet 1: 904–907.

5. Khan MA, Ball EJ (2002) Genetic aspects of ankylosing spondylitis. Best Pract Res Clin Rheumatol 16: 675–690.
6. Guo ZS, Li C, Lin ZM, Huang JX, Wei QJ, et al. (2010) Association of IL-1 gene complex members with ankylosing spondylitis in Chinese Han population. Int J Immunogenet 37: 33–37.
7. Safrany E, Pazar B, Csongei V, Jaromi L, Polgar N, et al. (2009) Variants of the IL23R gene are associated with ankylosing spondylitis but not with Sjogren syndrome in Hungarian population samples. Scand J Immunol 70: 68–74.
8. Wei JC, Tsai WC, Lin HS, Tsai CY, Chou CT (2004) HLA-B60 and B61 are strongly associated with ankylosing spondylitis in HLA-B27-negative Taiwan Chinese patients. Rheumatology (Oxford) 43: 839–842.

9. Reveille JD, Sims AM, Danoy P, Evans DM, Leo P, et al. (2010) Genome-wide association study of ankylosing spondylitis identifies non-MHC susceptibility loci. Nat Genet 42: 123–127.

10. Assassi S, Reveille JD, Arnett FC, Weisman MH, Ward MM, et al. (2011) Whole-blood gene expression profiling in ankylosing spondylitis shows upregulation of toll-like receptor 4 and 5. J Rheumatol 38: 87–98.

11. Sanchez A, Szczypiorska M, Juanola X, Bartolome N, Gratacos J, et al. (2010) Association of the intergenic single-nucleotide polymorphism rs10865331 (2p15) with ankylosing spondylitis in a Spanish population. J Rheumatol 37: 2345–2347.

12. Furuichi T, Maeda K, Chou CT, Liu YF, Liu TC, et al. (2008) Association of the MSX2 gene polymorphisms with ankylosing spondylitis in Japanese. J Hum Genet 53: 419–424.

13. Chen C, Zhang X, Wang Y (2010) Analysis of JAK2 and STAT3 polymorphisms in patients with ankylosing spondylitis in Chinese Han population. Clin Immunol 136: 442–446.

14. Berridge MJ, Bootman MD, Roderick HL (2003) Calcium signalling: dynamics, homeostasis and remodelling. Nat Rev Mol Cell Biol 4: 517–529.

15. Hogan PG, Lewis RS, Rao A (2010) Molecular basis of calcium signaling in lymphocytes: STIM and ORAI. Annu Rev Immunol 28: 491–533.

16. Penna A, Demuro A, Yeromin AV, Zhang SL, Safrina O, et al. (2008) The CRAC channel consists of a tetramer formed by Stim-induced dimerization of Orai dimers. Nature 456: 116–120.

17. Vig M, DeHaven WI, Bird GS, Billingsley JM, Wang H, et al. (2008) Defective mast cell effector functions in mice lacking the CRACM1 pore subunit of store-operated calcium release-activated calcium channels. Nat Immunol 9: 89–96.

18. Feske S, Gwack Y, Prakriya M, Srikanth S, Puppel SH, et al. (2006) A mutation in Orai1 causes immune deficiency by abrogating CRAC channel function. Nature 441: 179–185.

19. Parekh AB, Putney JW, Jr. (2005) Store-operated calcium channels. Physiol Rev 85: 757–810.

20. van der Linden S, Valkenburg HA, Cats A (1984) Evaluation of diagnostic criteria for ankylosing spondylitis. A proposal for modification of the New York criteria. Arthritis Rheum 27: 361–368.

21. Wei JC, Wong RH, Huang JH, Yu CT, Chou CT, et al. (2007) Evaluation of internal consistency and re-test reliability of Bath ankylosing spondylitis indices in a large cohort of adult and juvenile spondylitis patients in Taiwan. Clin Rheumatol 26: 1685–1691.

22. Chou CT, Tsai YF, Liu J, Wei JC, Liao TS, et al. (2001) The detection of the HLA-B27 antigen by immunomagnetic separation and enzyme-linked immunosorbent assay-comparison with a flow cytometric procedure. J Immunol Methods 255: 15–22.

23. Barrett JC, Fry B, Maller J, Daly MJ (2005) Haploview: analysis and visualization of LD and haplotype maps. Bioinformatics 21: 263–265.

24. Rudwaleit M, Siegert S, Yin Z, Eick J, Thiel A, et al. (2001) Low T cell production of TNFalpha and IFNgamma in ankylosing spondylitis: its relation to HLA-B27 and influence of the TNF-308 gene polymorphism. Ann Rheum Dis 60: 36–42.

25. Nilsen TW (2007) Mechanisms of microRNA-mediated gene regulation in animal cells. Trends Genet 23: 243–249.

26. Chatzikyriakidou A, Voulgari PV, Georgiou I, Drosos AA (2010) The role of microRNA-146a (miR-146a) and its target IL-1R-associated kinase (IRAK1) in psoriatic arthritis susceptibility. Scand J Immunol 71: 382–385.

27. Lopez D, Garcia-Hoyo R, Lopez de Castro JA (1994) Clonal analysis of alloreactive T cell responses against the closely related B*2705 and B*2703 subtypes. Implications for HLA-B27 association to spondyloarthropathy. J Immunol 152: 5557–5571.

28. Colotta F, Re F, Muzio M, Bertini R, Polentarutti N, et al. (1993) Interleukin-1 type II receptor: a decoy target for IL-1 that is regulated by IL-4. Science 261: 472–475.

29. Chou CT, Timms AE, Wei JC, Tsai WC, Wordsworth BP, et al. (2006) Replication of association of IL1 gene complex members with ankylosing spondylitis in Taiwanese Chinese. Ann Rheum Dis 65: 1106–1109.

30. Shiau MY, Lo MK, Chang CP, Yang TP, Ho KT, et al. (2007) Association of tumour necrosis factor alpha promoter polymorphisms with ankylosing spondylitis in Taiwan. Ann Rheum Dis 66: 562–563.

31. Duncan DJ, Yang Z, Hopkins PM, Steele DS, Harrison SM (2010) TNF-alpha and IL-1beta increase Ca2+ leak from the sarcoplasmic reticulum and susceptibility to arrhythmia in rat ventricular myocytes. Cell Calcium 47: 378–386.

32. Lee SK, Lee JO, Kim JH, Jung JH, You GY, et al. (2010) C-peptide stimulates nitrites generation via the calcium-JAK2/STAT1 pathway in murine macrophage Raw264.7 cells. Life Sci 86: 863–868.

33. Roberts-Thomson SJ, Peters AA, Grice DM, Monteith GR (2010) ORAI-mediated calcium entry: mechanism and roles, diseases and pharmacology. Pharmacol Ther 127: 121–130.

34. Schindl R, Frischauf I, Bergsmann J, Muik M, Derler I, et al. (2009) Plasticity in Ca2+ selectivity of Orai1/Orai3 heteromeric channel. Proc Natl Acad Sci U S A 106: 19623–19628.

35. Abdullaev IF, Bisaillon JM, Potier M, Gonzalez JC, Motiani RK, et al. (2008) Stim1 and Orai1 mediate CRAC currents and store-operated calcium entry important for endothelial cell proliferation. Circ Res 103: 1289–1299.

36. Trebak M (2009) STIM1/Orai1, ICRAC, and endothelial SOC. Circ Res 104: e56–57.

37. DeHaven WI, Smyth JT, Boyles RR, Putney JW, Jr. (2007) Calcium inhibition and calcium potentiation of Orai1, Orai2, and Orai3 calcium release-activated calcium channels. J Biol Chem 282: 17548–17556.

38. Li Z, Lu J, Xu P, Xie X, Chen L, et al. (2007) Mapping the interacting domains of STIM1 and Orai1 in Ca2+ release-activated Ca2+ channel activation. J Biol Chem 282: 29448–29456.

# 5

# Association between Polymorphism of the Vitamin D Metabolism Gene CYP27B1 and HLA-B27-Associated Uveitis. Is a State of Relative Immunodeficiency Pathogenic in HLA B27-Positive Uveitis?

Gernot Steinwender[1], Ewald Lindner[2], Martin Weger[1], Sophie Plainer[2], Wilfried Renner[3], Navid Ardjomand[1], Yosuf El-Shabrawi[2]*

1 Department of Ophthalmology, Auenbrugger University Graz, Graz, Austria, 2 Department of Ophthalmology, Klinikum Klagenfurt, Klagenfurt, Austria, 3 Clinical Institute of Medical and Chemical Laboratory Diagnostics, Medical University Graz, Graz, Austria

## Abstract

*Objective:* Polymorphisms of the vitamin D metabolism gene CYP27B1 showed associations with multiple autoimmune diseases. The aim of this study was to investigate a possible association between the rs703842 A>G polymorphism of the CYP27B1 gene and HLA-B27-associated uveitis.

*Design:* One hundred fifty-nine patients with HLA-B27-associated uveitis, 138 HLA-B27-negative controls and 100 HLA-B27-positive controls were recruited for this retrospective case-control study. Main outcome parameters were genotype distribution and allelic frequencies determined by polymerase chain reaction.

*Results:* Carriers of the rs703842G allele were found significantly more often in patients with HLA-B27-associated uveitis than in HLA-B27-positive controls ($p = 0.03$). Between patients and HLA-B27-negative controls no significant difference in the genotype distribution of the rs703842 A>G polymorphism was found ($p = 0.97$).

*Conclusions:* Our data suggest that the rs703842 A>G polymorphism may play a role in HLA-B27-associated uveitis.

**Editor:** Andreas Wedrich, Medical University Graz, Austria

**Funding:** The authors have no support or funding to report.

**Competing Interests:** The authors have declared that no competing interests exist.

* E-mail: yosuf.elshabrawi@kabeg.at

## Introduction

The by far most common type of uveitis is acute anterior uveitis (AAU). It is an important cause of visual impairment in western populations [1,2]. About 50% of all cases of AAU are associated with a positive Human leukocyte antigen (HLA) B27 haplotype [3,4]. HLA-B27-associated AAU represents a well-defined clinical entity and occurs usually unilateral, but both eyes may be affected sequentially.

HLA-B27 is closely linked not just with AAU but a spectrum of seronegative spondyloarthropathies (SpA) [5]. Development of these systemic inflammatory diseases is seen in almost half of patients suffering from HLA-B27-associated AAU [3]. The strongest disease association of HLA-B27 positivity is demonstrated in ankylosing spondylitis (AS) with around 90% of patients possessing the HLA-B27 haplotype. Other HLA-B27-associated systemic inflammatory diseases include reactive arthritis, psoriatic arthropathy, inflammatory bowel disease, and undifferentiated SpA [6].

Since only 2% of the individuals carrying the HLA-B27 haplotype (7–8% in Caucasians) will eventually develop SpAs or an AAU [2,7,8], additional environmental and genetic factors contributing to disease development have been suggested. In particular, bacterial triggers have been shown to play a critical role in the development of HLA-B27+-associated AAU and SpA. After genitourinary or gastrointestinal tract infection with Gram-negative bacteria microbe-derived antigens may trigger a CD8-restricted T lymphocyte immune response that cross-reacts with self-tissue antigens, resulting in an autoimmune tissue inflammation [3,9]. In addition, it has been proposed that the HLA-B27 haplotype plays an immunmodulatory role. Its presence has been correlated to an enhanced intracellular invasion or impaired intracellular elimination of gram-negative bacteria [10–13]. Thus it is feasible that the reduced ability to clear off intracellular antigens, as a result of the down-regulated inflammatory response, may result in the induction of chronic auto-inflammatory disease in HLA-B27+ individuals.

The established association between vitamin D deficiency and many autoimmune diseases [14–16] encouraged us to investigate a possible role of the vitamin D metabolism gene CYP27B1 (cytochrome P450 family 27 subfamily B peptide 1) in the development of HLA-B27-associated AAU. Large genome-wide

**Table 1.** Demographic Characteristics of Patients and Controls.

| | Patients with HLA-B27-Associated AAU (n = 159) | HLA-B27-Negative Controls (n = 138) | HLA-B27-Positive Controls (n = 100) |
|---|---|---|---|
| Male | 88 (55.3) | 97 (70.3) | 49 (49.0) |
| Female | 71 (44.7) | 41 (29.7) | 51 (51.0) |
| Mean Age±SD (yrs) | 44.8±14.3 | 35.3±12.5 | 38.2±4.2 |

AAU = Acute Anterior Uveitis
SD = Standard Deviation
Values are n (%) unless otherwise indicated. The mean age for the patient group states the age of onset of the disease.

association studies (GWAS) detected SNPs (single nucleotide polymorphisms) within this gene associated with type 1 diabetes [17,18], Hashimotòs thyroiditis, Gravès disease [19] and multiple sclerosis (MS) [20,21]. CYP27B1 encodes the enzyme 25-hydroxy-vitamin D-1 alpha hydroxylase, which hydroxylates the precursor of vitamin D3, 25-OHD$_3$, in its more bioactive form, 1,25(OH)$_2$D$_3$. Besides regulating calcium metabolism through binding to the vitamin D receptor (VDR), vitamin D3 also plays an important role in the innate and adaptive immune system [22]. In particular, 25-OHD$_3$ stimulates the expression of cathelicidin, an antibacterial peptide with critical influence on innate immune defense against invasive bacterial infection [23]. Furthermore, 1,25(OH)$_2$D$_3$ suppresses the adaptive immune response by enhancing the development of anti-inflammatory T helper cells type 2 (Th2) as well as inhibiting the development of T helper cells type 1 (Th1) [24,25].

In a recent GWAS rs703842 was identified as the strongest MS-associated polymorphism of the CYP27B1 gene [20]. The G-allele of rs703842 was shown to be significantly associated with lower

levels of 25-OHD$_3$ in a Canadian twin-study [26]. To the best of our knowledge CYP27B1 polymorphisms have not yet been studied in HLA-B27-associated AAU. Therefore, the purpose of this study was to investigate a possible association between the rs703842 A>G polymorphism and HLA-B27-associated AAU. In that context our group found significant associations with gene polymorphisms of monocyte chemoattractant protein-1 (MCP-1) and tumor necrosis factor-α (TNF-α) promoter [27,28]. The influence of those SNPs on AAU-susceptibility might be explained with a state of relative immunodeficiency in HLA-B27-positive individuals, leading to a prolonged bacterial persistence. This notion would be further supported in case of a correlation of HLA-B27-associated AAU and the G-allele of rs703842.

## Materials and Methods

In the present retrospective case-control study 159 patients with acute HLA-B27-associated uveitis, 138 HLA-B27-negative controls and 100 HLA-B27-positive controls were enrolled. Written informed consent was obtained from all participants prior to enrolment. The study was conducted in compliance of the principles of the Declaration of Helsinki and has been approved by the Ethics Committee of the Medical University Graz.

The following data were collected from all participants: gender, age at presentation, age at onset of anterior uveitis, diagnosis of associated systemic disease, number and duration of flares, and severe ocular complications (vitreous inflammation≥2+cells, cataract ≥2+opacity, secondary glaucoma, clinically significant macular edema as visualized by optic coherence tomography or fluorescein angiography). Patients with Fuchs̀ heterochromic iridocyclitis, sarcoidosis, or any history of malignancy were excluded from our investigation. All participants underwent an examination by a rheumatologist, including radiographs of the sacroiliac joints and the spine in presence of symptoms compatible with spondyloarthropathy.

The control cohort included 138 random, unrelated, healthy individuals who visited our clinic for reasons other than ocular inflammation. Subjects positive for HLA-B27, or with any history of ocular inflammation, autoimmune diseases, lower back pain or malignancy were not included as HLA-B27-negative control patients. 100 HLA-B27-positive, healthy, unrelated blood donors, whose DNA was provided by the Department of Blood Serology and Transfusion Medicine, served as the HLA-B27-positive control group.

### Laboratory methods

Blood samples from all subjects were collected in vaccutainers containing EDTA and stored at −20°C. Genomic DNA was isolated using the QIAmp Blood Mini kit (Quiagen GmbH, Hilden, Germany). Genotyping was performed by high-resolution

**Table 2.** Baseline Ocular and Systemic Parameters.

| Ocular parameters: | |
|---|---|
| One eye affected | 96 (60.4) |
| Both eyes alternating | 54 (34.0) |
| Both eyes concomitant | 9 (5.6) |
| Mean number of flares±SD | 7.19±9.24 |
| Mean duration of flares±SD (weeks) | 4.09±2.74 |
| Mean duration between flares±SD (months) | 20.95±18.31 |
| Secondary cataract | 17 (10.7) |
| Secondary glaucoma | 5 (3.1) |
| Posterior segment inflammation | 31 (19.5) |
| Macular edema | 21 (13.2) |
| Systemic parameters: | |
| Ankylosing spondylitis | 71 (44.7) |
| Juvenile idiopathic arthritis | 1 (0.6) |
| Undifferentiated spondylarthritis | 24 (15.1) |
| Reactive arthritis | 6 (3.8) |
| Crohns disease | 1 (0.6) |
| Psoriatic arthritis | 15 (9.4) |
| Overall systemic manifestation | 118 (74.2) |

SD = Standard Deviation
Values are n (%) unless otherwise indicated.

**Table 3.** Distribution of the rs703842 A>G Gene Polymorphism in Patients and Controls.

|    | Patients with HLA-B27-Associated AAU (n = 159) | HLA-B27-Negative Controls*(n = 138) | HLA-B27-Positive Controls**(n = 100) |
|----|---|---|---|
| GG | 14(8.8) | 6(4.3) | 5(5.0) |
| GA | 66(41.5) | 70(50.7) | 31(31.0) |
| AA | 79(49.7) | 62(44.9) | 64(64.0) |

AAU = Acute Anterior Uveitis, OR = Odds Ratio, CI = Confidence Interval, Values are n (%) unless otherwise indicated.
*HLA-B27-associated patients vs. HLA-B27-negative control subjects *p* = 0.97* (OR = 1.01, 95% CI 0.70–1.46)
**HLA-B27-associated patients vs. HLA-B27-positive control subjects *p* = 0.03** (OR = 0.62, 95% CI 0.41–0.94)

melting (LightCycler® 480 System, Roche Diagnostics, Vienna, Austria) following a protocol previously described [29]. Gene scanning software version 1.5 (Roche Applied Science, Mannheim, Germany) was used to determine sequence variations.

## Statistics

SPSS 15.0 for Windows (SPSS Inc., Chicago, IL) was used to analyze data. Genotype and allele frequencies were compared between patients and controls using the $\chi 2$ test. Logistic regression analysis was performed to calculate Odds ratios (OR) and 95% confidence intervals (95% CI). A *P*-value<0.05 was considered statistically significant.

## Results

Baseline characteristics of patients and controls are presented in Table 1, while the clinical characteristics of the patients are shown in Table 2. Ankylosing spondylitis (AS), the most common systemic manifestation in our cohort, was found in 71 (44.7%) out of 159 patients. 24 (15.1%) patients suffered from undifferentiated spondyloarthritis, 6 (3.8%) from reactive arthritis (ReA), 15 (9.4%) from psoriatic arthritis (PsA), and 1 (0.6%) patient suffered from Crohn's disease.

Table 3 shows the genotype distribution of the rs703842 A>G polymorphism in patients with HLA-B27-associated AAU and the two control groups. All allele and genotype frequencies were in Hardy-Weinberg-equilibrium. Carriers of the rs703842G allele were found significantly more often in patients with HLA-B27-associated AAU compared to healthy HLA-B27-positive individuals (OR = 0.62, 95% CI 0.41–0.94; p = 0.03). As the CYP27B1 gene is located on chromosome 12 and the gene for MHC-class I molecule HLA-B27 lies on chromosome 17 a linkage in the inheritance of these two genes is rather unlikely.

No statistically significant difference in the distribution of the rs703842 A>G polymorphism was observed between HLA-B27-positive and HLA-B27-negative controls (p = 0.54). The frequency of the minor allele also did not significantly differ between patients and healthy HLA-B27-negative subjects (p = 0.97).

There was no significant association between rs703842 A>G genotypes and recurrence of uveitis flare, and we did not find any association between rs703842 and underlying systemic diseases in our patient cohort. No significant difference in the genotype distribution of rs703842 in AAU-patients suffering from AS compared to AAU-patients without AS was observed (OR = 0.97, 95% CI 0.59–1.59; p = 0.89).

## Discussion

In the present study, we investigated the association of the CYP27B1 gene polymorphism rs703842 A>G with HLA-B27-

associated AAU in a central European population. We observed a significant higher prevalence of the G-allele in HLA-B27-associated AAU patients compared to healthy HLA-B27-positive controls.

Recently, immunomodulatory actions of vitamin D and an association between vitamin D deficiency and many autoimmune diseases have been reported [14–16]. Besides suppressing the adaptive immune response by enhancing the development of anti-inflammatory Th2-cells and inhibiting the development of Th1-cells [24,25], vitamin D3 also plays an important role in the innate immune response. It has been shown that vitamin D supplementation in vivo can enhance the expression of cathelicidin, an antibacterial peptide [23]. Cathelicidin was identified several years ago as a target for transcriptional regulation by 1,25(OH)2D3-liganded vitamin D receptor (VDR) [30,31] and has a critical influence on the innate immune defense against invasive bacterial infection [23].

Lower levels of 25-OHD$_3$, which were reported to be significantly associated with the G-allele of rs703842 [26], are thought to result in a reduced expression of the antibacterial protein cathelicidin, with a consecutive impaired pathogen elimination [23]. The finding of our study, where we find a higher prevalence of the G-allele in HLA-B27-associated AAU patients, suggests that a state of a relative immune deficiency in HLAB27$^+$ patients, is pathognomic in HLA B27$^+$ associated diseases, is in accordance with those of a recent gene expression profiling study [32]. Duan et al. described gene expression patterns in white blood cells in AS patients, an immunosuppressive phenotype [32].

Thus, a possible explanation for the increased AAU-susceptibility in HLA-B27-positive individuals harboring the minor G-allele is a further reduction of the already impaired ability of HLA-B27-positive individuals to clear off intracellular pathogens [10–13] through an additional immunosuppressive function of the investigated rs703842-SNP, ultimately leading to chronic autoinflammatory response of the immune system.

The results of the present study, also recapitulate previous findings of our group and thus supports the relevance of the investigated rs703842-SNP. Recently, we identified polymorphisms in the MCP-1 gene, which influence the susceptibility for HLA-B27-associated AAU via the aforementioned inefficient clearance of infectious agents [27]. We were also able to show that SNPs of the TNF-α promoter, leading to an increased transcription of TNF-α, an important factor in early stages of the innate immune response, had a protective effect against HLA-B27-associated AAU [28].

This is the first study to examine the role of the CYP27B1 gene in HLA-B27-associated AAU. The limitations of this study are those inherent to any other retrospective study. Genetic factors, however, unlike many other biologic parameters, are not influenced during lifetime.

In conclusion, our data suggest an association between the rs703842 A>G polymorphism and the risk for HLA-B27-associated AAU. Further research will be required to elucidate the underlying mechanisms of pathogenesis more precisely.

## References

1. Chang JH, Wakefield D. (2002) Uveitis: A global perspective. Ocul Immunol Inflamm 10: 263–279.
2. Wakefield D, Chang JH. (2005) Epidemiology of uveitis. Int Ophthalmol Clin 45: 1–13.
3. Chang JH, McCluskey PJ, Wakefield D. (2005) Acute anterior uveitis and HLA-B27. Surv Ophthalmol 50: 364–388.
4. Suhler EB, Martin TM, Rosenbaum JT. (2003) HLA-B27-associated uveitis: Overview and current perspectives. Curr Opin Ophthalmol 14: 378–383.
5. Linssen A, Rothova A, Valkenburg HA, Dekker-Saeys AJ, Luyendijk L, et al. (1991) The lifetime cumulative incidence of acute anterior uveitis in a normal population and its relation to ankylosing spondylitis and histocompatibility antigen HLA-B27. Invest Ophthalmol Vis Sci 32: 2568–2578.
6. Brewerton DA, Hart FD, Nicholls A, Caffrey M, James DC, et al. (1973) Ankylosing spondylitis and HL-A 27. Lancet 1: 904–907.
7. van der Linden SM, Valkenburg HA, de Jongh BM, Cats A. (1984) The risk of developing ankylosing spondylitis in HLA-B27 positive individuals. A comparison of relatives of spondylitis patients with the general population. Arthritis Rheum 27: 241–249.
8. Martin TM, Rosenbaum JT. (2011) An update on the genetics of HLA B27-associated acute anterior uveitis. Ocul Immunol Inflamm 19: 108–114.
9. Dougados M, Baeten D. (2011) Spondyloarthritis. Lancet 377: 2127–2137.
10. Saarinen M, Ekman P, Ikeda M, Virtala M, Gronberg A, et al. (2002) Invasion of salmonella into human intestinal epithelial cells is modulated by HLA-B27. Rheumatology (Oxford) 41: 651–657.
11. Laitio P, Virtala M, Salmi M, Pelliniemi LJ, Yu DT, et al. (1997) HLA-B27 modulates intracellular survival of salmonella enteritidis in human monocytic cells. Eur J Immunol 27: 1331–1338.
12. Virtala M, Kirveskari J, Granfors K. (1997) HLA-B27 modulates the survival of salmonella enteritidis in transfected L cells, possibly by impaired nitric oxide production. Infect Immun 65: 4236–4242.
13. Falgarone G, Blanchard HS, Riot B, Simonet M, Breban M. (1999) Cytotoxic T-cell-mediated response against yersinia pseudotuberculosis in HLA-B27 transgenic rat. Infect Immun 67: 3773–3779.
14. Pelajo CF, Lopez-Benitez JM, Miller LC. (2010) Vitamin D and autoimmune rheumatologic disorders. Autoimmun Rev 9: 507–510.
15. Maruotti N, Cantatore FP. (2010) Vitamin D and the immune system. J Rheumatol 37: 491–495.
16. Arnson Y, Amital H, Shoenfeld Y. (2007) Vitamin D and autoimmunity: New aetiological and therapeutic considerations. Ann Rheum Dis 66: 1137–1142.
17. Bailey R, Cooper JD, Zeitels L, Smyth DJ, Yang JH, et al. (2007) Association of the vitamin D metabolism gene CYP27B1 with type 1 diabetes. Diabetes 56: 2616–2621.
18. Lopez ER, Regulla K, Pani MA, Krause M, Usadel KH, et al. (2004) CYP27B1 polymorphisms variants are associated with type 1 diabetes mellitus in germans. J Steroid Biochem Mol Biol 89–90: 155–157.
19. Lopez ER, Zwermann O, Segni M, Meyer G, Reincke M, et al. (2004) A promoter polymorphism of the CYP27B1 gene is associated with addison's disease, hashimoto's thyroiditis, graves' disease and type 1 diabetes mellitus in germans. Eur J Endocrinol 151: 193–197.
20. Australia and New Zealand Multiple Sclerosis Genetics Consortium (ANZgene). (2009) Genome-wide association study identifies new multiple sclerosis susceptibility loci on chromosomes 12 and 20. Nat Genet 41: 824–828.
21. Sundqvist E, Baarnhielm M, Alfredsson L, Hillert J, Olsson T, et al. (2010) Confirmation of association between multiple sclerosis and CYP27B1. Eur J Hum Genet 18: 1349–1352.
22. Hewison M. (2010) Vitamin D and the immune system: New perspectives on an old theme. Endocrinol Metab Clin North Am 39: 365–79, , table of contents
23. Adams JS, Ren S, Liu PT, Chun RF, Lagishetty V, et al. (2009) Vitamin d-directed rheostatic regulation of monocyte antibacterial responses. J Immunol 182: 4289–4295.
24. Boonstra A, Barrat FJ, Crain C, Heath VL, Savelkoul HF, et al. (2001) 1alpha,25-dihydroxyvitamin d3 has a direct effect on naive CD4(+) T cells to enhance the development of Th2 cells. J Immunol 167: 4974–4980.
25. Daniel C, Sartory NA, Zahn N, Radeke HH, Stein JM. (2008) Immune modulatory treatment of trinitrobenzene sulfonic acid colitis with calcitriol is associated with a change of a T helper (th) 1/Th17 to a Th2 and regulatory T cell profile. J Pharmacol Exp Ther 324: 23–33.
26. Orton SM, Morris AP, Herrera BM, Ramagopalan SV, Lincoln MR, et al. (2008) Evidence for genetic regulation of vitamin D status in twins with multiple sclerosis. Am J Clin Nutr 88: 441–447.
27. Wegscheider BJ, Weger M, Renner W, Posch U, Ulrich S, et al. (2005) Role of the CCL2/MCP-1 -2518A>G gene polymorphism in HLA-B27 associated uveitis. Mol Vis 11: 896–900.
28. El-Shabrawi Y, Wegscheider BJ, Weger M, Renner W, Posch U, et al. (2006) Polymorphisms within the tumor necrosis factor-alpha promoter region in patients with HLA-B27-associated uveitis: Association with susceptibility and clinical manifestations. Ophthalmology 113: 695–700.
29. Lindner E, Weger M, Steinwender G, Griesbacher A, Posch U, et al. (2011) IL2RA gene polymorphism rs2104286 A>G seen in multiple sclerosis is associated with intermediate uveitis: Possible parallel pathways? Invest Ophthalmol Vis Sci 52: 8295–8299.
30. Gombart AF, Borregaard N, Koeffler HP. (2005) Human cathelicidin antimicrobial peptide (CAMP) gene is a direct target of the vitamin D receptor and is strongly up-regulated in myeloid cells by 1,25-dihydroxyvitamin D3. FASEB J 19: 1067–1077.
31. Wang TT, Nestel FP, Bourdeau V, Nagai Y, Wang Q, et al. (2004) Cutting edge: 1,25-dihydroxyvitamin D3 is a direct inducer of antimicrobial peptide gene expression. J Immunol 173: 2909–2912.
32. Duan R, Leo P, Bradbury L, Brown MA, Thomas G. (2010) Gene expression profiling reveals a downregulation in immune-associated genes in patients with AS. Ann Rheum Dis 69: 1724–1729.

## Author Contributions

Conceived and designed the experiments: GS MW WR YE. Performed the experiments: YE. Analyzed the data: EL GS SP MW NA. Contributed reagents/materials/analysis tools: WR YE. Wrote the paper: GS MW NA YE.

# 6

# Increased Levels of IgG Antibodies against Human HSP60 in Patients with Spondyloarthritis

**Astrid Hjelholt**[1]*, **Thomas Carlsen**[2], **Bent Deleuran**[1,3], **Anne Grethe Jurik**[4], **Berit Schiøttz-Christensen**[5], **Gunna Christiansen**[1,6], **Svend Birkelund**[2,6]

1 Department of Biomedicine – Medical Microbiology and Immunology, Aarhus University, Aarhus, Denmark, 2 Department of Health Science and Technology, Aalborg University, Aalborg, Denmark, 3 Department of Rheumatology, Aarhus University Hospital, Aarhus, Denmark, 4 Department of Radiology, Aarhus University Hospital, Aarhus, Denmark, 5 Aarhus Clinic for Rheumatic Diseases, Aarhus, Denmark, 6 Loke Diagnostics, Risskov, Denmark

## Abstract

Spondyloarthritis (SpA) comprises a heterogeneous group of inflammatory diseases, with strong association to human leukocyte antigen (HLA)-B27. A triggering bacterial infection has been considered as the cause of SpA, and bacterial heat shock protein (HSP) seems to be a strong T cell antigen. Since bacterial and human HSP60, also named HSPD1, are highly homologous, cross-reactivity has been suggested in disease initiation. In this study, levels of antibodies against bacterial and human HSP60 were analysed in SpA patients and healthy controls, and the association between such antibodies and disease severity in relation to HLA-B27 was evaluated. Serum samples from 82 patients and 50 controls were analysed by enzyme-linked immunosorbent assay (ELISA) for immunoglobulin (Ig)G1, IgG2, IgG3 and IgG4 antibodies against human HSP60 and HSP60 from *Chlamydia trachomatis*, *Salmonella enteritidis* and *Campylobacter jejuni*. Disease severity was assessed by the clinical scorings Bath Ankylosing Spondylitis Disease Activity Index (BASDAI), Bath Ankylosing Spondylitis Functional Index (BASFI) and Bath Ankylosing Spondylitis Metrology Index (BASMI). Levels of IgG1 and IgG3 antibodies against human HSP60, but not antibodies against bacterial HSP60, were elevated in the SpA group compared with the control group. Association between IgG3 antibodies against human HSP60 and BASMI was shown in HLA-B27$^+$ patients. Only weak correlation between antibodies against bacterial and human HSP60 was seen, and there was no indication of cross-reaction. These results suggest that antibodies against human HSP60 is associated with SpA, however, the theory that antibodies against human HSP60 is a specific part of the aetiology, through cross-reaction to bacterial HSP60, cannot be supported by results from this study. We suggest that the association between elevated levels of antibodies against human HSP60 and disease may reflect a general activation of the immune system and an increased expression of human HSP60 in the synovium of patients with SpA.

**Editor:** Anna Carla Goldberg, Albert Einstein Institute for Research and Education, Brazil

**Funding:** The study was supported by the EuroPathoGenomics –'EPG' (contract no. LSHB-CT-2005-512061), The Lundbeck Foundation (contract no. R19-A2023), Danish Rheumatism Association (contract no. R80-A1287), The Institute of Clinical Medicine Aarhus University and Jens Aage Sørensens and wife Edit Sørensens Foundation. The funders had no role in study design, data collection and analysis, decision to publish, or preparation of the manuscript.

**Competing Interests:** SB and GC are shareholders in Loke Diagnostics, Risskov, Denmark, which provided the HSP60 used in this study.

* E-mail: astrid.hjelholt@studmed.au.dk

## Introduction

Spondyloarthritis (SpA) comprises a heterogeneous group of chronic inflammatory diseases, including reactive arthritis, ankylosing spondylitis, psoriatic arthritis, inflammatory bowel disease (IBD) associated arthritis and undifferentiated spondyloarthritis. The clinical picture of these diseases is similar and characterized by inflammation of joints and entheses, predominantly in the spine and pelvis [1]. Assessments of disease activity, the physical function and the spinal mobility of ankylosing spondylitis patients are performed by the Bath Ankylosing Spondylitis Disease Activity Index (BASDAI), the Bath Ankylosing Spondylitis Functional Index (BASFI) and the Bath Ankylosing Spondylitis Metrology Index (BASMI), respectively. These indexes are based on clinical measurements (BASMI) along with questions pertaining degree of functional limitation and symptoms (BASDAI and BASFI) [2]. In this study BASDAI, BASFI and BASMI are considered parameters of experienced disease severity.

The pathogenesis of SpA is not fully elucidated, however, there is a remarkable hereditary component, and several MHC class I genes have been linked to disease. Best characterized is the association with human leukocyte antigen (HLA)-B27. The frequency of HLA-B27 varies in different spondyloarthritides [3]. The mechanisms underlying the influence of HLA-B27 on disease susceptibility are poorly understood. However, an interaction between HLA-B27 and a triggering bacterium as part of disease initiation has been suggested, partly based on animal studies [1,3]. In such a study HLA-B27 transgenic rats developed spondyloarthritis-like features, only if bred in a non-germ-free environment [4]. Moreover, reactive arthritis is in humans triggered by infection with urogenital or gastrointestinal bacteria such as *Salmonella enterica*, *Campylobacter jejuni*, *Yersinia enterocolitica* and *Chlamydia trachomatis* [5]. However, evidence supporting a preceding bacterial infection in other spondyloarthritides is limited [1], and the potential interplay between HLA-B27 and bacteria in the development of SpA in humans remains to be proven.

Bacterial heat shock protein (HSP) 60 has been shown to generate a strong immune response in patients suffering from reactive arthritis [6,7]. In humans, HSP60 is also named HSPD1 [8]. HSPs are a group of functionally related chaperones found in both eukaryotic and prokaryotic organisms. They are stress-proteins, and their expression is significantly up-regulated when cells are exposed to stressors, such as increased temperature, oxidative stress or inflammation [9]. Over the last few years it has been established that in addition to their function as intracellular chaperones, HSPs are also found in the cell membrane and outside the cell, presumably acting as indicators of the stressful conditions, activating other cells, particularly cells of the immune system [10]. It is assumed that circulating HSPs can have immunostimulating as well as immunosuppressing effects, depending on the circumstances by which they interact with other cells [10].

HSPs are highly conserved throughout evolution with considerable sequence homology between various species, and cross-reactivity between bacterial and human HSP60 has been connected with a number of inflammatory disorders [11,12]. Rheumatologic studies have primarily focused on the role of HSP60 in rheumatoid arthritis [13], whereas less studies are done on SpA. However, autoimmunity against HSP60 has also been suggested as a part of the aetiology in this group of diseases [14].

The aim of this study was to analyse serum levels of antibodies against bacterial and human HSP60 in SpA patients compared with an age and gender matched control group. Though other studies have examined the association between bacterial HSP60 and SpA [15,16,17], only one previous study has measured antibodies to human HSP60 in SpA patients [17]. Previous studies measuring IgG against HSP60 did not determine subclass specificity. However, since the significance of different IgG subclasses in relation to other inflammatory diseases has been described [18], this study evaluates the IgG subclasses to bacterial and human HSP60. In addition to the analyses of antibody levels in SpA patients compared with healthy controls, the association between antibody levels and disease severity assessed by the disease parameters BASDAI, BASFI and BASMI in relation to HLA-B27 status was evaluated.

## Materials and Methods

### Serum samples

Serum samples from SpA patients with symptoms restricted to the axial skeleton (n = 82) were obtained, together with HLA-B27 status and the clinical scorings, BASDAI, BASFI and BASMI. All patients met the European Spondyloarthropathy Study Group (ESSG) criteria [19]. Serum from age and gender matched normal healthy volunteers (n = 50) served as controls (control group) (Table 1).

The patients were enrolled in the study and serum was collected from the outpatient clinic at Aarhus University Hospital after informed written consent was given, according to the Danish Data Protection Agency, the Local Ethics Committee (project number 20050046) and the Declaration of Helsinki.

### Characteristics of the patients

Characteristics of the patient group are shown in Table 1. The age and gender of the patient and control group were comparable. As expected, the number of HLA-B27 positive persons was higher in the patient group (57%) than in the control group (8% in Caucasians) [20]. The average disease duration was eight years. Most of the patients did not receive any treatment at the time of enrolment in the study in agreement with their CRP being within the normal range (Table 1).

### Enzyme-linked immunosorbent assay (ELISA)

Prevalence of antibodies was determined by enzyme-linked immunosorbent assay (ELISA) using IgG subclass-specific secondary antibodies.

*cHSP60-IgG-ELISA* plates (Medac, Hamburg, Germany) [21] were used for *C. trachomatis* HSP60. The ELISA for *Campylobacter jejuni*, *Salmonella enteritidis* and human HSP60 were performed as described [22]. ELISA plates were coated with 4 µg/ml human HSP60, *C. jejuni* HSP60 or *S. enteritidis* HSP60.

Full length human HSP60 was obtained from Loke Diagnostics (Risskov, Denmark). *C. jejuni* and *S. enteritidis* HSP60 genes were cloned in pET30ek-LIC vector (Invitrogen, Carlsbad, CA, USA). The *C. jejuni* HSP60 gene was amplified with the forward primer 5′GACGACGACAACATGGCAAAAGAAATTATTTTTTCA-GATGAAGC3′ and reverse primer 5′GAGGAGAAGCCCGG-TTTACATCATTCCTCCCATGCC3′. For *S. enteritidis* HSP60 gene, the primers 5′GACGACGACAAGATGGCAGCTAAA-GACGTAAAATTCGG3′ and 5′GAGGAGAAGCCCGGTT-TACATCATGCCGCCC3′ were used. The PCR products were cloned into pET30ek-LIC by ligase independent cloning, according to the manufacturer's instructions. The proteins were expressed in *Escherichia coli* BL21 (DE3) using 1 mM isopropyl-β-D-thio-galactoside (IPTG) for two hrs. The recombinant HSP60 proteins were purified by $Ni^{2+}$ affinity chromatography under native conditions according to Schmitt et al. (1993) [23].

The human sera were diluted 1:50 in Bac-dil (Medac) before use. The secondary anti-human IgG antibodies used were horseradish peroxidase (HRP) conjugated, sheep-anti-human IgG1, IgG2, IgG3 and IgG4, (Binding site, Birmingham, UK), diluted 1:10,000 in Bac-dil. The dilutions were chosen so that the $OD_{450 nm}$ levels were within the linear part of the standard curve.

For quantification of IgG subclasses, NUNC MaxiSorp plates were coated with dilution series of native IgG1, IgG2, IgG3 and IgG4 from human myeloma plasma (EMD Biosciences, San Diego, CA, USA) in CCB-buffer (50 mM $NaHCO_3$, pH 9.6). The respective secondary antibodies were added to the dilutions.

In this study, inter-assay and intra-assay variability were less than 10% and 5%, respectively.

### Statistical analysis

The data were analysed by GraphPad Prism version 5.0a for Mac OS X (Graphpad Software Inc., La Jolla, CA, USA), using individual samples as experimental unit. Mann-Whitney U-test was used to analyse the differences between antibody levels in the two groups (SpA and control group) and between IgG1 and IgG3 antibody levels. Spearman nonparametric correlation was used to analyse the correlation between antibody levels, and between antibody levels and the disease parameters BASDAI, BASFI and BASMI. Probabilities <0.01 were considered as significant. The detection limits were calculated as the standard deviations (SD) of the blanks (wells incubated without sample) times two [cut-off = SD (Blanks) * 2].

## Results

### Antibodies against bacterial and human HSP60 in SpA patients and healthy controls

The levels of antibodies against bacterial HSP60 in the SpA group did not differ from the control group (Figure 1A, 1B, 1C). IgG1 and IgG3 antibodies against HSP60 from all three bacteria were frequently detected in both groups. The level of IgG1 was significantly higher than the IgG3 level (Figure 1A, 1B, 1C). Medians and interquartile ranges (IQR) of IgG1 and IgG3

**Table 1.** Characteristics of SpA patients, analysed in total and divided in the HLA-B27$^+$- and the HLA-B27$^-$-group, and healthy controls.

| Characteristics | SpA patients (n = 82) | | | Controls (n = 50) |
|---|---|---|---|---|
| | Total (n = 82) | HLA-B27$^+$ (n = 47) | HLA-B27$^-$ (n = 30) | |
| Age, years, mean (CI) | 37 (35;39) | 36 (34;39) | 37 (34;41) | 38 (21;65) |
| Gender, females, no. (%) | 55 (57) | 22 (47) | 22 (73) | 28 (56) |
| Disease duration, years, mean (CI) | 8 (7;9) | 9 (7;10) | 7 (6;8) | NA |
| Treatment | | | | |
| None, no. (%) | 64 (78) | 36 (77) | 24 (80) | NA |
| Methotrexate, no. (%) | 8 (10) | 4 (9) | 3 (10) | NA |
| Salazopyrin, no. (%) | 9 (11) | 6 (13) | 3 (10) | NA |
| Anti-TNF, no. (%) | 6 (7) | 5 (11) | 0 (0) | NA |
| CRP mg/L (CI) | 2.2 (1.5;3.9) | 5.5 (2.2;9.1) | 2.1 (1.5;2.7) | - |
| BASDAI, mean (CI) | 32 (27;37) | 27 (20;34) | 39 (30;49) | NA |
| BASMI, mean (CI) | 5 (2;8) | 8 (3;12) | 1 (0;3) | NA |
| BASFI, mean (CI) | 20 (16;25) | 17 (11;23) | 25 (16;34) | NA |

SpA spondyloarthritis, CRP C-reactive protein, BASDAI Bath Ankylosing Spondylitis Disease Activity Index, BASMI Bath Ankylosing Spondylitis Metrology index, BASFI Bath Ankylosing Functional index, CI confidence interval.

antibody levels (µg/mL) against human and bacterial HSP60 in the SpA group are shown in Table 2.

IgG2 antibodies were only demonstrated against HSP60 from S. enteritidis and C. jejuni in a few SpA patients (n = 5 and n = 1, respectively, data not shown). IgG4 antibodies were below detection limit (0.03 µg/ml) in all individuals.

IgG antibodies against human HSP60 were detected in both SpA patients and healthy controls. However, serum levels of both IgG1 and IgG3 antibodies against human HSP60 were higher in the SpA group compared with the control group (p<0.0001, Figure 1D). As demonstrated for bacterial HSP60, the IgG subclasses produced against human HSP60 were IgG1 and IgG3, whereas no IgG2 and IgG4 were detected (detection limit 0.03 µg/ml). There was no significant difference between levels of IgG1 and IgG3, however a trend towards a higher IgG3 level was observed (Figure 1D, Table 2). There was no correlation between serum levels of IgG1 and IgG3 against human HSP60.

Weak correlations between IgG1 antibodies against human HSP60 and IgG1 against HSP60 from the three bacteria species were found, whereas there was no correlation between IgG3 against human and bacterial HSP60 (Table 3). Also, correlation between IgG1 against the three bacterial HSP60, as well as IgG3 against the three bacterial HSP60, was observed (data not shown). The strongest correlation was between IgG1 against HSP60 from C. trachomatis and C. jejuni (r = 0.49, p<0.0001, data not shown).

No association was found between antibody levels and the patients' age, sex or treatment.

## Association between antibody levels, HLA-B27 status and the clinical parameters BASDAI, BASFI and BASMI

IgG3, but not IgG1, antibodies against human HSP60 were correlated with BASMI (Spearman r = 0.34, p = 0.003, Table 4), whereas no connection was found to BASDAI and BASFI. There was no association between antibodies against bacterial HSP60 and BASDAI, BASFI, or BASMI.

Patients were divided into two groups based on HLA-B27 status (HLA-B27$^+$, n = 47; HLA-B27$^-$, n = 30, Table 4). There was no difference in antibody levels in the two groups (Figure S1). A larger

part of the patients in the HLA-B27$^-$ group had a BASMI score of zero compared with the patients in the HLA-B27$^+$ group, and a tendency towards a higher mean BASMI score was seen in the HLA-B27$^+$ group compared with the HLA-B27$^-$ group (p = 0.02). Contrary to this, the mean value of BASFI (p = 0.13) and BASDAI (p = 0.05) tended to be higher in the HLA-B27$^-$ group (Table 1a). However, no significant differences in BASDAI, BASFI and BASMI scores were observed between the two groups (Table 1). In the HLA-B27$^+$ group the correlation between IgG3 against human HSP60 and BASMI was recognized again, and the association was stronger than observed in the total group of patients (Spearman r = 0.48, p = 0.001, Table 4). There was no correlation to bacterial HSP60. In the HLA-B27$^-$ group, no correlations were observed to neither bacterial nor human HSP60.

## Discussion

In this study, elevated levels of antibodies to human HSP60 but not bacterial HSP60 were found in patients with SpA. Correlation between antibodies against HSP60 from different bacteria was demonstrated, but no evidence of cross-reaction to human HSP60 was found, since only limited correlation occurred between antibodies to human and bacterial HSP60. Furthermore, the predominant IgG subclasses produced in response to human and bacterial HSP60 were different, IgG3 and IgG1, respectively.

The connection between antibodies against human HSP60 and SpA, reflected by the elevated antibody levels, was further supported by the fact that also the disease severity assessed by the clinical disease index, BASMI, was positively associated with antibodies against human HSP60. This association indicates that a higher antibody level against human HSP60 is connected to more severe disease. BASMI evaluates the mobility of the spine and more severe disease is therefore likely to reflect a higher degree of inflammation in joints and entheses. Altogether, this suggests that the level of antibodies against human HSP60 is related to the degree of inflammation.

The analysis of the HLA-B27$^+$- and the HLA-B27$^-$-group showed that the association between antibodies to human HSP60 and BASMI was restricted to HLA-B27 positive patients, whereas

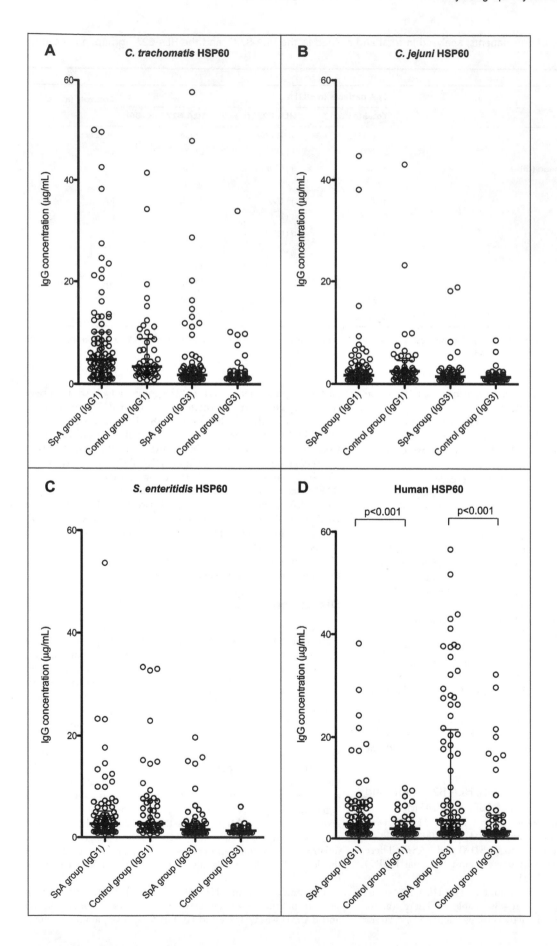

**Figure 1. Antibody levels in the SpA group and the control group.** Serum levels (µg/mL) of IgG1 and IgG3 antibodies against *C. trachomatis* HSP60 (A), *C. jejuni* HSP60 (B), *S. enteritidis* HSP60 (C) and human HSP60 (D) in the SpA group and the control group. No differences in serum levels of antibodies against the bacterial HSP60 were found between the two groups (A–C). Levels of anti-human HSP60 IgG1 and IgG3 were elevated in the SpA group compared with the control group (D). The two groups are compared using the non-parametric Mann-Whitney rank sum test. Bars represent medians with interquartile ranges (IQR).

no correlation was seen in the HLA-B27⁻ group. No difference in antibody levels between the two groups was evident, demonstrating that HLA-B27 is not essential in the generation of antibodies against human HSP60. However, the results suggest that the HLA-B27 allele may facilitate the association between antibodies to human HSP60 and joint inflammation. This is possibly reflecting a difference in the pathogenesis between the SpA diseases, since the frequency of HLA-B27 varies in the different diseases comprising the SpA group [3]. For example, in ankylosing spondylitis 96% of patients are HLA-B27 positive [25], whereas in IBD associated arthritis the frequency of the HLA-B27 allele is 40–60% [26,27]. Consequently, among HLA-B27 positive patients, ankylosing spondylitis is likely to be overrepresented compared with IBD associated arthritis. The association to the HLA-B27 allele may, however, be explained by the fact that a larger part of the HLA-B27 negative patients had a BASMI score of zero, compared with the HLA-B27 positive patients, though no significant difference between the two groups was evident.

A potential association between HLA-B27 and generation of antibodies is supported by findings from previous studies reporting an increased level of antibodies to bacterial HSP60 in HLA-B27 positive individuals [15,16]. Many hypothesises regarding the correlation to HLA-B27 have been suggested, including molecular mimicry, the arthritogenic peptide hypothesis, which postulates that HLA molecules act as a peptide-binding molecule for infectious agents, or that HLA-B27 may simply represent a marker locus, closely linked to a yet unidentified true immune response gene responsible for the inflammatory response [3]. Previous published results are ambiguous. In one study, association between antibodies to HSP60 from yersinia enterocolitica in patients suffering from uveitis was found primarily in HLA-B27 positive patients [28], whereas in another study, no difference in levels of IgA antibodies against *C. pneumoniae* HSP60 between HLA-B27 –positive and negative patients with uveitis was found [29]. In order to clarify a potential connection between HLA-B27 and the role of human HSP60, more studies, focusing on HLA-B27, need to be done.

One other study has analysed antibodies against human HSP60 in relation to a group of inflammatory diseases, including reactive arthritis [17]. This study measured total IgG against human HSP60 and reported a similar elevation of antibodies in patients

with reactive arthritis. In addition, elevated levels of antibodies to *E. coli* HSP60 and positive correlation between antibodies to human and bacterial HSP60 were reported [17]. The possible link between an eliciting bacterial infection, generation of antibodies against human HSP60 and the development of SpA was not demonstrated in the present study. First, the positive correlations between IgG1 antibodies against human HSP60 and antibodies against *S. enteritidis*, *C. jejuni* and *C. trachomatis* HSP60 were weak and no correlation to IgG3 antibodies, which was the predominant subclass to human HSP60, was observed. Second, the fact that bacterial HSP60 induced an IgG1 dominated response while IgG3 was the main IgG subclass against human HSP60 makes cross-reaction unlikely. Third, even though both IgG1 and IgG3 antibodies to human HSP60 were associated with SpA, no elevation in serum levels of antibodies against HSP60 from *S. enteritidis*, *C. jejuni* and *C. trachomatis* was seen in the SpA group compared with the healthy controls. These results imply that the SpA patients, as a group, do not have a history of more frequent or severe infections with *S. enteritidis*, *C. jejuni* and *C. trachomatis*, leading to a higher antibody level, compared with the background population. This suggests that a potential causality between infection and disease is not straightforward, and that the risk of developing SpA after infection may vary between individuals. This could possibly be due to a hereditary vulnerability. However, this may also reflect the fact, that the SpA patients was analysed as a group. The group of SpA comprises a number of heterogeneous diseases, possibly with different pathogeneses and so far, only an association between reactive arthritis and bacterial infection is evident [5].

In addition, the importance of other bacteria needs to be considered. Higher levels of antibodies to HSP60 from *E. coli* and *Klebsiella pneumoniae* have been reported in patients with ankylosing spondylitis compared with a control group [15,16]. In the present study, antibodies against HSP60 from *E. coli* and *K. pneumoniae* were not measured. The HSP60 amino acid sequences from these bacteria are almost identical to HSP60 from *S. enteritidis* (98.4% and 96.2% respectively) [30]. Consequently, the antibody epitopes are considered to be very similar, and it is not expected that measurement of antibodies against HSP60 from *E. coli* and *K. pneumoniae* would reveal a different result. HSP60 from *S. enteritidis* was chosen because at the time when most of the SpA cases

**Table 2.** Medians and interquartile ranges (IQR) of IgG1 and IgG3 antibody levels (µg/mL) against human and bacterial HSP60 in the SpA group.

| | Median (IQR) | | Statistical result of the Mann Whitney U test (p-value) |
| --- | --- | --- | --- |
| | IgG1 | IgG3 | |
| Human HSP60 | 2.91 (1.71;6.53) | 3.38 (1.31;21.42) | P = 0.53 |
| *C. trachomatis* HSP60 | 5.50 (3.07;10.81) | 1.52 (1.07;3.08) | p<0.0001 |
| *C. jejuni* HSP60 | 2.14 (1.64;3.22) | 1.64 (1.41;2.08) | P = 0.0001 |
| *S. enteritidis* HSP60 | 3.22 (2.00;6.03) | 1.55 (1.12;2.31) | p<0.0001 |

The two groups are compared using the non-parametric Mann-Whitney rank sum test.

**Table 3.** The Spearman rank correlation coefficient, r, for the correlation between levels of IgG1 and IgG3 against bacterial and human HSP60.

|  | C. trachomatis (IgG1) | C. trachomatis (IgG3) | S. enteritidis (IgG1) | S. enteritidis (IgG3) | C. jejuni (IgG1) | C. jejuni (IgG3) |
|---|---|---|---|---|---|---|
| Human (IgG1) | 0.32** | 0.01 | 0.26* | 0.06 | 0.26* | 0.01 |
| Human (IgG3) | 0.02 | 0.12 | −0.02 | 0.19 | −0.06 | 0.12 |

**p<0.001;
*p<0.01.

developed, a high number of *S. enteritidis* infections were seen in Denmark [31]. Furthermore, *S. enteritidis* is shown to be strongly associated with reactive joints symptoms [32].

Altogether, indications supporting cross-reacting antibodies were not evident from this study. This is supported by our findings in a previous study on patients with tubal factor infertility after *C. trachomatis* infection, in which we found no indications of cross-reaction between antibodies against HSP60 from *C. trachomatis* and human HSP60 either [33].

It was evident from the present study, that the IgG antibodies produced against bacterial and human HSP60 were IgG1 and IgG3, respectively. A similar IgG subclass distribution in response to self-antigens has been demonstrated in other inflammatory diseases, including rheumatoid arthritis [18] and lupus erythematosus [34]. However, also IgG2 and IgG4 has been demonstrated to be of importance in inflammatory diseases, such as vasculitis and [18] and myasthenia gravis [35].

The main function of IgG1 and IgG3 antibodies are complement activation and opsonisation of invading microbes through FC receptor binding on macrophages. IgG3 is the strongest complement activator [36], and furthermore, IgG3 is more flexible as a result of a longer hinge region [37]. In this study, we observed a significantly higher serum level of IgG1 against bacterial HSP60 compared with the level of IgG3. Contrary, a trend towards a higher level of IgG3 compared with IgG1 antibodies against human HSP60 was observed. This is remarkable, since the general content of IgG1 in the blood is higher than IgG3 (65% and 7%, respectively) [38,39], and the half-life of IgG3 is three times shorter than IgG1 [40]. This suggests that IgG3 is the most significant IgG subclass produced against human HSP60 in relation to SpA. Furthermore, this indicates, that IgG3 is generated continuously, possibly as a result of ongoing inflammation, whereas, IgG1 may have been generated years ago, during infection. It is possible, that

**Table 4.** The Spearman rank correlation coefficient, r, for the correlation between levels of IgG1 and IgG3 against human HSP60 and BASDAI, BASMI and BASMI in the total group of SpA patients, the group of HLA-B27 positive patients (HLA-B27$^+$) and the group of HLA-B27 negative patients (HLA-B27$^-$).

|  | Total SpA group | | HLA-B27$^+$ | | HLA-B27$^-$ | |
|---|---|---|---|---|---|---|
|  | IgG1 | IgG3 | IgG1 | IgG3 | IgG1 | IgG3 |
| BASDAI | 0.13 | 0.05 | 0.18 | 0.05 | 0.05 | 0.02 |
| BASFI | −0.03 | 0.01 | 0.08 | 0.00 | −0.27 | −0.13 |
| BASMI | 0.16 | 0.34* | 0.29 | 0.48** | −0.13 | 0.05 |

**p<0.001;
*p<0.01.

the flexibility and shorter half-life of IgG3 may be of critical value for regulatory responses that can be quickly up- and down regulated.

The isotype switching and secretion of IgG subclasses are stimulated by CD4+ Th cell subsets and their cytokines [41]. However, the knowledge about the ability of specific cytokines to induce B-cells production of different IgG subclasses is controversial. This is partly because of methodological differences in the identification of B- and T cell subtypes, making comparison difficult. Furthermore, the complexity of the cytokine environment in the lymph nodes makes *in vitro* studies a rather inaccurate approximation but the inaccessibility of this B-cell compartment in humans makes *in vivo* studies difficult [42]. In studies using CD40L activated human B cells, IL-4 stimulation was predominantly associated with IgG1 expression, whereas stimulation with IL-21 primarily generated IgG3$^+$ B-cells [43], indicating that these cytokines influence the IgG subclass switch. The different IgG response observed in this study may be explained by a different balance of T-cell regulatory factors at the site of antigen presentation, which is likely to occur in the joints for human HSP60, and in the gastrointestinal and urogenital tract for bacterial HSP60.

Stressed cells and tumor cells have been shown to express and release human HSP60 [44,45]. Likewise, increased expression of human HSP60 in the synovium of patients with rheumatoid arthritis has been demonstrated [24,46]. A similar upregulation is likely to happen in the synovium of SpA patients, which could be the explanation of the increased levels of antibodies against human HSP60 in SpA patients compared with healthy controls seen in the current study. Because of the joint inflammation related to SpA, we expect expression of human HSP60 to be increased and as a consequence, levels of antibodies may thereby be elevated. This could also explain the association between antibody levels and disease severity, demonstrated in this study. Though higher levels of antibodies and circulating HSP60 have been associated with disease, antibodies against HSP60 were also measured in the control group, just like expression of human HSP60 was found in normal synovium [46] and circulating HSP60 was detected in healthy subjects [12]. Furthermore, human HSP60 is not disease specific, but is found to be associated with a number of inflammatory diseases besides SpA. Moreover, not all patients produced antibodies against human HSP60. This indicates that an immune response against human HSP60 may not be the cause of SpA, but rather a marker reflecting inflammation. Human HSP60 is considered an immunomodulating agent, capable of interacting with the cells of the immune system [10,47], and thereby having the potential to down- as well as up-regulate inflammation. The role of the increased expression of human HSP60 in SpA and other inflammatory diseases is still to be discovered.

In conclusion, the results of the present study support an association between SpA and a humoral immunological response towards human HSP60. No elevation of serum levels of antibodies against HSP60 from *S. enteritidis*, *C. jejuni* and *C. trachomatis* was seen in the SpA patients. Furthermore, the hypothesis regarding cross-reacting antibodies as a causal factor in SpA could not be supported. The antibody level was positively correlated with disease severity, possibly reflecting the degree of inflammation. Altogether, the theory that antibodies against human HSP60 is a specific part of the aetiology, through cross-reaction to bacterial HSP60, cannot be supported by the results from this study. However, we suggest that the association between elevated levels of antibodies against human HSP60 and disease may reflect a general activation of the immune system and an increased expression of human HSP60 in the synovium of patients with SpA.

## Supporting Information

**Figure S1    Levels of antibodies against human HSP60 in the HLA-B27$^+$- and the HLA-B27$^-$group.** Serum levels (μg/mL) of IgG1 and IgG3 antibodies against human HSP60 in SpA patient divided into an HLA-B27$^+$- and an HLA-B27$^-$-group. No

difference in levels of anti-human HSP60 IgG1 and IgG3 was seen between the two groups. The groups are compared using the nonparametric Mann-Whitney rank sum test. Bars represent medians with interquartile ranges (IQR).

## Acknowledgments

We are grateful to Karin Skovgaard Sørensen and Ahmed Bassim Abduljabar for excellent and skilful technical assistance. Furthermore, we'd like to thank Lisbet Wellejus Pedersen, Thomas Johannesson and Karin H. Jensen for proofreading.

## Author Contributions

Conceived and designed the experiments: AH SB GC. Performed the experiments: AH TC. Analyzed the data: AH. Contributed reagents/materials/analysis tools: SB GC AGJ BSC BD. Wrote the paper: AH SB GC TC.

## References

1. Braun J, Sieper J (2007) Ankylosing spondylitis. Lancet 369: 1379–1390.
2. Barr A, Keat A (2010) Spondyloarthritides: evolving therapies. Arthritis Res Ther 12: 221.
3. McMichael A, Bowness P (2002) HLA-B27: natural function and pathogenic role in spondyloarthritis. Arthritis Res 4 Suppl 3: S153–158.
4. Taurog JD, Richardson JA, Croft JT, Simmons WA, Zhou M, et al. (1994) The germfree state prevents development of gut and joint inflammatory disease in HLA-B27 transgenic rats. J Exp Med 180: 2359–2364.
5. Townes JM (2010) Reactive arthritis after enteric infections in the United States: the problem of definition. Clin Infect Dis 50: 247–254.
6. Sieper J, Braun J, Kingsley GH (2000) Report on the Fourth International Workshop on Reactive Arthritis. Arthritis Rheum 43: 720–734.
7. Zeidler H, Kuipers J, Kohler L (2004) Chlamydia-induced arthritis. Curr Opin Rheumatol 16: 380–392.
8. Kampinga HH, Hageman J, Vos MJ, Kubota H, Tanguay RM, et al. (2009) Guidelines for the nomenclature of the human heat shock proteins. Cell Stress Chaperones 14: 105–111.
9. Zugel U, Kaufmann SH (1999) Role of heat shock proteins in protection from and pathogenesis of infectious diseases. Clin Microbiol Rev 12: 19–39.
10. De Maio A (2011) Extracellular heat shock proteins, cellular export vesicles, and the Stress Observation System: a form of communication during injury, infection, and cell damage. It is never known how far a controversial finding will go! Dedicated to Ferruccio Ritossa. Cell Stress Chaperones 16: 235–249.
11. Raska M, Weigl E (2005) Heat shock proteins in autoimmune diseases. Biomed Pap Med Fac Univ Palacky Olomouc Czech Repub 149: 243–249.
12. Pockley AG, Bulmer J, Hanks BM, Wright BH (1999) Identification of human heat shock protein 60 (Hsp60) and anti-Hsp60 antibodies in the peripheral circulation of normal individuals. Cell Stress Chaperones 4: 29–35.
13. Huang MN, Yu H, Moudgil KD (2010) The involvement of heat-shock proteins in the pathogenesis of autoimmune arthritis: a critical appraisal. Semin Arthritis Rheum 40: 164–175.
14. Gaston JS (1998) Heat shock proteins as potential targets in the therapy of inflammatory arthritis. Biotherapy 10: 197–203.
15. Dominguez-Lopez ML, Ortega-Ortega Y, Manriquez-Raya JC, Burgos-Vargas R, Vega-Lopez A, et al. (2009) Antibodies against recombinant heat shock proteins of 60 kDa from enterobacteria in the sera and synovial fluid of HLA-B27 positive ankylosing spondylitis patients. Clin Exp Rheumatol 27: 626–632.
16. Dominguez-Lopez ML, Burgos-Vargas R, Galicia-Serrano H, Bonilla-Sanchez MT, Rangel-Acosta HH, et al. (2002) IgG antibodies to enterobacteria 60 kDa heat shock proteins in the sera of HLA-B27 positive ankylosing spondylitis patients. Scand J Rheumatol 31: 260–265.
17. Handley HH, Yu J, Yu DT, Singh B, Gupta RS, et al. (1996) Autoantibodies to human heat shock protein (hsp)60 may be induced by Escherichia coli groEL. Clin Exp Immunol 103: 429–435.
18. Cambridge G, Williams M, Leaker B, Corbett M, Smith CR (1994) Anti-myeloperoxidase antibodies in patients with rheumatoid arthritis: prevalence, clinical correlates, and IgG subclass. Ann Rheum Dis 53: 24–29.
19. Dougados M, van der Linden S, Juhlin R, Huitfeldt B, Amor B, et al. (1991) The European Spondylarthropathy Study Group preliminary criteria for the classification of spondylarthropathy. Arthritis Rheum 34: 1218–1227.
20. Bowness P (2002) HLA B27 in health and disease: a double-edged sword? Rheumatology (Oxford) 41: 857–868.
21. Bax CJ, Dorr PJ, Trimbos JB, Spaargaren J, Oostvogel PM, et al. (2004) Chlamydia trachomatis heat shock protein 60 (cHSP60) antibodies in women without and with tubal pathology using a new commercially available assay. Sex Transm Infect 80: 415–416.
22. Drasbek M, Nielsen PK, Persson K, Birkelund S, Christiansen G (2004) Immune response to Mycoplasma pneumoniae P1 and P116 in patients with atypical pneumonia analyzed by ELISA. BMC Microbiol 4: 7.
23. Schmitt J, Hess H, Stunnenberg HG (1993) Affinity purification of histidine-tagged proteins. Mol Biol Rep 18: 223–230.
24. Schett G, Tohidast-Akrad M, Steiner G, Smolen J (2001) The stressed synovium. Arthritis Res 3: 80–86.
25. Benjamin R, Parham P (1990) Guilt by association: HLA-B27 and ankylosing spondylitis. Immunol Today 11: 137–142.
26. Fitzgerald O, Winchester R (2009) Psoriatic arthritis: from pathogenesis to therapy. Arthritis Res Ther 11: 214.
27. Rashid T, Ebringer A (2011) Gut-mediated and HLA-B27-associated arthritis: an emphasis on ankylosing spondylitis and Crohn's disease with a proposal for the use of new treatment. Discov Med 12: 187–194.
28. Cancino-Diaz JC, Vargas-Rodriguez L, Grinberg-Zylberbaum N, Reyes-Lopez MA, Dominguez-Lopez ML, et al. (2004) High levels of IgG class antibodies to recombinant HSP60 kDa of Yersinia enterocolitica in sera of patients with uveitis. Br J Ophthalmol 88: 247–250.
29. Huhtinen M, Puolakkainen M, Laasila K, Sarvas M, Karma A, et al. (2001) Chlamydial antibodies in patients with previous acute anterior uveitis. Invest Ophthalmol Vis Sci 42: 1816–1819.
30. Needleman SB, Wunsch CD (1970) A general method applicable to the search for similarities in the amino acid sequence of two proteins. J Mol Biol 48: 443–453.
31. Wegener HC, Hald T, Lo Fo Wong D, Madsen M, Korsgaard H, et al. (2003) Salmonella control programs in Denmark. Emerg Infect Dis 9: 774–780.
32. Locht H, Molbak K, Krogfelt KA (2002) High frequency of reactive joint symptoms after an outbreak of Salmonella enteritidis. J Rheumatol 29: 767–771.
33. Hjelholt A, Christiansen G, Johannesson TG, Ingerslev HJ, Birkelund S (2011) Tubal factor infertility is associated with antibodies against Chlamydia trachomatis heat shock protein 60 (HSP60) but not human HSP60. Hum Reprod 26: 2069–2076.
34. Manolova I, Dancheva M, Halacheva K (2002) Predominance of IgG1 and IgG3 subclasses of autoantibodies to neutrophil cytoplasmic antigens in patients with systemic lupus erythematosus. Rheumatol Int 21: 227–233.
35. Liu Y, Wang W, Li J (2011) Evaluation of serum IgG subclass concentrations in myasthenia gravis patients. Int J Neurosci 121: 570–574.
36. Spiegelberg HL (1974) Biological activities of immunoglobulins of different classes and subclasses. Adv Immunol 19: 259–294.
37. Adlersberg JB, Franklin EC, Frangione B (1975) Repetitive hinge region sequences in human IgG3: isolation of an 11,000-dalton fragment. Proc Natl Acad Sci U S A 72: 723–727.
38. Schroeder HW Jr, Cavacini L (2010) Structure and function of immunoglobulins. J Allergy Clin Immunol 125: S41–52.
39. Morell A, Skvaril F, Steinberg AG, Van Loghem E, Terry WD (1972) Correlations between the concentrations of the four sub-classes of IgG and Gm Allotypes in normal human sera. J Immunol 108: 195–206.
40. Morell A, Terry WD, Waldmann TA (1970) Metabolic properties of IgG subclasses in man. J Clin Invest 49: 673–680.
41. Stevens TL, Bossie A, Sanders VM, Fernandez-Botran R, Coffman RL, et al. (1988) Regulation of antibody isotype secretion by subsets of antigen-specific helper T cells. Nature 334: 255–258.
42. Garraud O, Borhis G, Badr G, Degrelle S, Pozzetto B, et al. (2012) Revisiting the B-cell compartment in mouse and humans: more than one B-cell subset exists in the marginal zone and beyond. BMC Immunol 13: 63.

43. Avery DT, Bryant VL, Ma CS, de Waal Malefyt R, Tangye SG (2008) IL-21-induced isotype switching to IgG and IgA by human naive B cells is differentially regulated by IL-4. J Immunol 181: 1767–1779.
44. Pfister G, Stroh CM, Perschinka H, Kind M, Knoflach M, et al. (2005) Detection of HSP60 on the membrane surface of stressed human endothelial cells by atomic force and confocal microscopy. J Cell Sci 118: 1587–1594.
45. Merendino AM, Bucchieri F, Campanella C, Marciano V, Ribbene A, et al. (2010) Hsp60 is actively secreted by human tumor cells. PLoS One 5: e9247.
46. Sharif M, Worrall JG, Singh B, Gupta RS, Lydyard PM, et al. (1992) The development of monoclonal antibodies to the human mitochondrial 60-kd heat-shock protein, and their use in studying the expression of the protein in rheumatoid arthritis. Arthritis Rheum 35: 1427–1433.
47. Thiel A, Wu P, Lauster R, Braun J, Radbruch A, et al. (2000) Analysis of the antigen-specific T cell response in reactive arthritis by flow cytometry. Arthritis Rheum 43: 2834–2842.

# 7

# Circulating Protein Fragments of Cartilage and Connective Tissue Degradation Are Diagnostic and Prognostic Markers of Rheumatoid Arthritis and Ankylosing Spondylitis

**Anne C. Bay-Jensen[1]\*, Stephanie Wichuk[2], Inger Byrjalsen[1], Diana J. Leeming[1], Nathalie Morency[2], Claus Christiansen[1], Morten A. Karsdal[1], Walter P. Maksymowych[2]**

1 Rheumatology, Nordic Bioscience, Herlev, Denmark, 2 Division of Rheumatology, University of Alberta, Edmonton, Alberta, Canada

## Abstract

Inflammation driven connective tissue turnover is key in rheumatic diseases, such as ankylosing spondylitis (AS). Few biomarkers are available for measuring disease prognosis or the efficacy of interventions applied in these tissue-related conditions. Type II collagen is the primary structural protein of cartilage and type III collagen of connective tissues, and obvious targets for the collagenalytic, which increase during tissue inflammation. The objective of the study was to investigate the diagnostic and prognostic utility of cartilage, C2M, and synovial, C3M, turnover biomarkers in AS. Serum samples were retrieved from patients suffering from AS (n = 103), RA (n = 47) and healthy controls (n = 56). AS progressors were defined as having new vertebral syndesmophytes or more that 3 unit change in mSASSS over a two-year period. Type II collagen degradation markers in serum were measured by the C2M ELISA, and type III collagen degradation by the C3M ELISA. Logistic regression and dichotomized decision tree were used to analyze the prognostic value of the markers individually or in combination. Both C2M and C3M levels were significantly higher in RA patients than in healthy controls (p<0.0001). Diagnostic utility was analyzed by ROC and areas under the curve (AUCs) were 72% and 89% for C2M and C3M, respectively. Both C2M and C3M, were significantly higher in serum samples from AS patient than from healthy controls (p<0.0001). The AUCs of C2M and C3M, respectively, were 70% and 81% for AS. A combination of C2M and C3M, dichotomized according to best cut-offs for individual markers, could correctly identify 80% of the progressors and 61% of the non-progressors. The present study is the first to show that specific biomarkers of cartilage and connective tissue degradation facilitate both diagnosis and prediction of progression of RA and AS.

**Editor:** Masataka Kuwana, Keio University School of Medicine, Japan

**Funding:** The study was partly supported by the Danish Research Foundation and partly by the research budgets of the departments of ACBJ and WP at Nordic Bioscience and University of Alberta, respectively. The funders had no role in study design, data collection and analysis, decision to publish, or preparation of the manuscript.

**Competing Interests:** ACBJ, IB, DJL and MK are full time employees at, and CC and MK hold stocks in, Nordic Bioscience. This study was partly funded by Nordic Bioscience. Nordic Bioscience is a privately-owned; small-medium size enterprise partly focused the development of biomarkers for rheumatic and fibrotic diseases. The two biomarkers described in the manuscript are patented by Nordic Bioscience (C2M, "ASSAY FOR A TYPE II COLLAGEN BIOMARKER" Patent Application WO/2012/038331; C3M, "FIBROSIS BIOMARKER ASSAY" Patent Application WO/2010/115749 & United States Patent Application 20100209940). Further research on the markers will be conducted which may lead to commercialization. There are no further patents, products in development or marketed products to declare. None of the authors received fees, bonuses or other benefits for the work described in the manuscript. WP, SW and NM have no financial or competing interest to declare. WP is a Medical Scientist of the Alberta Heritage Foundation for Medical Research.

\* E-mail: acbj@nordicbioscience.com

## Introduction

Ankylosing spondylitis (AS) and rheumatoid arthritis (RA) are both chronic inflammatory arthropathies that are associated with excessive turnover of connective tissues, such as cartilage and ligaments, in and surrounding the affected joint [1]. RA is a systemic autoimmune disease that primarily attacks synovial joints leading to deterioration and loss of mobility. Moreover synovial inflammation and fibrosis are key events in the pathogenesis of RA [1]. Bone changes such as erosions, bone marrow lesions, and osteitis are also common pathological features of RA [2]. AS is also a systemic disease characterized by chronic inflammation of the

sacroiliac joints, entheses, bone marrow, and structural lesions such as, syndesmophytes and joint ankylosis [3–5]. Accordingly, a common denominator of RA and AS is an elevated, inflammation-dependent turnover of connective tissue, specifically the extracellular matrix (ECM), in cartilage and synovium. ECM composition varies between connective tissues. The major ECM protein of cartilage is type II collagen, while type III collagen is the key protein of soft tissue (such as the synovium and entheses). Monitoring the turnover of these collagens may aid the understanding of the pathogenesis of RA and AS.

In pathological situations, such as RA and AS, inflammation disturbs the normal repair response leading to excessive remodeling and tissue turnover. The consequence of this heightened ECM remodeling is the release of a range of protein-degradation products generated by the proteases expressed locally in the pathologically affected area. The degradation fragments result in the exposure of *de novo* sites in the proteins, referred to as neo-epitopes. These protein degradation fragments may be specific for the tissue of origin and for the involved enzymes, and may consequently be used for the identification of molecular biochemical markers [6]. Recently, neo-epitope-based biochemical markers measured in serum have received increased attention for their diagnostic and prognostic potential in rheumatic diseases [7]. In slowly progressing diseases, such as osteoporosis and osteoarthritis (OA), bone resorption and cartilage degradation markers have been studied extensively [8].

It has been shown that cartilage degradation is highly elevated in RA patients, as measured by C-terminal telopeptide of type II collagen (CTX-II) in urine and *in situ* histological assessments [9]. These specific activities are precisely coordinated under physiological situations, with a specified sequence of events resulting in controlled tissue turnover.

Only a few serological biomarkers with diagnostic and prognostic properties are available for rheumatic diseases [10]. Most available biomarkers measure systemic and inflammatory factors, which do not reflect pathogenesis in the affected tissue. There is also a lack of sensitive biomarkers that can be used to predict those patients who will progress and those who will respond to treatment. One of the few examples of a prognostic biomarker is MMP3 measured in serum [11], which was elevated in patients who had an mSASSS change of more than 3 over a 3-year period. We recently developed two neo-epitope biomarkers C2M [12] and C3M [13], which directly measure tissue remodeling, and ultimately might be used to predict progression in inflammatory diseases. C2M is a serum biomarker that measures a matrix metalloproteinase (MMP)-generated neo-epitope of type II collagen and correlates with the severity of knee OA. C2M therefore reflects cartilage degradation [14]. C3M is a biomarker of soft tissue turnover associated with inflammation [15–17], which has been shown to be elevated in liver, skin and lung fibrosis. We recently reported that both biomarkers were highly elevated in AS and that the diagnostic utility for the combination of these two biomarkers was high (AUC 0.87, *p<0.0001*) [14]. The primary aims of the present study were to (i) to compare the diagnostic utility of these markers in AS versus RA and (ii) to investigate the prognostic potential of these novel connective tissue turnover markers in patients with AS.

## Methods

### Serum samples from healthy individuals and patients

Serum samples from controls were retrieved from two separate studies [12,14]. Subjects were all lean (BMI<25 kg/m2), between 21 and 72 years of age, had no history of rheumatic or arthritic disease or treatment for such. All subjects felt healthy and had no reported pain or symptoms of any disease. All patients signed an informed consent. Baseline characteristics are shown in Table 1.

Serum samples were collected from patients suffering from AS (n = 106). Of the 106 patients, 94 had 2-year radiographic follow-up. All patients had an established diagnosis of AS according to the modified New York Criteria [18]. Patients had received standard care, including physical therapy and treatment with a non-steroidal anti-inflammatory drug (NSAID), but were naïve to biologics at baseline. For progression analysis, patients were separated into two groups based on the presence (Yes/No) of a new syndesmophyte at 2-year follow-up. Bath AS Disease Activity

Index (BASDAI) [19] and modified Stoke AS Spinal Score (mSASSS)[20] were recorded for each AS patient. Baseline characteristics are shown in Table 1.

Serum samples from RA patients (n = 47) were retrieved prior to the start of treatment with biologics. Patients are eligible for biologics in the Province of Alberta, Canada, if they had active disease despite treatment with methotrexate, a methotrexate combination with a second disease-modifying agent, or leflunomide. Baseline characteristics are shown in Table 1.

The retrieval of serum samples from healthy subjects and patients was approved by the Danish national Committee on Biomedical Research ethics (approval no KA 2006–0054), and by the Ethical board of University of Alberta, Edmonton, Canada. The study was conducted in the countries of residence of the authors, Denmark and Canada respectively.

### Biomarker assays

Cartilage degradation and connective tissue inflammation were measured in all serum samples, whether from controls or patients with AS or RA, using competitive enzyme-linked immune sorbent assays (ELISAs) for C2M [12] and C3M [15], respectively. The C2M ELISA measures type II collagen fragments generated by MMPs in cartilage. Briefly, a streptavidin-coated microtiter plate was coated with 4 ng/mL biotinylated peptide. Unbound peptide was washed off and 20 µL 1:2 prediluted serum samples were added, followed by 100 µL of 60 ng/mL peroxidase-labeled monoclonal antibody (MAb-C2M-3C1). The plate was incubated at 4C for 18 hours, washed and developed using 3,3',5,5'-Tetramethylbenzidine (TMB) and stopped with sulfuric acid. The plate was read on a standard plate reader at 450 nm. The C3M ELISA measures type III collagen fragments generated by MMPs in connective tissue. Briefly, a streptavidin-coated microtiter plate was coated with 1.25 ng/mL biotinylated peptide. Unbound peptide was washed off and 20 µL 1:4 prediluted serum samples were added, followed by 100 µL 25 ng/mL peroxidase-labeled monoclonal antibody (MAb-C3M-610T1). The plate was incubated at 20°C for 1 hour, washed and developed using the TMB and stopped with sulfuric acid. The plate was read on a standard plate reader at 450 nm. Technical performances of the assays were assessed according to in-house standard operating procedures and final inspections included tests on detection range, sample stability and linearity, a sample and assay stress test, matrix and interference test, prolonged storage of the assays and normal range tests. In addition, analyte stability was investigated in terms of freeze-thaw, ambient temperatures, prolonged storage, etc. Serum C-reactive protein (CRP) levels were assessed by standard measures. The final inspection results concerning serum testing are summarized in Table 2.

### Statistics

Statistical analyses of correlations and logistic regression were performed using MedCalc® version 12 and GraphPad Prism® version 5. The primary objectives were to investigate: i) the serum levels of the two novel biomarkers, C2M and C3M, in RA and AS patients as compared to controls, and ii) whether there was an association between the biomarkers and progression of AS over a 2-year period. Comparison between the log transformed mean levels of the markers was performed using the Student's t-test (fig. 1, 2). Data was shown as the geometric mean with 95% confidence intervals (95%-CI), which depicts the principal distribution of the biomarker levels. The diagnostic power were investigated by area under the receiver-operator curve (AUROC) giving the AUC with 95%-CI (fig. 1, 2). Using the principle of Z-score normalization, cut-off values for the diagnostic test were set

**Table 1.** Baseline demographics and clinical assessment scores for the healthy controls, RA and AS patients.

| | Controls Mean (SD) | RA patients Mean (SD) | AS patients Mean (SD) |
|---|---|---|---|
| N | 56 | 47 | 103 |
| Mean age (SD), years | 42.8 (10.5) | 55.3 (12.4) | 42.0 (13.6) |
| Number of Female/male | 21/35 | 12/35 | 30/94 |
| NSAID users, % | 0 | 17 | 84 |
| Disease duration, years | – | 14.4 (10.7) | 18.0 (11.9) |
| RF positive, % | – | 86 | 0 |
| Mean ESR (SD), mm/hour | – | 40 (29) | 22 (20) |
| CRP (mg/L) | – | 33.5 (45.1) | 14.2 (22.2) |
| BASDAI | – | – | 5.6 (2.2) |
| mSASSS | – | – | 14.2 (18.5) |
| DAS28 | – | 6.6 (1.2) | – |
| HAQ | – | 1.9 (0.8) | – |
| TJC | – | 18.2 (7.9) | – |
| SJC | – | 13.5 (5.9) | – |

as 1 standard deviation (SD) above the mean of the controls which will include 84% below this cut-off assuming a normal distribution. Using these cut-off values the number of patients below and above the cut-off was counted and put into a 2×2 contingency table. From this the odds ratios (ORs), sensitivity, specificity and likelihood ratios were calculated by Fisher's exact test (fig. 1, 2).

**Table 2.** ELISA technical performance.

| | C2M | C3M |
|---|---|---|
| *Assay specifications* | | |
| Slope of Standard curve (CV %) | 1.10 (6.6) | 1.03 (10.8) |
| IC50, nmol/L (CV %) | 0.45 (3.8) | 5.22 (11.9) |
| Intra-assay variation, CV% | 6.2 | 6.7 |
| Inter-assay variation, CV% | 7.3 | 12.1 |
| Lower limit of detection, nmol/L | 0.037 | 0.28 |
| Quantifiable range, nmol/L | 0.274–4.36 | 0.54–42.1 |
| | | |
| *Analyte recovery* | | |
| Serum dilution linearity (analyte recovery) | Neat to 1:4; >82% | 1:4 to 1:64; >88% |
| Freeze-thaw | > 7 cycles | > 10 cycles |
| On-table stability | >48hours | >48hours |
| | | |
| *Interference* | | |
| Hemoglobin | <11% | <7% |
| Lipidimia | <6% | <2% |
| Biotin | <0.1% | <0.1% |
| Rheumatoid factor | <0.1% | <0.1% |
| HAMA | <0.1% | <0.1% |
| *Biological variation* | | |
| Correlation to age, R, *p-value* | 0.083, *ns* | 0.13, *ns* |
| Gender difference, Difference, *p-value* | 0.055, *ns* | 3.12, *ns* |

Univariate correlation analyses between the biomarkers and clinical scores, or between the individual biomarkers, were analyzed by non-parametric Spearman's test (table 3, 4).

The prognostic utility was investigated by a decision tree approach by asking following questions: how many AS progressors were we able to select and how many patients were we able to deselect by measuring the two biomarkers in question. The biomarkers for disease progression (NewSynd) was calculated using dichotomized values for the markers by discriminating high biomarker levels by Classification and Regression Tree Analysis (using the 2×2 diagnostic contingency table). Sensitivity (fraction progressors) and specificity (fraction non-progressors) values were produced. Data were considered significant when the P-value was below 0.05.

## Results

### Technical performance of the C2M and C3M ELISAs

The technical performance of the C2M and the C3M ELISAs was assessed before serum levels were measured in patients with RA, AS and healthy controls. Table 2 describes the basic technical characteristics of the two assays, both of which had good technical performance. Intra- and inter-assay coefficients of variation were less than 7% and 13%, respectively. The data analyte recovery, interference (hemoglobin, lipidimia, and biotin, rheumatoid factor (RF) and human anti-mouse antibody (HAMA)) and biological variation are shown in Table 2. None of the markers were significantly correlated to age. There was no gender difference for either marker investigated by Mann-Whitney test.

### The level of cartilage and connective tissue degradation fragments in serum of RA patients

Both serum C2M and C3M levels were significantly higher in RA patients than in healthy controls ($p < 0.0001$, fig. 1). Diagnostic utility, as analyzed by ROC and the AUCs, was 72% and 89% for C2M and C3M, respectively (fig. 1C). The odds ratio (OR) for identifying RA patients were 6.3 and 16 for C2M and C3M respectively (fig. 1C). Serum C2M levels were not associated with age, disease duration or any of the clinical outcome scores (Table 3). In contrast, serum C3M levels were highly correlated

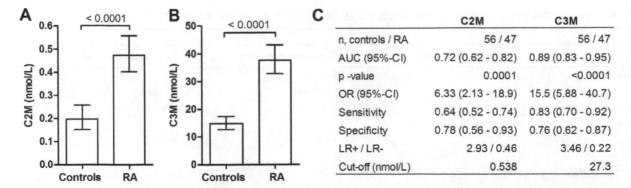

| | C2M | C3M |
|---|---|---|
| n, controls / RA | 56 / 47 | 56 / 47 |
| AUC (95%-CI) | 0.72 (0.62 - 0.82) | 0.89 (0.83 - 0.95) |
| p -value | 0.0001 | <0.0001 |
| OR (95%-CI) | 6.33 (2.13 - 18.9) | 15.5 (5.88 - 40.7) |
| Sensitivity | 0.64 (0.52 - 0.74) | 0.83 (0.70 - 0.92) |
| Specificity | 0.78 (0.56 - 0.93) | 0.76 (0.62 - 0.87) |
| LR+ / LR- | 2.93 / 0.46 | 3.46 / 0.22 |
| Cut-off (nmol/L) | 0.538 | 27.3 |

**Figure 1. The level of the cartilage degradation and connective tissue inflammation in RA patients (n = 47) and healthy controls (n = 56).** A) Cartilage degradation measured by C2M in serum. B) Connective tissue degradation measured by C3M in serum. C) The diagnostic utility depicted as area under the curve (AUC), odds ratio (OR), sensitivity, specificity and likelihood ratio (LR). Cut-off values were set as 1 SD above the mean of the healthy controls. Comparison of RA patients and controls was performed on log transformed data with student's t-test. Results are shown as geometric mean with 95% CI. Diagnostic utility was calculated by a contingency table applying Fisher's exact test.

with disease activity score (DAS), health assessment questionnaire (HAQ), erythrocyte sedimentation rate (ESR), C-reactive protein (CRP), swollen (SJC) and tender joint count (TJC). There was no correlation (table 3) between serum C2M and C3M.

### The level of cartilage and connective tissue degradation in serum of AS patients

Both C2M and C3M levels were significantly higher in AS patients than in healthy controls (fig. 1A and 1B). The diagnostic utility of C2M in discriminating between controls and AS patients was 70% (*p<0.0001*) (Fig. 2C) and thereby similar to that in the RA analysis (Fig. 1C). A high C2M level could correctly identify 40% of the AS patients and 80% of the healthy controls. A high C3M value could correctly identify 46% of the AS patients and 82% of the healthy controls. Thus the sensitivity was markedly lower for AS than for RA. The diagnostic utility of C3M was 81% (*p<0.0001*, Fig. 2C), which was 10% lower than the utility in RA patients (Fig. 1C). The ORs for AS were 3.4 (*p = 0.003*) and 4.7 (*p<0.0001*) for C2M and C3M, respectively (Fig. 2C).

The evaluation of all patients collectively showed C2M correlated with neither of the disease scores; Disease duration, ESR, CRP, mSASSS or BASDAI (table 4). Serum C3M was

significantly correlated with ESR (*p<0.0001*) and CRP (*p<0.0001*), as well as with mSASSS (*p = 0.0006*), but was of only borderline significant correlation (*p = 0.054*) with BASDAI (table 4). No correlation was observed between the two biomarkers C2M and C3M when measured in either AS patients, or RA patients (data not shown).

### Clinical predictive utility of measuring serum C2M and C3M

An abnormally high serum C2M level, defined as one SD above the mean of that found in healthy controls, could positively predict 44% of the progressors of AS and exclude 70% of the non-progressors (table 5). High serum C3M levels could positively predict 59% of the progressors and excluded 55% of the non-progressors. A high serum level of both C2M and C3M could predict 80% of the progressors and 61% of the non-progressors.

### Discussion

In the current study we firstly validated the diagnostic utility of the two novel markers, C2M and C3M, in RA and found that the serum levels of the markers were elevated in patients compared

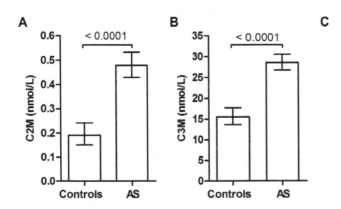

| | C2M | C3M |
|---|---|---|
| n, controls / AS | 56 / 106 | 56 / 106 |
| AUC (95%-CI) | 0.70 (0.61 - 0.79) | 0.81 (0.73 - 0.88) |
| p -value | <0.0001 | <0.0001 |
| OR (95%-CI) | 4.05 (1.48 - 11.1) | 4.02 (1.92 - 8.43) |
| Sensitivity | 0.40 (0.31 - 0.49) | 0.46 (0.36 - 0.56) |
| Specificity | 0.86 (0.71 - 0.95) | 0.82 (0.72 - 0.91) |
| LR+ / LR- | 2.85 / 0.70 | 2.64 / 0.66 |
| Cut-off (nmol/L) | 0.538 | 27.3 |

**Figure 2. The level of the cartilage degradation and connective tissue inflammation in AS patients (n = 103) and controls (n = 56).** A) Cartilage degradation measured by C2M in serum. B) Connective tissue degradation measured by C3M in serum C) The diagnostic utility depicted as area under the curve (AUC), odds ratio (OR), sensitivity, specificity and likelihood ratio (LR). Cut-off values were set as 1 SD above the mean of the healthy controls. Comparison of AS patients and controls was performed on log transformed data with student's t-test. Results are shown as geometric mean with 95% CI. Diagnostic utility was calculated by a contingency table applying Fisher's exact test.

**Table 3.** Univariate analysis for C2M and C3M associations with age, disease duration and RA clinical characteristics; Disease activity score (DAS), health assessment questionnaire (HAQ), erythrocyte sedimentation rate (ESR), high sensitive C-reactive protein (CRP), tender joint count (TJC) and swollen joint count (SJC).

| | C2M | C3M |
|---|---|---|
| Age | −0.12, *ns* | 0.13, *ns* |
| Disease Duration | 0.16, *ns* | 0.18, *ns* |
| DAS | 0.09, *ns* | 0.54, *p<0.001* |
| HAQ | 0.01, *ns* | 0.52, *p<0.001* |
| ESR | 0.05, *ns* | 0.60, *p<0.0001* |
| CRP | −0.06, *ns* | 0.59, *p<0.0001* |
| TJC | −0.02, ns | 0.34, *p<0.05* |
| SJC | −0.10, *ns* | 0.18, *ns* |
| C2M | | −0.10, *ns* |

Data are shown as Spearman's correlation coefficient R and *p-value*.

**Table 4.** Univariate analysis for C2M and C3M associations with age, disease duration and AS clinical characteristics; erythrocyte sedimentation rate (ESR), high sensitive C-reactive protein (CRP), mSASSS and BASDAI.

| | C2M | C3M |
|---|---|---|
| Age | 0.06, *ns* | 0.17, *ns* |
| Disease duration | 0.01, *ns* | 0.14, *ns* |
| ESR | 0.03, *ns* | 0.40, *p<0.0001* |
| CRP | 0.06, *ns* | 0.55, *p<0.001* |
| mSASSS | 0.02, *ns* | 0.32, *p<0.001* |
| BASDAI | −0.04, *ns* | 0.19, *ns* |
| C2M | | 0.12, *ns* |

Data are shown as Spearman's correlation coefficient R and p-value.

with controls with an OR of more than 6. This is expected since RA is characterized by massive joint turnover, which includes cartilage degradation and connective tissue turnover, such as occurs during synovial inflammation. While elevated serum C2M did not seem to be correlated with any disease characteristics in RA, high serum C3M was highly correlated with DAS, HAQ and ESR, as well as TJC. These results support the concept that connective tissue degradation is indeed related to the inflammatory component of RA, whereas cartilage degradation seemed to be partly uncoupled from this component. This suggests that the two biomarkers contribute independent and additive information about the disease pathogenesis and maybe supplementary diagnostic tools for clinical diagnosis. These markers can not compete with diagnostic markers such as RF and CRP, however in stead they can provide additional information on tissue integrity, which may aid in the understanding of disease severity.

Secondly, we investigated whether these joint turnover markers could be used for AS. In contrast to RA, RF and CRP are not applicable diagnostic markers in AS. The present study supports a role of C2M and C3M as potential diagnostic biomarkers in AS. We also saw a strong correlation between connective tissue degradation as measured by serum C3M and the radiographic score, mSASSS. Cartilage degradation as measured by serum C2M levels was likewise elevated in AS patients compared with controls. But C2M did not correlate with the mSASSS. These results are interesting because they indicate that cartilage degradation and soft tissue turnover may provide independent information also in AS.

The first part of the study validated and supports the importance of monitoring connective tissue remodeling in the pathogenesis of rheumatic diseases. The second part of the study evaluated the prognostic potential of the markers. We demonstrated that a combination of these novel markers could identify 80% of the progressors in AS. This combination could be used to select only the likely progressors for clinical trials, and thus reduce the number of patients exposed to treatment in such studies. Furthermore, by identifying likely progressors in an AS population, one could test strategies aimed at early intervention to prevent deterioration of structural damage using anti-inflammatory therapies [21,22]. Our data also shows that the combination

of biomarkers may possess higher prognostic utility than individual biomarkers. We showed that cartilage and soft tissue turnover is indeed increased in AS patients, and that the level of increase is predictive of those who will progress–a potential which CRP does not possess [23].

There are considerable limitations to the information provided by standard clinical and laboratory parameters to guide treatment decisions. Consequently, there has been a particular interest in evaluating biomarkers in AS that reflect disease activity and predict structural progression [5,24,25]. Although CRP and ESR are sensitive detectors of disease activity in RA, they are not so in AS, probably because these markers are elevated in only about 50% of AS patients [23]. Unlike in RA, they also correlate poorly with clinical measures of AS, although good correlations have been noted with MRI assessment of inflammation in the spine [26–28]. In contrast to RA, CRP and ESR do not appear to predict progression of structural damage in AS although CRP does predict clinical response to anti-TNF therapy in both RA and AS [29,30].

Cartilage degradation and connective tissue turnover are hallmarks of most arthropathies. We have developed two new serological biomarkers of cartilage degradation (C2M) [12] and soft tissue turnover (C3M) [13,16]. Both biomarkers are MMP-mediated collagen fragments, which are also called collagen neo-epitopes. Assays for these two biomarkers are specific for the cleavage site in the respective collagens. Hence the assays do not measure full-size collagens, but only the pathogenic fingerprint of that collagen. We have previously demonstrated that serum C2M was associated with increased Kellgreen-Lawrence score in knee osteoarthritis [12], indicating a correlation with cartilage loss and joint deterioration. C3M is derived by degradation of type III collagen, which is a central component of most connective tissues. The turnover of both types II and III collagens is high [31]. There was a strong correlation between CRP and C3M in both RA and AS, which supports the concept that inflammation accelerates the turnover of connective tissue and thereby the release of C3M [14]. This may contribute to the increased levels of these biomarkers in AS which could arise from excessive remodeling of the joint. However, additional contributions may be derived from multiple organs of the body affected by inflammation.

A previous report showed that other markers of extracellular remodeling had limited association with baseline BASDAI and mSASSS [11]. Cartilage oligomeric protein and YKL-40 were both correlated with baseline mSASSS (p<0.05), but they were not associated with 2-year change in mSASSS. Interestingly that

**Table 5.** Clinical predictive utility of the serum markers.

| | High C2M (n = 94) | High C3M (n = 94) | High C2M & high C3M (n = 33) |
|---|---|---|---|
| Cut-offs | >0.538 nmol/L | >27.3 nmol/L | |
| Sensitivity (%) | 44.1 (28.6–61.7) | 58.8 (40.7–75.6) | 80.0 (51.9–95.7) |
| Specificity (%) | 70.0 (56.8–81.2) | 55.0 (41.6–67.9) | 61.1 (35.8–82.7) |
| Positive/Negative Likelihood ratio | 1.46/0.80 | 1.31/0.75 | 2.06/0.33 |
| Proportion of progressors with a positive test | 15/34 | 20/34 | 12/15 |
| Proportion of non-progressors with a negative test | 42/60 | 33/60 | 11/18 |

Progressors were defined as NewSynd Yes/No over at a two year period.

study showed a clear association between elevated MMP-3 and radiographic progression. MMP-3 is widely up-regulated by inflammation in the connective tissue surrounding the joints (e.g. synovial tissue). Thus MMP-3 might very well be one of the MMPs responsible for the degradation of type II and type III collagens. It would interesting to investigate the relationship between MMP-3 and type II and type III collagen turnover and potentially combine the markers in an algorithm for predicting inflammatory disease. This kind of investigation will increase our understanding of the role of MMPs in AS and the proteolytical products resulting from MMP activity.

## Conclusions

This is the first study to show the prognostic value of two novel biomarkers of MMP-mediated degradation of types II and III collagen. These two biomarkers, C2M and C3M, might be the best diagnostic [14] and prognostic markers available to date for AS. Further longitudinal study is needed to confirm these preliminary data. We speculate that markers measuring joint

tissue turnover and deterioration may assist better understanding of disease pathogenesis and eventually disease severity. In the era of personalized medicine markers that are direct measures of disease status and severity may aid in designing the best treatment for the individual patients.

## Acknowledgments

We would like to acknowledge our skilled technicians Kathrine Mikkelsen, Sedi Tavallaee, Maibritt Andersen and Trine Overgaard whom all contributed in the development of the ELISAs. Furthermore we would like to thank *Den Danske Forskningsfond*.

## Author Contributions

Conceived and designed the experiments: ACBJ SW MK WPM CC. Performed the experiments: ACBJ DJL SW NM. Analyzed the data: ACBJ SW MK WPM CC. Contributed reagents/materials/analysis tools: ACBJ SW IB DJL NM CC MK WPM. Wrote the paper: ACBJ SW MK WPM CC.

## References

1. Lories RJ, Baeten DL (2009) Differences in pathophysiology between rheumatoid arthritis and ankylosing spondylitis. Clin Exp Rheumatol 27: S10–S14.
2. Goldring SR (2003) Pathogenesis of bone and cartilage destruction in rheumatoid arthritis. Rheumatology (Oxford) 42: ii11–ii16.
3. Braun J, Pincus T (2002) Mortality, course of disease and prognosis of patients with ankylosing spondylitis. Clin Exp Rheumatol 20: S16–S22.
4. Tam LS, Gu J, Yu D (2010) Pathogenesis of ankylosing spondylitis. Nat Rev Rheumatol 6: 399–405.
5. Colbert RA, Deodhar AA, Fox D, Gravallese EM, Khan MA, et al. (2009) Entheses and bones in spondyloarthritis: 2008 Annual Research and Education Meeting of the Spondyloarthritis Research and Therapy Network (SPARTAN). J Rheumatol 36: 1527–1531.
6. Karsdal MA, Henriksen K, Leeming DJ, Mitchell P, Duffin K, et al. (2009) Biochemical markers and the FDA Critical Path: how biomarkers may contribute to the understanding of pathophysiology and provide unique and necessary tools for drug development. Biomarkers 14: 181–202.
7. Segovia-Silvestre T, Bonnefond C, Sondergaard BC, Christensen ST, Karsdal MA, et al. (2011) Identification of the Calcitonin receptor in osteoarthritic chondrocytes. BMC Res Notes 4: 407.
8. Schaller S, Henriksen K, Hoegh-Andersen P, Sondergaard BC, Sumer EU, et al. (2005) In vitro, ex vivo, and in vivo methodological approaches for studying therapeutic targets of osteoporosis and degenerative joint diseases: how biomarkers can assist? Assay Drug Dev Technol 3: 553–580.
9. Garnero P, Desmarais S, Charni N, Percival MD (2005) The CII fragments Helix-II and CTX-II reveal distinct enzymatic pathways of cartilage collagen degradation: diagnostic and therapeutic implications in rheumatoid arthritis and osteoarthritis. Arthritis Rheum 52: P51.
10. de VK (2010) Soluble and tissue biomarkers in ankylosing spondylitis. Best Pract Res Clin Rheumatol 24: 671–682.
11. Maksymowych WP, Landewe R, Conner-Spady B, Dougados M, Mielants H, et al. (2007) Serum matrix metalloproteinase 3 is an independent predictor of structural damage progression in patients with ankylosing spondylitis. Arthritis Rheum 56: 1846–1853.
12. Bay-Jensen AC, Liu Q, Byrjalsen I, Li Y, Wang J, et al. (2011) Enzyme-linked immunosorbent assay (ELISAs) for metalloproteinase derived type II collagen neoepitope, CIIM--increased serum CIIM in subjects with severe radiographic osteoarthritis. Clin Biochem 44: 423–429.
13. Barascuk N, Veidal SS, Larsen L, Larsen DV, Larsen MR, et al. (2010) A novel assay for extracellular matrix remodeling associated with liver fibrosis: An enzyme-linked immunosorbent assay (ELISA) for a MMP-9 proteolytically revealed neo-epitope of type III collagen. Clin Biochem In press.
14. Bay-Jensen AC, Leeming DJ, Kleyer A, Veidal SS, Schett G, et al. (2011) Ankylosing spondylitis is characterized by an increased turnover of several different metalloproteinase-derived collagen species: a cross-sectional study. Rheumatol Int.
15. Veidal SS, Vassiliadis E, Barascuk N, Zhang C, Segovia-Silvestre T, et al. (2010) Matrix metalloproteinase-9-mediated type III collagen degradation as a novel serological biochemical marker for liver fibrogenesis. Liver Int 30: 1293–1304.
16. Vassiliadis E, Larsen DV, Clausen RE, Veidal SS, Barascuk N, et al. (2011) Measurement of CO3-610, a Potential Liver Biomarker Derived from Matrix Metalloproteinase-9 Degradation of Collagen Type III, in a Rat Model of Reversible Carbon-Tetrachloride-Induced Fibrosis. Biomark Insights 6: 49–58.
17. Vassiliadis E, Veidal SS, Simonsen H, Larsen DV, Vainer B, et al. (2011) Immunological detection of the type V collagen propeptide fragment, PVCP-1230, in connective tissue remodeling associated with liver fibrosis. Biomarkers .
18. van der LS, Valkenburg HA, Cats A (1984) Evaluation of diagnostic criteria for ankylosing spondylitis. A proposal for modification of the New York criteria. Arthritis Rheum 27: 361–368.
19. Garrett S, Jenkinson T, Kennedy LG, Whitelock H, Gaisford P, et al. (1994) A new approach to defining disease status in ankylosing spondylitis: the Bath Ankylosing Spondylitis Disease Activity Index. J Rheumatol 21: 2286–2291.
20. Creemers MC, Franssen MJ, van't Hof MA, Gribnau FW, van de Putte LB, et al. (2005) Assessment of outcome in ankylosing spondylitis: an extended radiographic scoring system. Ann Rheum Dis 64: 127–129.

21. Maksymowych WP, Landewe R, Tak PP, Ritchlin CJ, Ostergaard M, et al. (2009) Reappraisal of OMERACT 8 draft validation criteria for a soluble biomarker reflecting structural damage endpoints in rheumatoid arthritis, psoriatic arthritis, and spondyloarthritis: the OMERACT 9 v2 criteria. J Rheumatol 36: 1785–1791.

22. Maksymowych WP, FitzGerald O, Wells GA, Gladman DD, Landewe R, et al. (2009) Proposal for levels of evidence schema for validation of a soluble biomarker reflecting damage endpoints in rheumatoid arthritis, psoriatic arthritis, and ankylosing spondylitis, and recommendations for study design. J Rheumatol 36: 1792–1799.

23. Ruof J, Stucki G (1999) Validity aspects of erythrocyte sedimentation rate and C-reactive protein in ankylosing spondylitis: a literature review. J Rheumatol 26: 966–970.

24. Schett G (2007) Joint remodelling in inflammatory disease. Ann Rheum Dis 66 Suppl 3: iii42–iii44.

25. Schett G, Sieper J (2009) Inflammation and repair mechanisms. Clin Exp Rheumatol 27: S33–S35.

26. Spoorenberg A, van der HD, de KE, Dougados M, de VK, et al. (1999) Relative value of erythrocyte sedimentation rate and C-reactive protein in assessment of disease activity in ankylosing spondylitis. J Rheumatol 26: 980–984.

27. Lukas C, Braun J, van der HD, Hermann KG, Rudwaleit M, et al. (2007) Scoring inflammatory activity of the spine by magnetic resonance imaging in ankylosing spondylitis: a multireader experiment. J Rheumatol 34: 862–870.

28. Maksymowych WP, Dhillon SS, Park R, Salonen D, Inman RD, et al. (2007) Validation of the spondyloarthritis research consortium of Canada magnetic resonance imaging spinal inflammation index: is it necessary to score the entire spine? Arthritis Rheum 57: 501–507.

29. Wanders AJ, Gorman JD, Davis JC, Landewe RB, van der Heijde DM (2004) Responsiveness and discriminative capacity of the assessments in ankylosing spondylitis disease-controlling antirheumatic therapy core set and other outcome measures in a trial of etanercept in ankylosing spondylitis. Arthritis Rheum 51: 1–8.

30. de Vries MK, van E, I, van der Horst-Bruinsma IE, Peters MJ, Nurmohamed MT, et al. (2009) Erythrocyte sedimentation rate, C-reactive protein level, and serum amyloid a protein for patient selection and monitoring of anti-tumor necrosis factor treatment in ankylosing spondylitis. Arthritis Rheum 61: 1484–1490.

31. Gelse K, Poschl E, Aigner T (2003) Collagens--structure, function, and biosynthesis. Advanced Drug Delivery Reviews 55: 1531–1546.

# 8

# Genetic Polymorphisms of *Stromal Interaction Molecule 1* Associated with the Erythrocyte Sedimentation Rate and C-Reactive Protein in HLA-B27 Positive Ankylosing Spondylitis Patients

James Cheng-Chung Wei[1,2], Kuo-Sheng Hung[3], Yu-Wen Hsu[4], Ruey-Hong Wong[5], Chun-Huang Huang[2], Ming-Shiou Jan[6], Shyh-Jong Wu[7], Yung-Shun Juan[8], Wei-Chiao Chang[4,9]*

1 Division of Allergy, Immunology and Rheumatology, Department of Medicine, Chung Shan Medical University Hospital, Taichung, Taiwan, 2 Institute of Medicine, Chung Shan Medical University, Taichung, Taiwan, 3 Department of Neurosurgery, Center of Excellence for Clinical Trial and Research, Graduate Institute of Injury Prevention and Control, Taipei Medical University, Wan Fang Medical Center, Taipei, Taiwan, 4 Department of Clinical Pharmacy, School of Pharmacy, Taipei Medical University, Taipei, Taiwan, 5 Department of Public Health, Chung Shan Medical University, Taichung, Taiwan, 6 Institute of Microbiology and Immunology, Chung Shan Medical University, Taichung, Taiwan, 7 Department of Medical Laboratory Science and Biotechnology, College of Health Sciences, Kaohsiung Medical University, Kaohsiung, Taiwan, 8 Department of Urology, Kaohsiung municipal Hsiao-Kang Hospital and College of Medicine, Kaohsiung Medical University, Kaohsiung, Taiwan, 9 Department of Pharmacy, Taipei Medical University-Wanfang Hospital, Taipei, Taiwan

## Abstract

Ankylosing spondylitis (AS) is a chronic inflammation of the sacroiliac joints, spine and peripheral joints. The development of ankylosing spondylitis is still unclear. Genetics factors such as human leukocyte antigen *HLA-B27* and *ERAP1* have been widely reported to associate to AS susceptibility. In this study, we enrolled 361 AS patients and selected four tagging single nucleotides polymorphisms (tSNPs) at *STIM1* gene. The correlation between *STIM1* genetic polymorphisms and AS activity index (BASDAI, BASFI, BAS-G) as well as laboratory parameters of inflammation (erythrocyte sedimentation rate (ESR) and C-reactive protein (CRP)) were tested. Our results indicated that HLA-B27 positive AS patients who are carrying the minor allele homozygous G/G genotype of SNP rs3750996 significantly associated with a higher level of ESR in serum. Furthermore, rs3750996/rs3750994 pairwise allele analysis indicated that G-C haplotypes also significantly correlated with higher level of ESR as well as CRP. These findings provide a better understanding of *STIM1* genetic contribution to the pathogenesis of AS.

**Editor:** Pierre Bobé, Institut Jacques Monod, France

**Funding:** The authors have no support or funding to report.

**Competing Interests:** The authors have declared that no competing interests exist.

* E-mail: wcc@tmu.edu.tw

## Introduction

Ankylosing spondylitis (AS) is a chronic inflammatory disorder of the lumbar spine and sacroiliac that can also affect the peripheral joints [1]. Males are affected more frequently than females [2]. AS strongly associates with the human leukocyte antigen (*HLA*)-*B27* gene [3], but *HLA-B27* accounts for only 16% of the genetic variability in AS [4]. HLA-B60, B61 and IL-1, and IL-23R genes also have been proven to be important in the pathogenesis of AS [5–7]. In 2010, Lee et al. [8] identified that *CTLA-4* +49A>G genotype associated with circulatory CRP level. These results indicated that the level of inflammation in AS subjects may be pre-determined by *CTLA-4* genotypes.

Our previous studies indicated a significant association between genetic polymorphisms of store-operated calcium channel, *ORAI1*, and the risk of inflammatory diseases such as HLA-B27 positive AS and calcium nephrolithiasis [9,10]. In non-excitable cells such as T cell and mast cell, calcium influx is mainly via store-operated calcium channels (SOC) [11]. SOC is involved in a variety of physiological processes such as gene transcription, enzyme

metabolism and inflammatory reaction. The regulation mechanism of store-operated calcium entry was unclear until 2005, Roos et al, firstly identified a molecule called Stromal interaction molecule 1 (STIM1) [12]. STIM1 is a calcium sensor that localized in the endoplasmic reticulum. Upon activation of IP$_3$ receptor, calcium concentration in the store falls, which triggers the aggregation of STIM1, that resulted in the activation of store-operated calcium channel. Aberrant expression of STIM1-mediated calcium signaling has been implicated in the development of human cancers [13,14]. Knockdown *STIM1* by siRNA which impairs $Ca^{2+}$ influx, prevents the translocation of transcription factors and subsequent inflammatory *COX-2* gene activation [15,16].

In this study, we investigated the association between *STIM1* genetic polymorphisms, AS activity index (BASDAI, BASFI, BAS-G) and inflammatory biochemical examines (ESR and CRP). Our results indicated that rs3750996 in the *STIM1* gene significantly associated with a higher level of ESR. Furthermore, G-C haplotypes (rs3750996/rs3750994) significantly correlated with higher level of ESR and CRP. These findings provide a better

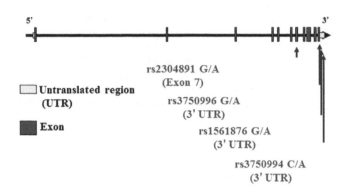

**Figure 1. Graphical overview of the genotyped human *STIM1* gene polymorphisms in relation to its exon/intron structure.**

understanding of *STIM1* genetic contribution to the pathogenesis of AS.

## Materials and Methods

### Patients studied

Patients were solicited sequentially at Chung Shan Medical University Hospital in Taichung, Taiwan. AS patients who met selection criteria were asked to participate in the study. Informed consent was obtained before any data was collected from the respondents. Three selection criteria were used to recruit AS patients: (a) patients aged 16–65 years; (b) AS diagnosis by the modified New York criteria [17]; and (c) cognitive performance not influenced by other diseases such as dementia. Sacroiliitis was confirmed by a qualified radiologist and AS diagnosis by a qualified rheumatologist. The detailed clinical history included age on initial symptom, family history of AS, and extraspinal manifestations. Age of AS symptom onset was defined as the time when the first symptom (axial symptom, peripheral arthritis, uveitis or enthesitis) had developed. Peripheral arthritis was defined as the presence of at least one swollen joint. Inflammatory bowel disease (IBD) (distinct from irritable bowel syndrome) was defined as the presence of the inflammatory condition of the colon and small intestine, including ulcerative colitis and Crohn's disease. Uveitis was defined as the presence of inflammation of the middle layer of the eye and involved patterns as unilateral, bilateral, or alternative. These symptoms were ascertained by the rheumatologist, ophthalmologist and gastroenterologist, and were recorded in medical record reviews. 100% of AS patients in this study have sacroiliitis. The design of the work and final report conformed to the Declaration of Helsinki and study was approved by the Institute Review Board of Chung Shan Medical University Hospital. All the subjects gave the written consent form.

### Bath Ankylosing Spondylitis Indices

The Bath Ankylosing Spondylitis Disease Activity Index (BASDAI), Bath Ankylosing Spondylitis Functional Index (BASFI) and Bath Ankylosing Spondylitis Global (BAS-G) were applied to evaluate the disease activity, physical function and global well-being, respectively. The modified Chinese versions of BASDAI, BASFI, and BAS-G have good intra-class correlation and Cronbach's alpha [18].

### Laboratory analyses

Peripheral blood was collected, and was centrifuged to separate the serum and the cells. Erythrocyte sedimentation rate (ESR), and C-reactive protein (CRP) were measured. HLA-B27 carriage was assessed by flow cytometry [19].

### DNA extraction

Blood cells were subjected to DNA extraction by treating them first with 0.5% SDS lysis buffer and then protease K (1 mg/ml) for digestion of nuclear protein for 4 h at 60°C. Total DNA was harvested by using the Gentra extraction kit followed by 70% alcohol precipitation.

**Table 1.** Basal characteristics and clinical features of patients with ankylosing spondylitis (AS).

| Characteristics | Patients with AS |
| --- | --- |
| Number of subjects | 361 |
| Gender:male, No (%) | 245 (67.9%) |
| Age (years)[a] | 33.5±12.8 |
| Range | 6–69 |
| HLA-B27(+) | 315 (87.3%) |
| BASDAI (0-10) | 4.1±2.3 |
| BASFI (0-10) | 1.9±2.2 |
| BAS-G (0-10) | 4.3±2.8 |

[a]Mean ± SD. SD:standard deviation.

**Table 2.** Difference in the scores of BASDAI, BASFI, and BAS-G among HLA-B27 positive AS patients stratified by different *STIM1* genotype.

| SNP | Genotype | Number (%) | BASDAI | BASFI | BAS-G |
| --- | --- | --- | --- | --- | --- |
| rs2304891 | GG | 58 (19.2) | 4.2±2.3[a] | 1.6±2.1 | 3.7±2.7 |
| | AG | 134 (44.4) | 4.3±2.4 | 2.1±2.4 | 4.5±2.9 |
| | AA | 110 (36.4) | 3.9±2.2 | 1.9±2.1 | 4.2±2.9 |
| Unadjusted *P*-value | | | 0.58 | 0.49 | 0.31 |
| Adjusted *P*-value | | | 0.58[†] | 0.52[§] | 0.31[†] |
| rs3750996 | GG | 13 (4.3) | 3.4±2.3 | 1.7±1.7 | 3.3±2.4 |
| | AG | 104 (34.6) | 4.2±2.2 | 1.9±2.2 | 4.5±2.8 |
| | AA | 184 (61.1) | 4.0±2.3 | 1.9±2.2 | 4.0±2.9 |
| Unadjusted *P*-value | | | 0.42 | 0.98 | 0.22 |
| Adjusted *P*-value | | | 0.43[†] | 0.97[§] | 0.21[†] |
| rs1561876 | GG | 23 (7.8) | 3.6±1.9 | 1.7±1.8 | 3.7±2.9 |
| | AG | 118 (40.0) | 4.3±2.3 | 2.4±2.5 | 4.7±3.0 |
| | AA | 154 (52.2) | 3.9±2.4 | 1.6±2.0 | 3.9±2.8 |
| Unadjusted *P*-value | | | 0.38 | 0.04* | 0.06 |
| Adjusted *P*-value | | | 0.38[†] | 0.03[§]* | 0.06[†] |
| rs3750994 | CC | 18 (5.9) | 3.9±2.6 | 1.9±2.2 | 4.5±3.1 |
| | AC | 116 (38.2) | 4.1±2.3 | 2.0±2.2 | 4.2±3.0 |
| | AA | 170 (55.9) | 4.1±2.3 | 1.9±2.3 | 4.3±2.7 |
| Unadjusted *P*-value | | | 0.93 | 0.92 | 0.90 |
| Adjusted *P*-value | | | 0.93[†] | 0.93[§] | 0.90[†] |

[a]Data represent means ± S.D..
[†]Adjusted the effects of age and sex.
[§]Adjusted the effects of age, sex and disease duration.
*Significant (*P*<0.05) values are in bold.

**Table 3.** Difference in the value of ESR and CRP among HLA-B27 positive AS patients stratified by different *STIM1* genotype.

| SNP | Genotype | Number (%) | ESR | CRP |
|---|---|---|---|---|
| rs2304891 | GG | 58 (19.2) | 20.4±14.9[a] | 0.8±1.3 |
| | AG | 134 (44.4) | 23.1±19.4 | 1.3±1.9 |
| | AA | 110 (36.4) | 25.2±20.2 | 1.5±2.3 |
| Unadjusted *P*-value | | | 0.38 | 0.14 |
| Adjusted *P*-value[†] | | | 0.38 | 0.12 |
| rs3750996 | GG | 13 (4.3) | 45.3±26.1 | 3.0±3.0 |
| | AG | 104 (34.6) | 22.3±19.7 | 1.2±2.0 |
| | AA | 184 (61.1) | 22.4±17.3 | 1.2±1.9 |
| Unadjusted *P*-value | | | **0.01*** | 0.06 |
| Adjusted *P*-value[†] | | | **0.01*** | 0.05 |
| rs1561876 | GG | 23 (7.8) | 25.8±17.7 | 1.1±1.9 |
| | AG | 118 (40.0) | 21.8±18.7 | 1.4±2.2 |
| | AA | 154 (52.2) | 24.4±18.9 | 1.2±1.9 |
| Unadjusted *P*-value | | | 0.53 | 0.80 |
| Adjusted *P*-value[†] | | | 0.53 | 0.79 |
| rs3750994 | CC | 18 (5.9) | 20.4±13.3 | 0.6±0.9 |
| | AC | 116 (38.2) | 21.8±18.4 | 1.2±2.0 |
| | AA | 170 (55.9) | 25.0±19.6 | 1.4±2.0 |
| Unadjusted *P*-value | | | 0.38 | 0.49 |
| Adjusted *P*-value[†] | | | 0.38 | 0.46 |

[a]Data represent means ± S.D..
[†]Adjusted the effects of age and sex.
*Significant (*P*<0.05) values are in bold.

## Genotyping

Four tagging SNPs of *STIM1* (rs2304891, rs3750996, rs1561876, rs3750994) with a minimum allele frequency of greater than 10% in the Han Chinese in Beijing population were selected from the HapMap database (http://hapmap.ncbi.nlm.nih.gov/). A graphical overview of genotyped polymorphisms is shown in **Figure 1**. One polymorphism (rs2304891) of *STIM1* located in the exon, other three polymorphisms are in the 3′ untranslated region (UTR).Genotyping was carried out using the TaqMan Allelic Discrimination Assay (Applied Biosystems, Foster city, CA) as our previous report [10]. The polymerase chain reaction (PCR) was performed by using a 96-well microplate with the ABI9700 Thermal Cycler. After PCR, fluorescence was detected and analyzed using the System SDS software version 1.2.3.

## Cell culture

THP-1 cells were bought from ATCC. Cells were cultured (37°C, 5% $CO_2$) in RPMI-1640 medium (GIBCO), supplemented with 10% fetal bovine serum and 10% penicillin-streptomycin.

## Reverse transcriptase PCR determination of TNF-α expression in THP-1 cells

Total RNA was extracted from THP-1 cells by RNeasy Mini Kit (Qiagen). A reverse transcriptase reaction was performed on 1 μg of extracted total RNA using reverse transcriptase reaction Kit (Applied Biosystems) according to the manufacturer's instructions. Following cDNA synthesis, Real-time PCR was performed in triplicate using a SYBR Green Master Mix. The specific primer

of TNF-α were forward primer: 5′-GACAAGCCTGTAGCC-CATGTTGTA-3′ and reverse primer: 5′-CAGCCTTGG-CCCTTGAAGA-3′. Each well contained the following reaction mix: 2 μl cDNA, 5 μl 10× Sensimix dT (Quantace, Watford, UK), 2.8 μl RNase-free water (QIAGEN), 0.1 μl forward primer, and 0.1 μl reverse primer. Universal cycling conditions were used (one cycle at 95°C for 15 min and 40 cycles at 90°C for 15 s and 60°C for 60 s). Relative gene expression was calculated using the comparative CT method. All values were normalized to the housekeeping gene.

## Transfection of siRNA

Cells were seeded in 6-well plates one day before transfection. The *STIM1* siRNA was purchased from santa cruz biotechnology, Inc. *STIM1* siRNA was transfected into cells by using lipofecta-mine 2000 (Invitrogen). Following transfection, the cells were cultured for 24 h and then prepare for Thapsigargin (2 uM) stimulation.

## Measurement of IL-6 and TNF-α

IL-6 (Invitrogen Corp. CA, USA) and TNF- α (Invitrogen Corp. CA, USA) assays were performed by using enzyme linked immuno sorbent assay method (ELISA) (Tecan Minilyser, Tecan Group Ltd. Mannedorf, Switzerland). IL-6 and TNF- α assay measurements were carried out at 450 nm optical density (OD). Samples were analyzed in triplicate, and mean concentrations were calculated for each sample.

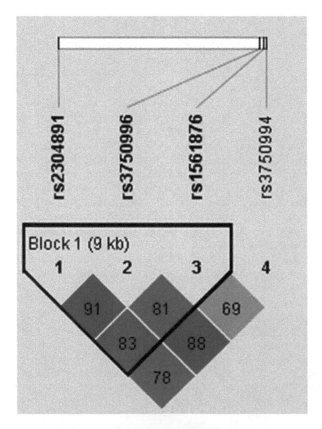

**Figure 2.** *STIM1* **gene LD and haplotype block structure in HLA-B27(+) AS.** The number on the cells is the LOD score of D′.

**Table 4.** Difference in the value of ESR among HLA-B27 positive AS patients stratified by different *STIM1* haplotypes.

| rs2304891/rs3750996 | ESR | rs3750996/rs1561876 | ESR | rs3750996/rs3750994 | ESR |
|---|---|---|---|---|---|
| G/G | 41.0±4.2[a] | G/G | 14.5±4.9 | G/C | 72.0 |
| A/G | 25.2±22.0 | A/G | 22.8±18.5 | G/A | 25.0±21.5 |
| G/A | 21.6±17.4 | G/A | 25.8±22.2 | A/C | 21.1±17.0 |
| A/A | 23.7±18.5 | A/A | 22.3±16.9 | A/A | 23.2±18.2 |
| Unadjusted *P*-value | 0.23 | Unadjusted *P*-value | 0.43 | Unadjusted *P*-value | **0.03*** |
| Adjusted *P*-value[†] | 0.23 | Adjusted *P*-value | 0.42 | Adjusted *P*-value[†] | **0.03*** |

[a]Data represent mean ± S.D..
[†]Adjusted the effects of age and sex.
*Significant (*P*<0.05) values are in bold.

## Statistical analysis

JMP 8.0 for Windows was used for analysis. Analysis of variance (ANOVA) was used to compare the mean of continuous variables (BASDAI, BASFI, BAS-G, ESR and CRP) among different genotypes in AS patients. Multiple regression analysis was used to adjust for age, sex and disease duration. A *P* value less than 0.05 is considered significant. Linkage disequilibrium (LD) was assessed for any pair of SNPs and haplotype blocks were defined using the default setting of the Haploview software 4.2 (Broad Institute, Cambridge, Massachusetts) and PHASE version 2.1.

## Results

### Basic and Clinical Characteristics of the Subjects

A total 361 AS patients were recruited in this study. **Table 1** showed the characteristics of the subjects. 67.9% of cases were male. The mean age (years) and standard deviation (S.D.) were 33.5±12.8. In AS subjects, 87.3% (315/361) were HLA-B27 positive and their mean BASDAI, mean BASFI, and mean BAS-G scores were 4.1±2.3, 1.9±2.2, and 4.3±2.8, respectively.

### Association of *STIM1* genetic polymorphisms with the rate of ESR in HLA-B27 positive AS patients

We analyzed the relationship between disease activity index (BASDAI, BASFI and BAS-G) and the four polymorphisms of *STIM1* among HLA-B27 positive AS patients. A borderline significant association between *STIM1* polymorphism rs1561876 and BASFI (*P*-value = 0.04) or BAS-G (*P*-value = 0.06) was found. However, we failed to improve the significance even after adjustment for the effects of ages and sex (**Table 2**). We further

analyzed the association between inflammatory biochemical examination (ESR and CRP) and *STIM1* gene polymorphisms. As shown in **Table 3**, rs3750996 homozygous G/G genotype significantly correlated with increased level of ESR compared with the A/G and A/A genotypes in HLA-B27 positive AS patients (*P*-value = 0.01). In addition, the risk G allele of rs3750996 in HLA-B27 positive AS patients was seen in a higher CRP level (*P*-value = 0.06).

### *STIM1* Haplotypes associated with ESR and CRP levels in HLA-B27 positive AS patients

We further calculated pairwise linkage disequilibrium (LD) (**Figure 2**) and analyzed two common haplotypes by using the Haploview 4.2 program and PHASE version 2.1. As shown in the **Table 4**, haplotypes of rs3750996/rs3750994 is significantly associated with ESR in the HLA-B27 positive AS patients (*P*= 0.03). In addition, rs3750996/rs3750994 haplotype G/C patients had higher CRP level (*P*= 0.001) (**Table 5**). After adjustment for the effects of age and gender, the significant association still exists (**Table 4 and Table 5**).

### Association of *STIM1* genotypes and cytokines (TNF-α and IL-6) levels

Gratacós et al., indicated that cytokines (TNF-α and IL-6) are increased in AS patients [20]. Expression level of IL-6 strongly correlated with clinical parameters of inflammation such as ESR and CRP. Thus, we further test the functional correlation between *STIM1* genotypes and cytokine (IL-6 and TNF-α). As shown in the **Fig. 3**, the AS patients with G/G or G/A genotypes of the *STIM1* showed a profound increase of serum IL-6 and TNF-α. AS

**Table 5.** Difference in the value of CRP among HLA-B27 positive AS patients stratified by different *STIM1* haplotypes.

| rs2304891/rs3750996 | CRP | rs3750996/rs1561876 | CRP | rs3750996/rs3750994 | CRP |
|---|---|---|---|---|---|
| G/G | 1.0±0.6[a] | G/G | 0.2±0.3 | G/C | 8.6 |
| A/G | 1.5±2.2 | A/G | 1.3±2.1 | G/A | 1.4±2.1 |
| G/A | 1.1±1.7 | G/A | 1.4±2.2 | A/C | 1.1±1.7 |
| A/A | 1.4±2.1 | A/A | 1.2±1.8 | A/A | 1.3±2.0 |
| Unadjusted *P*-value | 0.36 | Unadjusted *P*-value | 0.64 | Unadjusted *P*-value | **0.001*** |
| Adjusted *P*-value[†] | 0.32 | Adjusted *P*-value | 0.65 | Adjusted *P*-value[†] | **0.001*** |

[a]Data represent mean ± S.D..
[†]Adjusted the effects of age and sex.
*Significant (*P*<0.05) values are in bold.

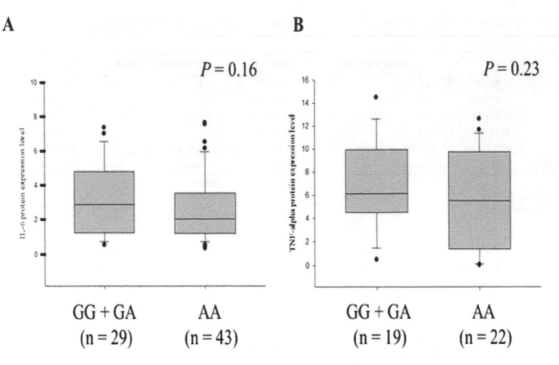

**Figure 3. Comparison of serum (A) IL-6 and (B) TNF-α levels among different genotypes of *STIM1* (rs3750996) in AS patients.**

patients with AA homozygote, however, has a lower level of IL-6 and TNF-α.

## Discussion

Acute phase reactants, including ESR and CRP, are generally used to evaluate AS patients and are also recommended core set endpoint for disease controlling antirheumatic therapy (DC-ART) [21]. Ruof et al. [22] observed a strong correlation between ESR and CRP. Yildirim et al., provided evidence for a close association between CRP and BASDAI [23]. In addition, in large prospective cohort study for in AS patients, ESR and CRP are served as powerful tools not only for monitoring the efficacy of anti-TNF therapy, but also for the selection of AS patients with a high likelihood of responding to anti-TNF treatment [24]. Therefore, the level of ESR and CRP has been widely used in the clinical diagnosis as well as treatment in AS patients.

The genetic polymorphism of Vitamin D receptor (*FokI*) was associated with the levels of ESR and CRP in AS patients [25]. In a Taiwanese population, Lee et al., reported that genotypes of *cytotoxic T lymphocyte-associated antigen-4 (CTLA-4)* associated with expression level of CRP in AS patients [8]. In this study, our results revealed a strong correlation between *STIM1* genotypes/haplotypes and the level of inflammatory factors (ESR and CRP). Since store-operated calcium entry is important in T cell-mediated autoimmunity [26], our results implied that polymorphisms of *STIM1* may influence store-operated calcium signals which in turn involve the regulation of cytokine release and ESR/CRP expression. Indeed, the AS patients with G/G and G/A genotypes of the *STIM1* polymorphism showed a higher level of serum IL-6 and TNF-α. Although the *P* value (0.16; 0.23) was still not significant, we attribute this result to the reduction of the sample size (only 72 cases with IL-6 data and 41 cases with TNF-α data).

In non-excitable cells such as T cells and mast cells, one major route for $Ca^{2+}$ entry is through store-operated $Ca^{2+}$ channels. Store-operated calcium entry has been reported to regulate

paracrine ($LTC_4$) signals in mast cells and autoimmunity in T cells [27,28]. In T cells [26,29], STIM1 is a key initiator that involves in the activation of store-operated $Ca^{2+}$ entry. Picard et al., reported a homozygous nonsense mutation in the *STIM1* gene the caused the deficiency of $Ca^{2+}$ entry which leads to immune dysfunction [30]. In B cells, STIM1-mediated calcium signals drive translocation of $Ca^{2+}$-dependent transcription factor NF-AT to the nucleus where it triggers *interleukin (IL)-10* gene [31]. Thus, STIM1 is an important regulator for cytokine production. Using cell-based experiments, our studies also indicated that knockdown *STIM1* resulted in the reduction of thapsigangin-mediated *TNF-α* expression (supplementary Fig 1). Therefore, polymorphisms of *STIM1* are very likely to involve in the regulation of immune system, which in turn control the ESR/CRP levels. Even so, the mechanism of stim1-mediated ESR/CRP pathways remains to be elucidated.

rs3750996 is located in the 3'UTR of *STIM1* gene. The mechanism by which miRNAs regulate *STIM1* gene expression is still unclear. By bioinformatics approaches from miRBase (http://www.mirbase.org), the allele variations on rs3750996 position may influence the binding affinity of miR223. The molecular mechanism of how miR223 regulates *STIM1* expression needs to be further investigated.

We also analyzed the relationship between genetic polymorphism rs3750996 and ESR in the HLA-B27 negative AS patients (46 HLA-B27 negative AS patients), however, no statistically significant association between genotypes and phenotypes were found (data not shown). We acknowledged that the tSNPs (exon and UTR) selected in this study may be not adequate to investigate the entire genetic polymorphisms of *STIM1*. Application of direct sequencing in a larger sample size may be helpful to identify novel polymorphisms of *STIM1*. In conclusion, our research indicated a significant association between genetic polymorphisms of *STIM1* and ESR/CRP in the HLA-B27 positive AS patients. Haplotypes of rs3750996/rs3750994 also further confirm the association.

## Author Contributions

Conceived and designed the experiments: JW KH YH HW WC. Performed the experiments: YH CH MJ SW. Analyzed the data: YH CH YJ KH HW WC. Contributed reagents/materials/analysis tools: WC YJ JW KH. Wrote the paper: WC HW JW YH.

## References

1. Braun J, Sieper J (2007) Ankylosing spondylitis. Lancet 369: 1379–1390.
2. Calin A, Brophy S, Blake D (1999) Impact of sex on inheritance of ankylosing spondylitis: a cohort study. Lancet 354: 1687–1690.
3. Brewerton DA, Hart FD, Nicholls A, Caffrey M, James DC, et al. (1973) Ankylosing spondylitis and HL-A 27. Lancet 1: 904–907.
4. Khan MA, Ball EJ (2002) Genetic aspects of ankylosing spondylitis. Best Pract Res Clin Rheumatol 16: 675–690.
5. Guo ZS, Li C, Lin ZM, Huang JX, Wei QJ, et al. (2010) Association of IL-1 gene complex members with ankylosing spondylitis in Chinese Han population. Int J Immunogenet 37: 33–37.
6. Safrany E, Pazar B, Csongei V, Jaromi L, Polgar N, et al. (2009) Variants of the IL23R gene are associated with ankylosing spondylitis but not with Sjogren syndrome in Hungarian population samples. Scand J Immunol 70: 68–74.
7. Wei JC, Tsai WC, Lin HS, Tsai CY, Chou CT (2004) HLA-B60 and B61 are strongly associated with ankylosing spondylitis in HLA-B27-negative Taiwan Chinese patients. Rheumatology (Oxford) 43: 839–842.
8. Lee WY, Chang YH, Lo MK, Chang CP, Yang SC, et al. (2010) Polymorphisms of cytotoxic T lymphocyte-associated antigen-4 and cytokine genes in Taiwanese patients with ankylosing spondylitis. Tissue Antigens 75: 119–126.
9. Wei JC, Yen JH, Juo SH, Chen WC, Wang YS, et al. (2011) Association of ORAI1 haplotypes with the risk of HLA-B27 positive ankylosing spondylitis. PLoS One 6: e20426.
10. Chou YH, Juo SH, Chiu YC, Liu ME, Chen WC, et al. (2011) A polymorphism of the ORAI1 gene is associated with the risk and recurrence of calcium nephrolithiasis. J Urol 185: 1742–1746.
11. Parekh AB, Putney JW, Jr. (2005) Store-operated calcium channels. Physiol Rev 85: 757–810.
12. Roos J, DiGregorio PJ, Yeromin AV, Ohlsen K, Lioudyno M, et al. (2005) STIM1, an essential and conserved component of store-operated Ca2+ channel function. J Cell Biol 169: 435–445.
13. Fedida-Metula S, Feldman B, Koshelev V, Levin-Gromiko U, Voronov E, et al. (2012) Lipid rafts couple store-operated Ca2+ entry to constitutive activation of PKB/Akt in a Ca2+/calmodulin-, Src- and PP2A-mediated pathway and promote melanoma tumor growth. Carcinogenesis 33: 740–750.
14. Chen YF, Chiu WT, Chen YT, Lin PY, Huang HJ, et al. (2011) Calcium store sensor stromal-interaction molecule 1-dependent signaling plays an important role in cervical cancer growth, migration, and angiogenesis. Proc Natl Acad Sci U S A 108: 15225–15230.
15. Huang WC, Chai CY, Chen WC, Hou MF, Wang YS, et al. (2011) Histamine regulates cyclooxygenase 2 gene activation through Orai1-mediated NFkappaB activation in lung cancer cells. Cell Calcium 50: 27–35.
16. Wang JY, Chen BK, Wang YS, Tsai YT, Chen WC, et al. (2012) Involvement of store-operated calcium signaling in EGF-mediated COX-2 gene activation in cancer cells. Cell Signal 24: 162–169.
17. van der Linden S, Valkenburg HA, Cats A (1984) Evaluation of diagnostic criteria for ankylosing spondylitis. A proposal for modification of the New York criteria. Arthritis Rheum 27: 361–368.
18. Wei JC, Wong RH, Huang JH, Yu CT, Chou CT, et al. (2007) Evaluation of internal consistency and re-test reliability of Bath ankylosing spondylitis indices in a large cohort of adult and juvenile spondylitis patients in Taiwan. Clin Rheumatol 26: 1685–1691.
19. Chou CT, Tsai YF, Liu J, Wei JC, Liao TS, et al. (2001) The detection of the HLA-B27 antigen by immunomagnetic separation and enzyme-linked immunosorbent assay-comparison with a flow cytometric procedure. J Immunol Methods 255: 15–22.
20. Gratacos J, Collado A, Filella X, Sanmarti R, Canete J, et al. (1994) Serum cytokines (IL-6, TNF-alpha, IL-1 beta and IFN-gamma) in ankylosing spondylitis: a close correlation between serum IL-6 and disease activity and severity. Br J Rheumatol 33: 927–931.
21. van der Heijde D, Bellamy N, Calin A, Dougados M, Khan MA, et al. (1997) Preliminary core sets for endpoints in ankylosing spondylitis. Assessments in Ankylosing Spondylitis Working Group. J Rheumatol 24: 2225–2229.
22. Ruof J, Stucki G (1999) Validity aspects of erythrocyte sedimentation rate and C-reactive protein in ankylosing spondylitis: a literature review. J Rheumatol 26: 966–970.
23. Yildirim K, Erdal A, Karatay S, Melikoglu MA, Ugur M, et al. (2004) Relationship between some acute phase reactants and the Bath Ankylosing Spondylitis Disease Activity Index in patients with ankylosing spondylitis. South Med J 97: 350–353.
24. de Vries MK, van Eijk IC, van der Horst-Bruinsma IE, Peters MJ, Nurmohamed MT, et al. (2009) Erythrocyte sedimentation rate, C-reactive protein level, and serum amyloid a protein for patient selection and monitoring of anti-tumor necrosis factor treatment in ankylosing spondylitis. Arthritis Rheum 61: 1484–1490.
25. Obermayer-Pietsch BM, Lange U, Tauber G, Fruhauf G, Fahrleitner A, et al. (2003) Vitamin D receptor initiation codon polymorphism, bone density and inflammatory activity of patients with ankylosing spondylitis. Osteoporos Int 14: 995–1000.
26. McCarl CA, Khalil S, Ma J, Oh-hora M, Yamashita M, et al. (2010) Store-operated Ca2+ entry through ORAI1 is critical for T cell-mediated autoimmunity and allograft rejection. J Immunol 185: 5845–5858.
27. Chang WC, Di Capite J, Singaravelu K, Nelson C, Halse V, et al. (2008) Local Ca2+ influx through Ca2+ release-activated Ca2+ (CRAC) channels stimulates production of an intracellular messenger and an intercellular pro-inflammatory signal. J Biol Chem 283: 4622–4631.
28. Chang WC, Nelson C, Parekh AB (2006) Ca2+ influx through CRAC channels activates cytosolic phospholipase A2, leukotriene C4 secretion, and expression of c-fos through ERK-dependent and -independent pathways in mast cells. FASEB J 20: 2381–2383.
29. Feske S (2011) Immunodeficiency due to defects in store-operated calcium entry. Ann N Y Acad Sci 1238: 74–90.
30. Picard C, McCarl CA, Papolos A, Khalil S, Luthy K, et al. (2009) STIM1 mutation associated with a syndrome of immunodeficiency and autoimmunity. N Engl J Med 360: 1971–1980.
31. Matsumoto M, Fujii Y, Baba A, Hikida M, Kurosaki T, et al. (2011) The calcium sensors STIM1 and STIM2 control B cell regulatory function through interleukin-10 production. Immunity 34: 703–714.

# 9

# Increased Soluble CD4 in Serum of Rheumatoid Arthritis Patients Is Generated by Matrix Metalloproteinase (MMP)-Like Proteinases

**Wen-Yi Tseng[1,2◯], Yi-Shu Huang[3◯], Nien-Yi Chiang[3], Yeh-Pin Chou[4,5], Yeong-Jian Jan Wu[1,4], Shue-Fen Luo[4,6], Chang-Fu Kuo[6], Ko-Ming Lin[7], Hsi-Hsien Lin[3,8]\***

1 Division of Rheumatology, Allergy and Immunology, Chang Gung Memorial Hospital at Keelung, Keelung, Taiwan, 2 Graduate Institute of Clinical Medicine, Chang Gung University, Tao-Yuan, Taiwan, 3 Graduate Institute of Biomedical Sciences, Chang Gung University, Tao-Yuan, Taiwan, 4 Department of Medicine, College of Medicine, Chang Gung University, Tao-Yuan, Taiwan, 5 Division of Hepato-Gastroenterology, Department of Internal Medicine, Chang Gung Memorial Hospital at Kaohsiung, Kaohsiung, Taiwan, 6 Division of Rheumatology, Allergy and Immunology, Chang Gung Memorial Hospital at Linkou, Linkou, Taiwan, 7 Division of Rheumatology, Allergy and Immunology, Chang Gung Memorial Hospital at Chiayi, Chiayi, Taiwan, 8 Department of Microbiology and Immunology, College of Medicine, Chang Gung University, Tao-Yuan, Taiwan

## Abstract

Higher soluble CD4 (sCD4) levels in serum have been detected in patients of infectious and chronic inflammatory diseases. However, how and why sCD4 is produced remains poorly understood. We establish sensitive ELISA and WB assays for sCD4 detection in conditioned medium of *in vitro* cell culture system and serum of chronic inflammatory patients. Serum samples from patients with systemic lupus erythematosus (SLE) (n = 79), rheumatoid arthritis (RA) (n = 59), ankylosing spondylitis (AS) (n = 25), gout (n = 31), and normal controls (n = 99) were analyzed using ELISA for sCD4 detection. Results from each assay were analyzed by the Kruskal-Wallis test. Dunn's multiple comparison post-test was then applied between groups. We confirm that cells expressing exogenous CD4 produce sCD4 in a constitutive and PMA-induced manner. Importantly, sCD4 production in a heterologous expression system is inhibited by GM6001 and TAPI-0, suggesting receptor shedding by matrix metalloproteinase (MMP)-like proteinases. Moreover, similar findings are recapitulated in human primary CD4+ T cells. Finally, we show that serum sCD4 levels are increased in patients of chronic inflammatory diseases including RA and SLE, but not in those with gout. Intriguingly, sCD4 levels in RA patients are correlated positively with the disease activities and higher sCD4 levels seem to associate with poor prognosis. Taken together, we conclude that CD4 is shed from cell surface by a MMP-like sheddase and sCD4 level is closely related with the inflammatory condition in certain chronic diseases. Hence, sCD4 might be considered an important parameter for RA disease progression with potential diagnostic importance.

**Editor:** Paul Proost, University of Leuven, Rega Institute, Belgium

**Funding:** This study was supported by grants from National Science Council, Taiwan (NSC98-2320-B-182-028-MY3 and NSC101-2320-B-182-029-MY3 to H.-H. Lin), and Chang Gung Memorial Hospital (CMRPG670381 and CMRPG280431 to W.-Y. Tseng, CMRPG891331 to Y.-P. Chou, and CMRPD190553 to H.-H. Lin). The funders had no role in study design, data collection and analysis, decision to publish, or preparation of the manuscript.

**Competing Interests:** The authors have declared that no competing interests exist.

\* E-mail: hhlin@mail.cgu.edu.tw

◯ These authors contributed equally to this work.

## Introduction

CD4 is a 60-kDa glycoprotein of the immunoglobulin super-family (IgSF), containing four extracellular Ig-like domains, a hydrophobic transmembrane region and a 40-residue cytoplasmic tail [1]. CD4 is expressed in many immune cells including T cells, monocytes, macrophages and dendritic cells. The role of CD4 in T cells is multifaceted so that it is involved in T cell differentiation and development as well as T cell activation by interacting with antigen-presenting cells (APCs). The cytoplasmic tail of CD4 associates with the Lck kinase, which in turn activates the signaling components of the T cell receptor (TCR)-CD3 complexes [2,3,4]. As such, one of the major functions of CD4 is to augment the TCR signaling during T cell-APC interaction by acting as a co-receptor.

In fact, due to its functional significance as a co-receptor, CD4 has been clinically tried as a major target in T cell-targeted

therapies for the treatment of T cell-mediated autoimmune diseases such as rheumatoid arthritis (RA). Indeed, CD4-specific monoclonal antibodies (mAb) were among the first biologic therapies developed for rheumatic diseases [5]. Both depleting and non-depleting mAbs against CD4 have been administrated in RA patients in an attempt to interrupt T cell functions, but were determined to be ineffective in randomized clinical trials [6,7]. The underlying mechanisms for the unfavorable clinical outcome following CD4 mAb treatment are multifaceted and complex [6,7].

CD4 also is the high-affinity entry receptor for human immunodeficiency virus (HIV) by binding to the viral envelope glycoprotein gp120 [8]. HIV apparently escapes the effect of neutralizing antibodies by generating new variants, but infection of T cells still requires gp120-CD4 interaction. Therefore, one approach to block HIV infection is to use the soluble form of CD4 (sCD4) to inhibit virus attachment to target cells. Indeed, recombinant sCD4 was shown effective in blocking HIV binding to CD4$^+$ T cells *in vitro*, and hence was considered a potential target for anti-HIV therapy [9,10].

Interestingly, elevated serum sCD4 has been found in patients of viral infections, such as HIV [11] and Epstein-Barr virus [12]. In addition, serum sCD4 was also identified in patients of chronic inflammatory diseases such as RA [13], Sjogren's syndrome [14], systemic lupus erythematosus (SLE) [14], common variable immunodeficiency [15], osteoarthritis (OA) [13], chronic renal failure [16], and localized scleroderma [17]. In prospective sequential studies of RA patients, serum sCD4 levels were found to correlate positively with the clinical disease status [13]. Therefore, unveiling the mechanism of sCD4 generation is of important relevance to understanding the role of CD4 receptor in these diseases. Delineation of the relationship between sCD4 and cellular CD4 receptor might also help explain the ineffective effect of CD4 mAbs in the RA clinical trials.

Soluble forms of transmembrane proteins, including adhesion molecules and receptors, which still retain biological activities have been identified in various extracellular compartments. At least three independent cellular processes are known to be involved in their production: First, soluble cytokine receptors can be generated by alternative splicing of mRNA transcripts; Second, cytokines and soluble cytokine receptors can be released as membrane components of cellular vesicles such as exosomes that are small membrane-enclosed entities (typically <100 nm in diameter); Third, extracellular proteinases such as matrix metalloproteinases (MMPs) actively target and shed the extracellular domain of cell surface proteins [18,19].

Previous studies have failed to detect any CD4 transcripts with deletion/premature termination at/around the transmembrane region, suggesting that sCD4 is unlikely resulted from alternatively-spliced mRNAs [20]. Through the use of flow cytometry, ELISA, and Western blotting analyses in primary CD4$^+$ T cells and cells expressing exogenous CD4, herein we unequivocally show that sCD4 is produced mainly via receptor shedding by MMP-like proteinases. Moreover, we found that serum sCD4 levels in chronic inflammatory diseases such as SLE and RA, are strongly elevated. Most significantly, serum sCD4 levels of RA patients are positively correlated with the disease status defined by the 28-joint count disease activity score (DAS28). Hence, we conclude that CD4 shedding is predominantly mediated by MMPs and abnormal expression and activity of MMPs in certain chronic inflammatory diseases may enhance serum sCD4 levels, which can be considered as a potential diagnostic parameter for chronic inflammatory disease progression.

## Materials and Methods

### Reagents, Antibodies and Cell Culture

Unless otherwise specified, general reagents and antibodies (Abs) were obtained from Sigma-Aldrich (St. Louis, MO, USA). DNA and protein reagents were obtained from Clontech (CA, USA), Invitrogen (Carlsbad, CA), Qiagen (Valencia, CA), Fermentas (ON, Canada) or New England Biolabs (MA, USA). Monoclonal Abs (mAbs) used in the study are: EMR2 stalk-specific 2A1 and anti-CD4 (1F6) from AbD Serotec (Kidlington, UK); anti-CD4 (OKT4) and biotin-conjugated anti-CD4 (RPA-T4) from eBioscience (San Diego, CA, USA); Anti-c-myc (9E10) from Invitrogen; PE-conjugated anti-CD4, anti-CD62L, anti-CD69 and mouse IgG$_1$ isotype control were from BD Systems (MN, USA). Cell culture media and supplements including 10% heat inactivated fetal calf serum (FCS), 2 mM L-glutamine, 50 IU/ml

penicillin and 50 μg/ml streptomycin were purchased from Invitrogen. CHO-K1 and primary CD4$^+$ T cells were cultured in Ham's F-12 and RPMI medium, respectively.

### Human CD4 Expression Construct

The human full-length CD4 expression construct, hCD4-myc, was generated using the full-length CD4 cDNA PCR-amplified from pooled human peripheral leukocytes total RNA (BD Biosciences-Clontech), and subcloned into the *Hin*dIII-*Xho*I sites of pcDNA3.1myc-His C (Invitrogen). The fidelity of the coding sequence was confirmed by DNA sequencing.

### Patients

This study was approved by the Chang Gung Memorial Hospital Ethics Committee (CGMF IRB No.: 97-1457B and 98-2805B) and all procedures were performed according to the guideline set by the Committee. The number of patients recruited for this study include: systemic lupus erythematosus (SLE), 79; rheumatoid arthritis (RA), 59; Ankylosing spondylitis (AS), 25; and gout, 31. A total of ninety-nine healthy volunteers are also included. All participants were recruited from the outpatient clinics of Chang Gung Memorial Hospital (Taiwan) from 2008 to 2010. Patients were screened to meet the criteria set by American College of Rheumatology for the diagnosis of SLE, RA or gout, and the modified New York criteria for AS. All were evaluated by specific validated disease activity indexes such as Systemic Lupus Erythematosus Activity Index (SLEDAI) (median: 4, interquartile range: 2–8), DAS28 (median:4.55, interquartile range: 2.90–5.85), Bath Ankylosing Spondylitis Disease Activity Index (BASDAI) (median: 2.7, interquartile range: 1.9–5.4) or Bath Ankylosing Spondylitis Functional Index (BASFI) (median: 1.55, interquartile range: 0.59–5.425) at the outpatient clinic from signs and symptoms as well as the results of laboratory tests. All gout patients recruited in this study had at least one episode of acute gouty arthritis attack in past one week. At the time of inclusion, 59 of 79 SLE patients were being treated with corticosteroids (prednisolone 2.5–30 mg/day). Almost all RA patients were already receiving at least one disease modifying anti-rheumatic drug and coricosteroids at inclusion (38 patients with MTX 5 mg-15 mg/week, 7 patients with lefluomide 10–20 mg/day, 31 patients with sulfasalazine 1–2 gm/day, 40 patients with hydroxycholroquine 200–400 mg/day and 44 patients with prednisolone 5–15 mg/day) and part of them also receiving biologic agents (16 patient with tumor necrosis blockers and 1 patients with rituximab). Almost all AS patients were treated with non-steroid anti-inflammatory drugs and some of them were treated with sulfasalazine (17 patients with sulfasalazine 1–2 gm/day) at inclusion. Patients and healthy volunteers were informed about the nature of the experimental procedures and all have signed written informed consent. Serum samples (~10 ml) were taken from patients, prepared as described previously [21] and stored at −80°C until use.

### Transient Transfection and Drug Treatment

Transient transfection of expression constructs was performed using Lipofectamine$^{TM}$ (Invitrogen) as described previously [22]. Transfected cells were sub-cultured into 6-well plate and fed with fresh medium for 1–2 day for further drug treatment. Cells were cultured for 2 days in OPTI-MEM containing protease inhibitors (CALBIOCHEM, CA, USA) such as GM6001 (50 μM), E-64 (50 μM), Pepstatin A (50 μM), α$_2$ macroglobulin (50 μM), Furin protease inhibitor I (50 μM), TAPI-0 (10 μM), TAPI-1(10 μM), or TAPI-2 (10 μM). When necessary, cells were also treated with 12-*O*-tetradecanoylphorbol- 13-acetate (PMA) in OPTI-MEM as indicated. In addition, CD4$^+$ T cells were treated with PMA in serum-free RPMI medium.

## Immunoblotting Analysis

Cells were lysed in RIPA lysis buffer (20 mM TrisHCl pH7.4, 5 mM MgCl$_2$, 100 mM NaCl, 0.5% NP-40 and 1X Complete Protease Inhibitors) supplemented with 1 mM sodium orthovanadate, 1 mM AEBSF and 5 mM Levamisole. Proteins were quantified using the Bicinchoninic acid (BCA) protein assay kit (PIERCE, Rockford, USA). Conditioned medium (CM) of CHO-K1 cells transfected with hCD4FL-myc was collected and concentrated using Amicon Ultra centrifugal filters-10 kDa cutoff (Millipore, MA, USA). SDS-PAGE and western blot (WB) analyses were carried out using standard procedures as described previously [22,23].

## Flow Cytometry

After treatment, primary CD4$^+$ T cells were washed, and fixed with fresh prepared 2% paraformaldehyde solution in PBS at 4°C for 30 min. Cells were then blocked for 1 hr in ice-cold blocking buffer (PBS buffer containing 1% BSA/5% normal serum of the animal where the secondary Ab was derived from). Cells were subsequently incubated with the indicated primary Ab diluted in blocking buffer for 1 hr, and then washed three times by cold PBS

and subjected to analysis by FACScan flow cytometer (BD Biosciences).

## Detection of Soluble CD4 by ELISA

To analyze the concentration of soluble CD4 (sCD4) in serum and culture conditioned medium, an ELISA assay utilizing two noncompeting murine mAbs to the human CD4 protein are established in house. Briefly, anti-CD4 mAb (clone: OKT4; 2.5 μg/ml) was diluted in PBS and coated onto the 96 well plate (100 μl/well) by incubating at 37°C for 2 h. The mAb solution was then discarded and the wells incubated with blocking buffer (1% bovine serum albumin (BSA) in PBS) overnight at 4°C. Following extensive washes with PBS/0.1% (v/v) Tween-20, samples (100 μl/well) were added and incubated at RT for 1 h. Recombinant sCD4 proteins (~7–2000 pg/ml) diluted in blocking buffer were used as standard. After discarding samples, wells were extensively washed and 100 μl of biotin-conjugated second anti-CD4 mAb (clone: RPA-T4; 0.5 μg/ml) was added for incubation at RT for 1 h. Wells were again washed extensively and then incubated with 100 μl of avidin-HRP (Sigma-Aldrich) (1:200 diluted in blocking buffer) for 1 hr at RT. Finally, wells were washed and incubated with 100 μl of O-phenylenediamine (0.5 mg/ml) in citrate-phosphate buffer containing 0.01% (v/v) hydrogen peroxide (BD Biosciences) for 20 min at RT in the dark. The reaction was stopped by adding 50 μl of 2 N H$_2$SO$_4$ per well.

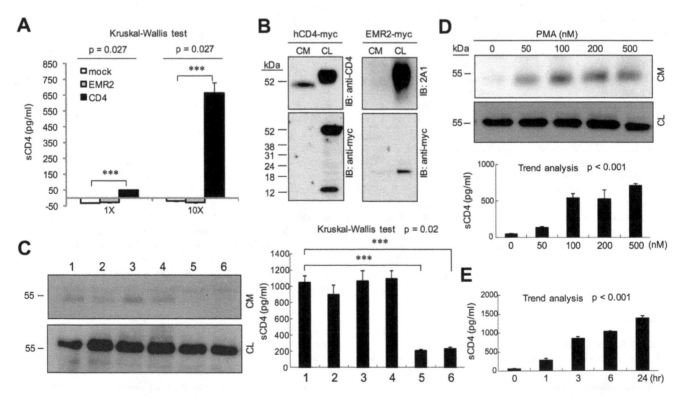

**Figure 1. CD4 is shed by MMP-like proteinases in transfected CHO-K1 cells.** (A, B) CHO-K1 cells were transiently transfected with the hCD4-myc or negative control EMR2-myc expression construct. Production of sCD4 is evaluated by ELISA (A) and WB (B) analysis. Conditioned medium (CM) and cell lysates (CL) were probed with 2A1 (specific to EMR2), anti-CD4 and anti-myc mAbs in WB analysis. Kruskal-Wallis test across all three groups of 1X and 10X concentration shows p = 0.027. Dunn's multiple comparisons post-test p values between groups show ***P<0.001. (C) sCD4 production is inhibited by pan-MMP inhibitors, GM6001 and TAPI-0. CHO-K1 cells transiently transfected with the hCD4-myc construct were treated with various protease inhibitors (1, Control; 2, DMSO; 3, Furin protease inhibitor I; 4, Pepstatin A; 5, GM6001; 6, TAPI-0) then analyzed by WB (left panel) and ELISA (right panel). Kruskal-Wallis test across all six groups shows p = 0.02. Dunn's multiple comparisons post-test p values between groups show ***P<0.001. (D, E) CHO-K1 cells transiently transfected with the hCD4-myc construct were treated with PMA in various concentrations (D) for 1 hr or 50 nM PMA for different time periods (E) then analyzed by ELISA and WB. ELISA. Statistical significance was assessed by the trend analysis.

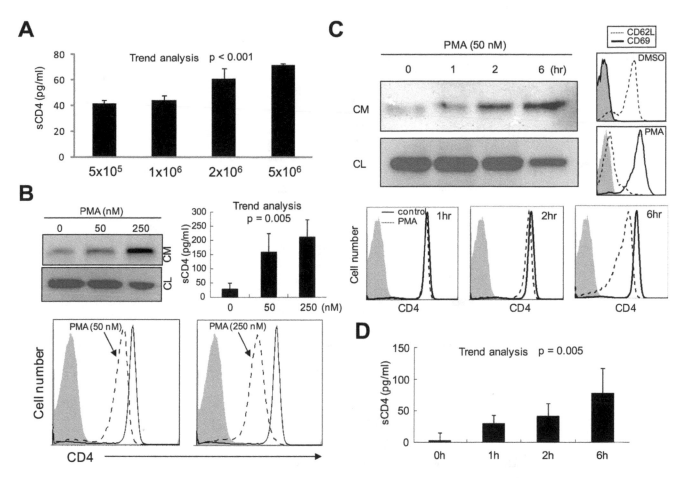

**Figure 2. sCD4 is also generated in primary CD4⁺ T cells.** (A) CD4⁺ T cells were purified from healthy volunteers and cultured in different cell densities as indicated. CM was then collected for ELISA analysis. (B-D) $1 \times 10^6$ CD4⁺ T cells were stimulated by PMA in different doses (B) for 3 hr or 50 nM PMA for different time periods (C and D) before collecting CM, CL and cells for ELISA, WB and FACS analysis. In addition, stimulated CD4⁺ T cells were stained with cell activation markers CD62L and CD69 and analyzed by FACS analysis (C). Statistical significance was assessed by the trend analysis.

The 450 nm OD reading of the plate was done in a Dynatech MR700 microplate reader (Tecan, Switzerland).

## CD4⁺ T Cell Purification

Peripheral blood monocytic cells (PBMCs) were isolated from fresh venous blood of healthy donors using a protocol approved by the institutional review board at Chang Gung Memorial Hospital (CGMF IRB No.: 97–1457B and 98–2805B). Written informed consent was signed by all participants. In short, fresh blood was collected and spun at 2000 rpm for 20 min at RT. Blood plasma at the upper fraction was discarded, while blood cells at the lower fraction were resuspended with equal volume of 1X PBS. Blood cells were overlaid onto a half volume of Ficoll Hypaque (Chalfont St Giles, UK), taking care not to destroy the interface between the two fractions. Cells were centrifuged at 2000 rpm for 20 min at RT, resulting in the generation of the PBMC fraction between serum and Ficoll Hypaque fractions for collection. Subsequently, CD4⁺ T cells were isolated from PBMCs by CD4⁺ T cell isolation kit II (MACS, Germany) according to the manufacturer's protocols. In brief, PBMCs were washed twice, counted, and resuspended in 2~5 mM cold EDTA buffer at the cell density of $1 \times 10^7$ cells/40 μl. Cells were mixed with 10 μl of biotin-Ab cocktail and incubated for 10 min at 4°C, followed by the addition of 30 μl of 2~5 mM cold EDTA buffer and 20 μl of anti-biotin

microbeads. The cell-Ab-microbead reaction mixture was incubated for 15 min at 4°C. Cells were then washed thoroughly with 1X cold PBS. Cells were resuspended in 1 ml of 2.5 mM cold EDTA buffer for CD4⁺ T cell purification using the LS (MACS) column.

## Statistical Analysis

The measured items and domain scores of the five study groups were presented as mean and standard deviation. All statistical tests were performed with the use of SPSS-19 software (SPSS Inc., USA). The ELISA data of *in vitro* cell culture systems and serum samples of patients did not fit a Gaussian distribution despite attempts at log transformation. Non-parametric Kruskal-Wallis test was therefore used analyze these data to determine if there was significant variation in the medians of the groups analyzed. If 95% significance was achieved, Dunn's multiple comparison post-test was then used to compare the assay results of one group with another. Correlations between sCD4 and gender, age and disease activity index of SLE (SLEDAI) and RA (DAS28) were analyzed according to Spearman's rank correlation coefficient. A trend analysis was used to compare the proportions of different kinds of outcomes between low level sCD4 (<0.125 ng/ml) and high level sCD4 (≥0.125 ng/ml) groups in RA patients, as well as the dose- and time-dependent response of PMA treatment. In all cases, a

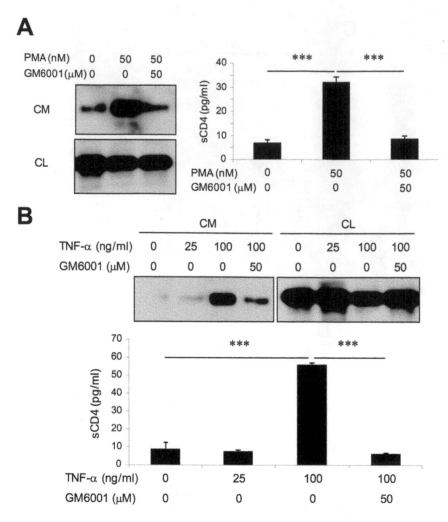

**Figure 3. Production of sCD4 by primary CD4⁺ T cells is mediated by MMP-like shedding.** (A, B) CD4⁺ T cells were stimulated by 50 nM PMA (A) or TNF-α (25 and 100 ng/ml) (B) in the absence or presence of GM6001 (50 μM) for 3 hr. CM and CL were collected for ELISA and WB analysis. Dunn's multiple comparisons post-test p values between groups show ***P<0.001.

p-value of <0.05 (two sided) was considered statistically significant. *P*-values are as follows: *P<0.05, **P<0.01 and ***P<0.001. The ELISA data of *in vitro* cell culture systems are means ± S.E.M. of 3 independent experiments performed in triplicate.

## Results

### Evidence that Soluble CD4 is Generated via Receptor Shedding

To date the molecular mechanism(s) whereby soluble CD4 (sCD4) is generated remains unclear. Previous studies have examined, but failed to detect novel CD4 RNA transcripts with deletion or premature termination signals at/before the transmembrane region. This suggested that RNA alternative splicing is unlikely the main cause for sCD4 [20]. Other alternatives include receptor exocytosis and shedding. To systematically investigate the potential mechanism(s) involved, we first established a sensitive sandwich ELISA assay to detect sCD4 in a heterologous cell expression system. Indeed, sCD4 can be readily detected by the ELISA assay in the conditioned medium (CM) of CHO-K1 cells expressing the full-length human CD4 with a C-terminal myc tag (hCD4-myc) (Fig. 1A). No signal was detected in the CM of mock-

transfected cells or cells expressing an unrelated EMR2 receptor (Fig. 1A).

Similarly, WB analysis identified sCD4 in the CM of hCD4-myc expressing cells, but no signal in the CM of cells expressing human EMR2, indicating the specific expression and generation of sCD4 (Fig. 1B). Most interestingly, the size of the sCD4 band found in CM (~50 kDa) is smaller than that detected in the whole cell lysate (CL) (~60 kDa), suggesting a possible shedding event. This idea is further strengthened by the fact that apart from the ~60 kDa full-length CD4 band, a ~13 kDa fragment is detected in the CL by anti-myc mAb (Fig. 1B and Fig. S1, S2). The ~13 kDa fragment most likely represents the C-terminal half of CD4 receptor including the transmembrane region and cytoplasmic tail. Hence, we conclude that a portion of the surface CD4 receptor is likely modified by ectodomain shedding to produce a smaller sCD4.

### CD4 Shedding is Mediated by Metalloproteinases (MMPs)

To identify the candidate sheddase(s) involved in the ectodomain shedding of CD4, transiently-transfected CHO-K1 cells were treated with various protease inhibitors. WB analysis shows that while most protease inhibitors show no apparent effect on CD4 shedding, GM6001 and TAPI-0 efficiently diminished the

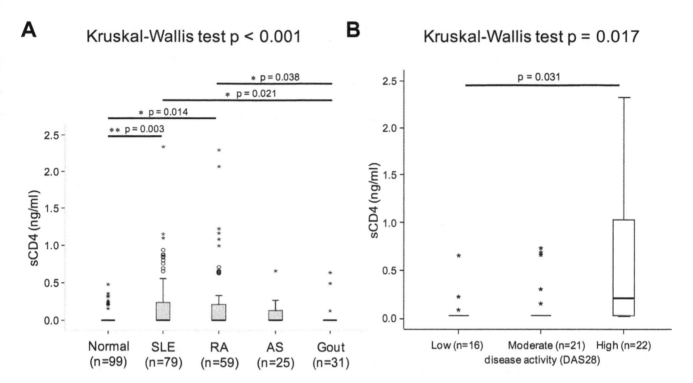

**Figure 4. Comparison of serum sCD4 levels in various chronic inflammatory diseases.** (A) Serum sCD4 levels in normal subjects groups, SLE, RA, AS, and gout. Data are shown as box plots. Each box represents the 25th to 75th percentiles. Lines inside the boxes represent the median. Lines outside the boxes represent the 10th and the 90th percentiles. Circles and asterisks indicate outliers and extreme values, respectively. Kruskal-Wallis test across all five groups shows p<0.001. Only significant Dunn's multiple comparisons post-test p values between groups are shown. (B) Comparison of serum sCD4 levels in RA patient groups classified by DAS28 as low-disease, moderate-disease, and high-disease activity. Data are shown as box plots. Each box represents the 25th to 75th percentiles. Lines inside the boxes represent the median. Lines outside the boxes represent the 10th and the 90th percentiles. Asterisks indicate extreme values. Kruskal-Wallis test across all three groups shows p=0.017. Only significant Dunn's multiple comparisons post-test p values between groups are shown.

production of sCD4 (Fig. 1C and Fig. S1, S2). This result strongly suggests that CD4 shedding is mediated by metalloproteinase(s) as both GM6001 and TAPI-0 are potent broad-spectrum hydroxamate inhibitors of metalloproteinases such as matrix metalloproteinases (MMPs) and members of a disintegrin and metalloprotease (ADAM) family [24]. To further verify this suggestion, cells were treated with 12-*O*-tetradecanoylphorbol- 13-acetate (PMA), which is well known to induce metalloproteinase activity [25]. As expected, PMA-treated CHO-K1 cells produce sCD4 in a dose- and time-dependent manner (Fig. 1D and E). Hence, we conclude that the ectodomain shedding of CD4 is mediated predominantly by MMPs.

## Primary CD4⁺ T cells also Produce sCD4 via MMP-like Mediated Ectodomain Shedding

To examine whether human primary CD4⁺ T cells also generate sCD4 by a similar mechanism(s), CD4⁺ T cells were isolated for analysis. ELISA analysis indicates that sCD4 is generated constitutively in a cell density-dependent manner (Fig. 2A). In addition, PMA-treated CD4⁺ T cells enhances the generation of sCD4 in a dose- and time-dependent manner (Fig. 2B, C and D). Consequently, reduced surface CD4 levels were found in PMA-treated T cells by FACS analysis (Fig. 2B and C). During T cell activation, CD69 is highly up-regulated while ADAM17-mediated CD62L shedding is enhanced [26,27,28,29,30]. Therefore, PMA-induced T cell activation is confirmed by reduced and enhanced surface expression of T cell

**Table 1.** Clinical characteristics and sCD4 levels of normal donors and subjects with SLE, RA, AS and gout.

| Variable | SLE (N = 79) | RA (N = 59) | AS (N = 25) | Gout (N = 30) | Normal donor (N = 99) |
|---|---|---|---|---|---|
| Age (y/o) | 42.85±11.65 | 54.92±10.43 | 41.44±14.53 | 50.13±16.14 | 48.31±10.87 |
| Male Sex no. (%) | 7 (8.86) | 8 (13.56) | 18 (72) | 30 (100) | 82 (82.83) |
| Soluble CD4 (ng/ml) median (IQR 25ᵗʰ–75ᵗʰ) | 0(0–0.272) | 0(0–0.22) | 0(0–0.134) | 0(0–0) | 0(0–0) |

Data are expressed as means ± SD and median (Interquartile range, 25ᵗʰ–75ᵗʰ).
SLE, systemic lupus erythematous; RA, rheumatoid arthritis; AS, ankylosing spondylitis;
IQR, interquartile range.

**Table 2.** Clinical characteristics and sCD4 levels of RA patients with low, moderate and high disease activity.

| | Low disease Activity (DAS28 ≤ 3.2) | Moderate disease activity (3.2<DAS28 ≤ 5.1) | High disease activity (DAS28>5.1) |
|---|---|---|---|
| Disease duration (yrs) | 4.53±5.41 | 4.77±6.08 | 9.40±8.55 |
| ESR (mm/hr) | 12.31±9.46 | 25.50±24.63 | 41.95±24.58 |
| CRP (mg/L) | 3.55±6.00 | 5.70±8.18 | 22.79±28.03 |
| Steroid dosage (mg/day) | 3.73±4.55 | 4.77±3.70 | 6.09±4.67 |
| Biologic agents usage | Etanercept (3) | Etanercept (1) Adalimumab(2) | Etanercept (3) Adalimumab(7) Mabthera (1) |
| Soluble CD4 (ng/ml) Median (IQR 25th–75th) | 0(0–0) | 0(0–0.06475) | 0.1839(0–1.016) |

Data are expressed as means ± SD and median (interquartile range 25th–75th).
DAS28, 28-joint count Disease Activity Score; ESR, erythrocyte sedimentation rate; CRP, C-reactive protein; IQR, interquartile range.

activation markers CD62L and CD69, respectively (Fig. 2C). Consistent with earlier results, WB and ELISA analyses showed that GM6001 treatment effectively inhibits PMA-induced CD4 shedding in T cells (Fig. 3A). Finally, sCD4 was detected in the CM of T cells activated by TNF-α in a dose-dependent manner that is inhibited by GM6001 (Fig. 3B). All together, these results indicate that CD4 receptor shedding occurs constitutively at a basal level in CD4$^+$ T cells, and T cell activation enhances CD4 shedding that is sensitive to GM6001.

## Serum sCD4 Levels are Elevated in Patients of Autoimmune Diseases

To determine whether the serum sCD4 level is relevant to disease progression, we screen patients of SLE, RA, and AS as these are well-known autoimmune diseases with typical chronic inflammation and leukocyte activation. Gout patients representing acute inflammation are also included for comparison. The concentrations of sCD4 in the serum of 194 patients with SLE, RA, AS and gout, as well as 99 normal subjects were assessed by the ELISA assay as described above. As shown in Fig. 4A and Table 1, patients with SLE and RA had significantly higher concentrations of sCD4 than the normal subjects. In the AS patient group, serum sCD4 levels were also elevated considerably though not statistically significant in comparison to controls. On the contrary, serum sCD4 level of 31 gout patients was not different from those of the normal control subjects.

The five patient groups differed significantly in sex and age when the demographic and clinical data are taken into consideration.

**Table 3.** Correlation between sCD4 levels in serum and clinical outcomes of RA patients after 3 months.

| Outcome | Low level sCD4 | High level sCD4 | P value |
|---|---|---|---|
| No response | 28 (68.3%) | 17 (94.4%) | |
| Moderate response | 10 (24.4%) | 1 (5.6%) | 0.034 |
| Good response | 3 (7.3%) | 0 (0.0%) | |

Data are expressed as number (%). All RA patients were assessed by DAS-28 again after 3 months and classified as no response, moderate response and good response according to EULAR response criteria. A low sCD4 level is defined as serum sCD4<0.125 ng/ml and a high sCD4 level is defined as serum sCD4 ≥ 0.125 ng/ml. Statistical significance was assessed by the trend analysis. DAS28, 28-joint count Disease Activity Score; EULAR, European League Against Rheumatism.

However, an examination of the effect of sex on serum sCD4 levels in the controls showed no significant differences between men and women. Similarly, no correlation was found between age and serum sCD4 levels (data not shown). Interestingly, significant correlation between serum sCD4 level and disease activity was found in the RA group but not in the SLE group. When the RA patients were divided into the low-disease activity (DAS28<3.2), moderate-disease activity (3.2 ≤ DAS28 ≤ 5.1) and high-disease activity (DAS28>5.1) groups, a significant elevation in serum sCD4 levels was noted in the high-disease activity group compared with the low-disease activity group (Fig. 4B and Table 2). The moderate-disease activity group also has higher sCD4 levels than the low-disease activity group, but the difference is not statistically significant.

To determine if there is a correlation between the sCD4 level and the outcome of RA patients, we assessed DAS28 of each RA patients again after 3 months and classified their clinical outcomes into no response, moderate response and good response based on the European League Against Rheumatism (EULAR) response criteria using DAS28. The ELISA data indicate the clinical outcomes are distinctively different between the patients with higher sCD4 levels (>0.125 ng/ml), which the cut off value is determined by the average background level of all normal subjects, and those with lower sCD4 levels (Table 3). Specifically, a significantly higher percentage of no responders is found among patients with the high serum sCD4 levels versus those with low sCD4 levels (94.4% versus 68.3%).

## Discussion

Our data indicate that sCD4 generated from transfected CHO-K1 cells and primary CD4$^+$ T cells is due to receptor shedding. This conclusion resonates with earlier reports showing that CD4 molecule can be cleaved by *Leishmaina*-derived peptidase gp63 and by bacteria exoproteases such as elastase and alkaline protease [31]. Most significantly, our results strongly suggest that endogenous cellular sheddases are also involved in the production of sCD4. While it is still unclear which specific sheddase is involved, the fact that the broad-spectrum metalloproteinase inhibitor, GM6001, efficiently inhibits CD4 shedding implicates members of MMP and/or ADAMs family as likely candidates. To further support this, it is noteworthy to know that gp63 is a MMP-like zinc-dependent endopeptidase, whose activity is inhibited by heavy metal ions and 1,10-phenanthroline, an inhibitor of metallopeptidases [31].

Previous studies have found evidence of overexpression of proteases by pathogens and cancer cells. This is thought to be beneficial for their own survival and growth by cleaving host cell-produced proteins in order to escape immune surveillance. Examples include acid protease secreted by bacteria for the proteolysis of $IgA_1$ and C5a, cysteine and alkaline proteases secreted by parasites for cytolysis, and metalloproteinases secreted by cancer cells for tumor metastasis, invasion, immune escape and angiogensis [32,33,34]. Indeed, CD4 proteolysis by bacteria- and parasite-derived proteases might represent a general means for enhancing their infectivity and/or survival via inhibition of T cell activation and hence the adaptive immune response [31].

However, it is less clear about the role of sCD4 in chronic inflammatory diseases and HIV infection. As recombinant sCD4 has been shown to inhibit HIV infection, replication and syncytium formation selectively, it is possible that the increased sCD4 found in HIV-infected patients might serve as a negative feedback mechanism for the inhibition of further HIV infection [11,35]. However, it is not known whether the endogenous sCD4 works similarly as recombinant sCD4. Similarly, the role of sCD4 in chronic inflammatory diseases might be a way to reduce $CD4^+$ T cell activation. High levels of sCD4 might be able to compete with cell surface CD4 receptor for the binding of depleting and non-depleting CD4 mAbs, affecting the efficacy of these therapeutic agents. Alternatively, CD4 mAb binding *in vivo* might potentially enhance CD4 shedding (stripping) as reported in the case of Keliximab [36]. In this scenario, sCD4 could be considered as an anti-infectious and anti-inflammatory agent. On the other hand, sCD4 has also been shown to act as a chemoattractant for polymorphonuclear cells (PMNs) [35]. In this case, production of sCD4 in inflamed tissues would potentially lead to more immune cell infiltration resulting in secretion of additional MMPs by PMNs and possibly more sCD4, essentially amplifying tissue inflammation. Interestingly, MMPs are known to be overexpressed in many chronic inflammatory diseases including RA and SLE [34,37,38]. Hence, it is likely that MMPs produced by infiltrated immune cells in chronic inflammatory conditions actively shed sCD4, which in turn cause continued inflammation by attracting more leukocytes.

Previous studies have found increased levels of serum sCD4 in RA and SLE patients, indicating a relevant link to disease activity [13,39,40]. In our analysis of clinical serum samples, significantly higher levels of serum sCD4 were found in RA and SLE patients, but not in those with gout. More importantly, serum sCD4 levels were shown to be positively correlated with the disease activities of RA patients and patients with higher serum sCD4 levels are more refractory to present treatment within three months. These findings not only confirm previous studies [13,20], but also seem to implicate sCD4 as an important parameter of disease severity/progression for certain chronic inflammatory diseases. The reason for the lack of correlation between sCD4 level and disease activities of SLE patients may be due to that the SLEDAI score gathered in this study is skewed to lower side and the heterogeneity of clinical manifestations in SLE patients also contributes to the difficulty in evaluating the relationship between soluble CD4 level and disease activities of SLE patients.

Hence, our results seem to suggest an association of sCD4 with a pro-inflammatory role in RA. The level of serum sCD4 has been considered as an indicator of T lymphocyte activation in various diseases [17,41]. Higher disease activities in RA patients usually mean more T cell activation, hence increased levels of serum sCD4. Our present study suggests that sCD4 not only serves as a parameter of T cell activation, but also is associated with a potential pro-inflammatory role in RA. With this in mind, the relationship of sCD4 levels and MMPs production/activity in the chronic inflammatory diseases will be of great interest in the future.

## Supporting Information

**Figure S1  GM6001 inhibits constitutive and PMA-induced CD4 shedding in transfected CHO-K1 cells. (A, B)** CHO-K1 cells transiently transfected with the hCD4-myc construct were treated with DMSO (lane 1), PMA (100 nM, lane2), GM6001 (50 µM, lane 3) and PMA plus GM6001 (lane 4) for 2 days (48 hours). 20X concentrated conditioned medium (A) and cell lysates (B) were analyzed by Western blotting using with anti-CD4 and anti-myc mAbs as indicated. The blotted membrane was stained with Ponceau S solution to confirm the equal loading of conditioned medium and cell lysate. In addition, equal loading of cell lysate is checked by Western blotting with anti-actin mAb staining. Protein band intensity was measured by a densitometer and normalized against the corresponding β-actin band.

**Figure S2  GM6001 inhibits constitutive and PMA-induced CD4 shedding in transfected CHO-K1 cells. (A, B)** CHO-K1 cells transiently transfected with the hCD4-myc construct were treated with DMSO (lane 1), PMA (50 nM, lane2), GM6001 (50 µM, lane 3), PMA plus 50 µM GM6001 (lane 4) or PMA plus 100 µM GM6001 (lane 5) for 36 hours. 20X concentrated conditioned medium (A) and cell lysates (B) were analyzed by Western blotting using with anti-CD4 and anti-myc mAbs as indicated. The blotted membrane was stained with Ponceau S solution to confirm the equal loading of conditioned medium and cell lysate. In addition, equal loading of cell lysate is checked by Western blotting with anti-actin mAb staining. Protein band intensity was measured by a densitometer and normalized against the corresponding β-actin band.

## Acknowledgments

We thank Dr. Martin Stacey (University of Leeds, UK) for helpful discussion and critical reading of the manuscript.

## Author Contributions

Conceived and designed the experiments: WYT YSH NYC HHL. Performed the experiments: WYT YSH NYC. Analyzed the data: WYT YSH NYC YPC CFK KML HHL. Contributed reagents/materials/analysis tools: WYT YSH NYC YPC CFK KML YJJW SFL. Wrote the paper: WYT YSH YJJW SFL HHL.

## References

1. Maddon PJ, Littman DR, Godfrey M, Maddon DE, Chess L, et al. (1985) The isolation and nucleotide sequence of a cDNA encoding the T cell surface protein T4: a new member of the immunoglobulin gene family. Cell 42: 93–104.

2. Rudd CE, Trevillyan JM, Dasgupta JD, Wong LL, Schlossman SF (1988) The CD4 receptor is complexed in detergent lysates to a protein-tyrosine kinase (pp58) from human T lymphocytes. Proc Natl Acad Sci U S A 85: 5190–5194.

3. Veillette A, Bookman MA, Horak EM, Bolen JB (1988) The CD4 and CD8 T cell surface antigens are associated with the internal membrane tyrosine-protein kinase p56lck. Cell 55: 301–308.

4. Veillette A, Bookman MA, Horak EM, Samelson LE, Bolen JB (1989) Signal transduction through the CD4 receptor involves the activation of the internal membrane tyrosine-protein kinase p56lck. Nature 338: 257–259.

5. Ridgeway W, Fathman C (1996) Anti-CD4 in the treatment of rheumatoid arthritis: A reappraisal. The Immunologist 4: 203–206.

6. Strand V, Kimberly R, Isaacs JD (2007) Biologic therapies in rheumatology: lessons learned, future directions. Nat Rev Drug Discov 6: 75–92.

7. Isaacs JD (2008) Therapeutic T-cell manipulation in rheumatoid arthritis: past, present and future. Rheumatology (Oxford) 47: 1461–1468.

8. Moore JP, Trkola A, Dragic T (1997) Co-receptors for HIV-1 entry. Curr Opin Immunol 9: 551–562.

9. Deen KC, McDougal JS, Inacker R, Folena-Wasserman G, Arthos J, et al. (1988) A soluble form of CD4 (T4) protein inhibits AIDS virus infection. Nature 331: 82–84.

10. Fisher RA, Bertonis JM, Meier W, Johnson VA, Costopoulos DS, et al. (1988) HIV infection is blocked in vitro by recombinant soluble CD4. Nature 331: 76–78.

11. Peakman M, Senaldi G, Foote N, McManus TJ, Vergani D (1992) Naturally occurring soluble CD4 in patients with human immunodeficiency virus infection. J Infect Dis 165: 799–804.

12. Yoneyama A, Nakahara K, Higashihara M, Kurokawa K (1995) Increased levels of soluble CD8 and CD4 in patients with infectious mononucleosis. Br J Haematol 89: 47–54.

13. Symons JA, McCulloch JF, Wood NC, Duff GW (1991) Soluble CD4 in patients with rheumatoid arthritis and osteoarthritis. Clin Immunol Immunopathol 60: 72–82.

14. Marcante R, Cavedon G (1991) Soluble CD4, CD8 and interleukin-2 receptor levels in patients with acute cytomegalovirus mononucleosis syndrome. Allergol Immunopathol (Madr) 19: 99–102.

15. North ME, Spickett GP, Webster AD, Farrant J (1991) Raised serum levels of CD8, CD25 and beta 2-microglobulin in common variable immunodeficiency. Clin Exp Immunol 86: 252–255.

16. Matsumoto Y, Shinzato T, Takai I, Nakai S, Miwa M, et al. (1998) Increased soluble CD4 and CD8 in chronic renal failure. Nephron 78: 490–491.

17. Sato S, Fujimoto M, Kikuchi K, Ihn H, Tamaki K, et al. (1996) Soluble CD4 and CD8 in serum from patients with localized scleroderma. Arch Dermatol Res 288: 358–362.

18. Levine SJ (2004) Mechanisms of soluble cytokine receptor generation. J Immunol 173: 5343–5348.

19. Levine SJ (2008) Molecular mechanisms of soluble cytokine receptor generation. J Biol Chem 283: 14177–14181.

20. Ohkubo T, Takei M, Mitamura K, Horie T, Fujiwara S, et al. (2001) Increased soluble CD4 molecules and the role of soluble CD4 production in patients with rheumatoid arthritis. J Int Med Res 29: 488–496.

21. Chen TY, Hwang TL, Lin CY, Lin TN, Lai HY, et al. EMR2 receptor ligation modulates cytokine secretion profiles and cell survival of lipopolysaccharide-treated neutrophils. Chang Gung Med J 34: 468–477.

22. Davies JQ, Chang GW, Yona S, Gordon S, Stacey M, et al. (2007) The role of receptor oligomerization in modulating the expression and function of leukocyte adhesion-G protein-coupled receptors. J Biol Chem 282: 27343–27353.

23. Lin HH, Chang GW, Davies JQ, Stacey M, Harris J, et al. (2004) Autocatalytic cleavage of the EMR2 receptor occurs at a conserved G protein-coupled receptor proteolytic site motif. J Biol Chem 279: 31823–31832.

24. Garton KJ, Gough PJ, Raines EW (2006) Emerging roles for ectodomain shedding in the regulation of inflammatory responses. J Leukoc Biol 79: 1105–1116.

25. Blobel CP (2005) ADAMs: key components in EGFR signalling and development. Nat Rev Mol Cell Biol 6: 32–43.

26. Hamann J, Fiebig H, Strauss M (1993) Expression cloning of the early activation antigen CD69, a type II integral membrane protein with a C-type lectin domain. J Immunol 150: 4920–4927.

27. Lopez-Cabrera M, Santis AG, Fernandez-Ruiz E, Blacher R, Esch F, et al. (1993) Molecular cloning, expression, and chromosomal localization of the human earliest lymphocyte activation antigen AIM/CD69, a new member of the C-type animal lectin superfamily of signal-transmitting receptors. J Exp Med 178: 537–547.

28. Ziegler SF, Ramsdell F, Hjerrild KA, Armitage RJ, Grabstein KH, et al. (1993) Molecular characterization of the early activation antigen CD69: a type II membrane glycoprotein related to a family of natural killer cell activation antigens. Eur J Immunol 23: 1643–1648.

29. Kahn J, Ingraham RH, Shirley F, Migaki GI, Kishimoto TK (1994) Membrane proximal cleavage of L-selectin: identification of the cleavage site and a 6-kD transmembrane peptide fragment of L-selectin. J Cell Biol 125: 461–470.

30. Zhao L, Shey M, Farnsworth M, Dailey MO (2001) Regulation of membrane metalloproteolytic cleavage of L-selectin (CD62l) by the epidermal growth factor domain. J Biol Chem 276: 30631–30640.

31. Hey AS, Theander TG, Hviid L, Hazrati SM, Kemp M, et al. (1994) The major surface glycoprotein (gp63) from Leishmania major and Leishmania donovani cleaves CD4 molecules on human T cells. J Immunol 152: 4542–4548.

32. Armstrong PB (2001) The contribution of proteinase inhibitors to immune defense. Trends Immunol 22: 47–52.

33. Yoon SO, Park SJ, Yun CH, Chung AS (2003) Roles of matrix metalloproteinases in tumor metastasis and angiogenesis. J Biochem Mol Biol 36: 128–137.

34. Amalinei C, Caruntu ID, Giusca SE, Balan RA Matrix metalloproteinases involvement in pathologic conditions. Rom J Morphol Embryol 51: 215–228.

35. Goto H, Gidlund M (1996) Soluble CD4: a link between specific immune mechanisms and non-specific inflammatory responses? Scand J Immunol 43: 690–692.

36. Hepburn TW, Totoritis MC, Davis CB (2003) Antibody-mediated stripping of CD4 from lymphocyte cell surface in patients with rheumatoid arthritis. Rheumatology (Oxford) 42: 54–61.

37. Burrage PS, Mix KS, Brinckerhoff CE (2006) Matrix metalloproteinases: role in arthritis. Front Biosci 11: 529–543.

38. Miller MC, Manning HB, Jain A, Troeberg L, Dudhia J, et al. (2009) Membrane type 1 matrix metalloproteinase is a crucial promoter of synovial invasion in human rheumatoid arthritis. Arthritis Rheum 60: 686–697.

39. Sawada S, Hashimoto H, Iijima S, Tokano Y, Takei M, et al. (1993) Immunologic significance of increased soluble CD8/CD4 molecules in patients with active systemic lupus erythematosus. J Clin Lab Anal 7: 141–146.

40. Sawada S, Sugai S, Iijima S, Takei M, Paredes E, et al. (1992) Increased soluble CD4 and decreased soluble CD8 molecules in patients with Sjogren's syndrome. Am J Med 92: 134–140.

41. Nadali G, Vinante F, Chilosi M, Pizzolo G (1997) Soluble molecules as biological markers in Hodgkin's disease. Leuk Lymphoma 26 Suppl 1: 99–105.

# 10

# Analysis of *PPARGC1B*, *RUNX3* and *TBKBP1* Polymorphisms in Chinese Han Patients with Ankylosing Spondylitis: A Case-Control Study

**Zijian Lian[1,2,3], Wei Chai[1], Lewis L. Shi[4], Chao Chen[1,3], Jingyi Liu[2], Yan Wang[1,2]***

**1** Department of Orthopaedics, Chinese People's Liberation Army General Hospital, Beijing, China, **2** Medical School of Nankai University, Tianjin, China, **3** Department of Orthopaedics, Tianjin Hospital, Tianjin, China, **4** Department of Orthopaedics, University of Chicago Hospital, Maryland Avenue, Chicago, Illinois, United States of America

## Abstract

***Background:*** Susceptibility to and severity of ankylosing spondylitis (AS) are largely genetically determined. *PPARGC1B*, *RUNX3* and *TBKBP1* have recently been found to be associated with AS in patients of western European descent. Our purpose is to examine the influence of *PPARGC1B*, *RUNX3* and *TBKBP1* polymorphisms on the susceptibility to and the severity of ankylosing spondylitis in Chinese ethnic majority Han population.

***Methods:*** Blood samples are drawn from 396 AS patients and 404 unrelated healthy controls. All the patients and the controls are Han Chinese and the patients are HLA-B27 positive. The AS patients are classified based on the severity of the disease. Twelve tag single nucleotide polymorphisms (tagSNPs) in *PPARGC1B*, *RUNX3* and *TBKBP1* are selected and genotyped. Frequencies of different genotypes and alleles are analyzed among the different severity AS patients and the controls.

***Results:*** After Bonferroni correction, the rs7379457 SNP in *PPARGC1B* shows significant difference when comparing all AS patients to controls (p = 0.005). This SNP also shows significant difference when comparing normal AS patients to controls (p = 0.002). The rs1395621 SNP in *RUNX3* shows significant difference when comparing severe AS patients to controls (p = 0.007). The rs9438876 SNP in *RUNX3* shows significant difference when comparing normal AS patients to controls (p = 0.007). The rs8070463 SNP in *TBKBP1* shows significant difference in genotype distribution when comparing severe AS patients to controls (p = 0.003).

***Conclusions:*** The rs7379457 SNP in *PPARGC1B* is related to susceptibility to AS in Chinese Han population. The rs7379457 SNP in *PPARGC1B*, the rs1395621 and rs9438876 SNPs in *RUNX3*, and the rs8070463 SNP in *TBKBP1* are related to the severity of AS in Chinese Han population.

**Editor:** Giuseppe Novelli, Tor Vergata University of Rome, Italy

**Funding:** Nature science founding of Beijing supports this research. The number is 7102146. The funders had no role in study design, data collection and analysis, decision to publish, or preparation of the manuscript.

**Competing Interests:** The authors have declared that no competing interests exist.

* E-mail: wangyaneasy@163.com

## Introduction

Ankylosing spondylitis (AS) is a chronic inflammatory disorder characterized by inflammation in the spine and sacroiliac joints causing initial bone and joint erosion and subsequent ankylosis [1]. Most patients develop first symptoms of AS younger than 30 years of age [2]. Significant radiographic progression occurs in the first 10 years of disease, and more recent studies have shown that structural damage at initial presentation is the best predictor of further damage [3–5].

AS patients' disease severity is largely genetically determined [6]. We aim to identify patients with susceptibility to AS before the appearance of significant deformities and disabilities, so we can intervene earlier. In genome-wide association studies (GWAS), rs11959820 in *PPARGC1B*, rs11249215 in *RUNX3*, and rs8070463 in *TBKBP1* are related to AS susceptibility in patients of western European descent [7–9]. These findings must be replicated and refined in different populations. Interpreting GWAS results at a gene-specific level is an important step towards understanding the molecular processes that lead to the disease [10].

We hypothesize that the *PPARGC1B*, *RUNX3*, and *TBKBP1* are related to AS in the Chinese ethnic majority Han population. Additionally, some single nucleotide polymorphisms (SNPs) of these genes may predict the severity of AS.

## Methods

### Study Population

In this work, 396 AS patients are recruited, along with 404 unrelated healthy controls who are age and sex-matched. All patients and controls are Han Chinese. All AS patients are HLA-B27 positive. All AS patients are treated by non-steroidal anti-inflammatory drug routinely; no other treatments are used for patients. Among the AS patients, there are 354 males (89.4%) and

42 females (10.6%); the average age is 29.6 years (range 16 to 60 years) (Table 1). Among the controls, there are 364 males (90.1%) and 40 females (9.9%); the average age is 30.0 years (range 16 to 60 years). Neither sex nor age distributions show significant differences between AS and control patients (p = 0.742, 0.518 respectively). The average duration since AS diagnosis is 11.5 years (range 8 to 18 years). The diagnosis of AS has been made by experienced rheumatologists; all diagnoses satisfy the modified New York criteria [11]. Subjects with inflammatory bowel disease, psoriasis, rheumatoid arthritis, or other autoimmune diseases are excluded from both the AS and the control groups.

## Basic Data Acquisition

The Bath AS function index (BASFI) and Bath AS disease activity index (BASDAI) are administered to the patients using questionnaires; these indices are the most widely used tools for the assessment of AS functional status and disease activity [12] [13]. The modified Stokes AS Spine Score (mSASSS) is a validated scoring system for quantification of chronic spinal changes [14]. Standard anteroposterior and lateral radiographs of the cervical and lumbar spine are obtained for each subject, and the lateral view is used to derive a mSASSS score for each patient [15] [16]. Three of the authors separately assigned the mSASSS scores, and the average is used.

## Severity Classification

There is a lack of consensus on how to classify AS severity [17]. In this work, we define severe subtype of AS as the disease form in those patients who require surgery within first ten years of diagnosis. The indications of surgery include inability to stand upright, inability to look straight ahead, and compression of the viscera due to kyphosis that manifests as pain [18]. Patients with the normal type of AS exhibit inflammation of sacroiliac joints, but their spine and other joints are relatively spared; these patients require only medical treatment. By this definition, 82 AS patients have the severe subtype, and 314 AS patients have the normal subtype. Clinical features comparing severe AS and normal AS are shown in Table 2.

## SNPs Selection

The SNPs in this study include five in *PPARGC1B*, five in *RUNX3* and two in *TBKBP1*. These three genes localize to chromosome 5, 1, and 17, respectively. The selected SNPs serve as

**Table 1.** Demographic data of AS patients and controls.

| Sex | | Cases (396) | Controls (404) | p-value |
|---|---|---|---|---|
| | male | 354 (89.4%) | 364 (90.1%) | 0.742 |
| | female | 42(10.6%) | 40 (9.9%) | |
| Age | | 29.6±8.5 | 30.0±9.4 | 0.518 |
| Duration of diagnosis | | 11.5±2.1 | N/A | |
| BASFI | | 3.97±1.49 | N/A | |
| BASDAI | | 3.95±1.05 | N/A | |
| mSASSS | | 12.6±13.4 | N/A | |

There is no significant difference in age and sex-distribution between AS patients and controls. Numerical values presented as mean±standard deviation. BASFI : Bath ankylosing spondylitis function index. BASDAI: Bath ankylosing spondylitis disease activity index. mSASSS: modified Stokes ankylosing spondylitis Spine Score.

**Table 2.** Clinical features comparing severe AS and normal AS.

| Sex | | severe AS (82) | normal AS (314) | p value |
|---|---|---|---|---|
| | male | 76(92.7%) | 276(87.9%) | 0.220 |
| | female | 6(7.3%) | 38(12.1%) | |
| Age | | 31.5±9.2 | 29.0±8.3 | 0.097 |
| Duration of diagnosis | | 11.2±3.0 | 11.6±1.8 | 0.290 |
| BASFI | | 6.03±2.06 | 3.43±0.55 | <0.001 |
| BASDAI | | 5.49±1.10 | 3.55±0.55 | <0.001 |
| mSASSS | | 37.1±13.3 | 6.21±1.06 | <0.001 |

There is no difference between severe AS patients and normal patients in age and sex distribution; however, the BASFI, BASDAI and mSASSS are higher in severe AS patients.

multi-marker tagging algorithm with criteria of $r^2$ more than 0.8 and for all SNPs with minor allele frequency more than 5% from the Han Chinese in Beijing population in the HapMap database. Haploview 4.2 software (Broad Institute, Cambridge, Massachusetts, USA) is used to select the tagSNPs. Figure 1 shows the positions of each tagSNP. The rs7379457 SNP is located in the promoter of *PPARGC1B*. The rs11249215 SNP is located in the promoter of *RUNX3*. The rs8070463 SNP is located in the promoter of *TBKBP1*. Other SNPs are located in the introns. Most SNPs in *TBKBP1* are in high linkage disequilibrium (LD), hence only two tagSNPs are selected.

## DNA Extraction and Genotyping Analysis

DNA is isolated from 2 ml whole blood samples using AxyPrep Blood Genomic DNA Miniprep kit (Axygen Biosciences, Union City, CA, USA). Detection of the SNPs is performed by MassARRAY system (Sequenom, San Diego, CA, USA). The chip-based matrix-assisted laser desorption ionization time-of-flight (MALDI-TOF) mass spectrometry technology is used in this procedure [19]. Most of the SNPs are successfully genotyped. The rs109077 SNP is 98.5% genotyped in case group and 97.5% in control group. The rs4648884 SNP is 98.5% genotyped in case group. The rs9438876 is 90.9% genotyped in case group and 95.5% in control group. In the other SNPs, more than 99.5% is genotyped in both case and control groups.

## Statistical Analysis

The Hardy-Weinberg equilibrium is tested for all 12 tagSNPs. The Pearson's chi-squared test and independent-samples t-test are used to compare the differences in age and sex between cases and controls. Comparisons of the distributions of the genotype, allele and haplotype frequencies are performed using the Pearson's chi-squared test. Especially, in the rs7379457 SNP the TT genotype is rare. Therefore, we use Fisher's exact test. Binary logistic regression analysis is used to adjust for age and sex. After Bonferroni correction, p-value less than 0.01 is considered significant. The last genotype of each SNP is the major genotype and the last allele is the major allele. The relative risks associated with the major genotypes or major alleles are estimated as an odds ratio (OR) with a 95% confidence interval (CI). The p-values of genotypes indicated in the result tables are used to estimate the significance of the distribution of genotype between cases and controls. All three genotypes of each SNP are compared, P-value

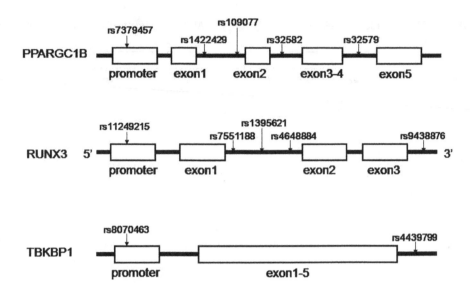

**Figure 1. Positions of each selected tagSNP on the genes.** The SNP rs7379457 is in the promoter of PPARGC1B. The SNP rs11249215 is in the promoter of RUNX3. The SNP rs8070463 is in the promoter of TBKBP1. Other SNPs are all in introns.

for individual genotypes are shown only if significant at 0.05 level (Table 3, details are shown in Table S1, Table S2 and Table S3). We compared the severe AS group to the entirety of the control group and then normal AS group to the entirety control group. Pearson's chi-squared test is used to compare the constructed haplotypes. The SNPs which show significant differences between AS patients and controls are considered to be related to susceptibility to AS. The SNPs which show significant differences between severe AS patients and controls but no differences between normal AS patients and controls are considered related to severity of AS. Moreover, SNPs show significant differences between normal AS patients and controls but no differences between severe AS patients and controls are considered related to severity of AS. Statistical analyses are carried out with SPSS v.17.0 software package (IBM, Armonk, New York, USA).

## Ethics Statement

The blood samples of both AS patients and controls used in this study are part of samples taken for diagnostic tests. During the collection and use of DNA samples, clinical data guidelines, regulations of the local Ethics Committee and the Helsinki Declaration in 1975 are followed. Written informed consents were obtained from all the patients and subjects (or their parents in the case of two patients less than 18 years old). The study procedure is approved by our Institutional Review Board.

## Results

### Clinical Features

The BASFI, BASDAI and mSASSS for the AS patients are recorded in Table 1. Among the 396 AS patients, the mean BASFI is $3.97\pm1.49$ (mean±standard deviation). The mean BASDAI is $3.95\pm1.05$. The mean mSASSS is $12.6\pm13.4$. When comparing the severe AS and the normal AS patient groups, there is no significant difference in sex, age, and disease duration (p-value = 0.220, 0.097, 0.290 respectively; Table 2). The BASFI is higher in severe AS group ($6.03\pm2.06$) than normal AS group ($3.43\pm0.55$) (p-value<0.001), reflecting poorer function of patients in the severe AS group. The BASDAI is similarly higher in the severe AS group ($5.49\pm1.10$) than normal AS group ($3.55\pm0.55$)

(p-value<0.001), reflecting higher disease activity. The pattern holds for mSASSS ($37.1\pm13.3$ versus $6.21\pm1.06$, p-value<0.001), signifying more radiographic changes in the severe AS patients.

### Genotype and Allele

We genotyped 12 SNPs, the detailed results are summarized in Table S1, Table S2, and Table S3. The genotype frequencies of these 12 tagSNPs are in Hardy-Weinberg equilibrium in all groups. Four of the 12 SNPs show significant difference in disease diagnosis and severity (Table 3). The genotype frequencies of these 12 tagSNPs are in Hardy-Weinberg equilibrium in all groups. After Bonferroni correction, the rs7379457 SNP in *PPARGC1B* shows significant difference when comparing all AS patients to controls, with TT genotype higher in AS than in controls (p = 0.005). This SNP also shows significant difference when comparing normal AS patients to controls, with TT genotype higher in normal AS than in controls (p = 0.002) and CC genotype higher in normal AS than in controls (p = 0.006). The rs1395621 SNP in *RUNX3* shows significant difference when comparing severe AS patients to controls, with AA genotype lower in severe AS patients than in controls (p = 0.007) and A allele is lower in severe AS patients than in controls (p = 0.003). The rs9438876 SNP in this gene shows significant difference when comparing normal AS patients to controls, with GG genotype lower in normal AS patients than in controls (p = 0.007). The rs8070463 SNP in *TBKBP1* shows significant difference in genotype distribution when comparing severe AS patients to controls, with CC genotype lower in severe AS patients than in controls (p = 0.003). This SNP also shows significant difference in C allele distribution when comparing severe AS patients to controls, with C allele lower in severe AS patients than in controls (p = 0.004).

### Haplotype

LD maps of the 12 tagSNPs of *PPARGC1B*, *TBKBP1* and *RUNX3* comparing all AS patients, severe AS patients, and normal AS patients to controls subjects are shown in Figure 2, Figure S1 and Figure S2, respectively. These figures have only a little difference, only Figure 2 is shown in the text comparing all AS patients to controls. Figure S1 and Figure S2 are shown in the

**Table 3.** Positive SNPs in *PPARGC1B RUNX3* and *TBKBP1* which are related to susceptibility to AS or severity of AS comparing all AS patients, severe AS patients and normal AS patients to the controls.

| | SNP | | All AS subjects cases/controls | | | Severe AS subjects cases/controls | | | Normal AS subjects cases/controls | | |
|---|---|---|---|---|---|---|---|---|---|---|---|
| | | | frequencies | OR(95% CI)[c] | p | frequencies | OR(95% CI) | p | frequencies | OR(95% CI) | p |
| *PPARGC1B* | **rs7379457** | All[a] | | | N/A | | | N/A | | | N/A |
| | Genotype | TT | 8/0 | 1.024(1.007~1.041) **0.005*** | | 0/0 | N/A | N/A | 8/0 | 1.029(1.009~1.050) **0.002*** | |
| | | CT | 50/72 | 0.671(0.453~0.993) 0.046# | | 18/72 | 1.292(0.714~2.339) | | 32/72 | 0.538(0.344~0.841) **0.006*** | |
| | | CC | 336/330 | 1[b] | | 64/330 | 1 | | 272/330 | 1 | |
| | Allele | T | 66/72 | 0.929(0.655~1.318) | | 18/72 | 1.253(0.726~2.164) | | 48/72 | 0.847(0.579~1.240) | |
| | | C | 722/732 | 1 | | 146/732 | 1 | | 576/732 | 1 | |
| *RUNX3* | **rs1395621** | All | | | 0.041# | | | **0.008*** | | | 0.147 |
| | Genotype | AA | 58/66 | 0.730(0.477~1.117) | | 6/66 | 0.408(0.178~0.934) **0.007*** | | 52/66 | 0.834(0.534~1.303) | |
| | | AG | 189/220 | 0.689(0.504~0.943) 0.015# | | 39/220 | 0.538(0.321~0.903) 0.025# | | 150/220 | 0.736(0.527~1.028) | |
| | | GG | 149/118 | 1 | | 37/118 | 1 | | 112/118 | 1 | |
| | Allele | A | 305/352 | 0.811(0.665~0.991) 0.040# | | 51/352 | 0.585(0.408~0.837) **0.003*** | | 254/352 | 0.880(0.712~1.087) | |
| | | G | 487/456 | 1 | | 113/456 | 1 | | 374/456 | 1 | |
| | **rs9438876** | All | | | 0.022# | | | 0.716 | | | **0.004*** |
| | Genotype | GG | 43/30 | 1.347(0.807~2.251) | | 4/30 | 0.556(0.180~1.713) | | 39/30 | 1.590(0.937~2.699) | |
| | | AG | 129/172 | 0.743(0.547~1.008) 0.047# | | 32/172 | 0.905(0.538~1.523) | | 97/172 | 0.701(0.504~0.974) 0.028# | |
| | | AA | 188/184 | 1 0.038# | | 38/184 | 1 | | 150/184 | 1 **0.007*** | |
| | Allele | G | 215/232 | 0.991(0.794~1.237) | | 40/232 | 0.862(0.581~1.278) | | 175/232 | 1.026(0.811~1.298) | |
| | | A | 505/540 | 1 | | 108/540 | 1 | | 397/540 | 1 | |
| *TBKBP1* | **rs8070463** | All | | | 0.187 | | | 0.014# | | | 0.415 |
| | Genotype | CC | 72/94 | 0.788(0.531~1.170) | | 8/94 | 0.400(0.186~0.861) **0.003*** | | 64/94 | 0.928(0.611~1.411) | |
| | | CT | 198/184 | 1.084(0.786~1.494) | | 40/184 | 0.815(0.483~1.376) | | 158/184 | 1.170(0.828~1.654) | |
| | | TT | 124/124 | 1 | | 34/124 | 1 | | 90/124 | 1 | |
| | Allele | C | 342/372 | 0.890(0.731~1.085) | | 56/372 | 0.602(0.424~0.856) **0.004*** | | 286/372 | 0.983(0.797~1.212) | |
| | | T | 446/432 | 1 | | 108/432 | 1 | | 338/432 | 1 | |

[a]"All" means the p value that we compare all the three genotype using 3×2 chi squared method. P-value for individual genotypes are shown only if significant at 0.05 level.

[b]The last lines of genotypes or alleles are the major genotypes or the major alleles. The other genotypes or alleles are compared to them. The relative risk associated with major genotypes and major alleles is estimated as an odds ratio (OR) with a 95% confidence interval (CI).

[c]OR (95% CI) are adjusted by age and sex using multiple regression analysis.

#indicates p-value is less than 0.05 but cannot pass Bonferroni correction which shows marginal significant difference.

*indicates p-value is less than 0.01 which shows significant difference after Bonferroni correction. The details of all the 12 SNPs are summarized in Table S1 (*PPARGC1B*) Table S2 (*RUNX3*) and Table S3 (*TBKBP1*).

supporting information comparing severe patients and normal patients to controls separately. Most of the SNPs are not in high linkage disequilibrium, with exception of one block in *RUNX3*. Analyses of constructed haplotypes for this block comparing all AS patients, severe AS patients, and normal AS patients to controls subjects are shown in Table 4. None of them is associated with the susceptibility to AS or severity of AS.

## Discussion

The pathogenesis of AS remains poorly understood. However, genetic factors play a significant role [20]. Changes in the spine involve syndesmophytes forming bony ankylosis of adjacent vertebrae or ankylosis of small vertebral joints. Some classification systems exist based on clinical and radiographic criteria [21] [22]. Most of our patients present with mild symptoms and do well with chronic medical treatments; however, some patients have more severe manifestations that require surgery within the first ten years of diagnosis. We use this criterion to define severe and normal AS

disease subtypes. We aim to find genetic markers for susceptibility to AS in general, as well as to the severe form of AS. This would provide powerful tools to clinicians and researchers to confirm the diagnosis of AS and predict for the development of severe form of AS. The ability to classify AS based on allelic differences would also have significant new therapies implications [23].

The human *PPARGC1B* gene (peroxisome proliferator-activated receptor-gamma coactivator 1 beta), encoding PGC-1β, localizes to chromosome 5q32, a region that shows linkage to type 2 diabetes [24]. Wirtenberger and colleagues found PGC-1β to be associated with familial breast cancer [25]. The mechanism that *PPARGC1B* relates to these diseases is still being investigated. Numerous publications indicate *PPARGC1B* plays a critical role in regulating multiple aspects of energy metabolism including mitochondrial biogenesis, thermogenesis, gluconeogenesis, and fatty acid β-oxidation [26–30]. Oxidative phosphorylation (OX-PHOS) dysfunction plays a critical pathogenic role in several human diseases [31]. Sarika found that PGC-1β over-expression

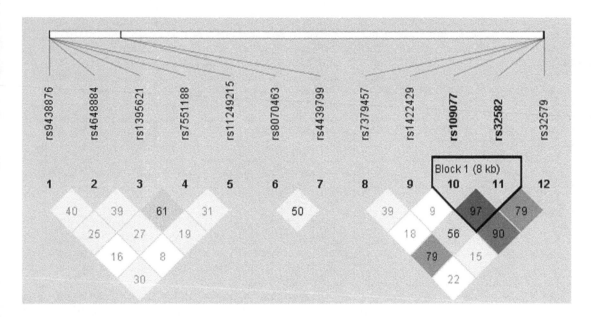

**Figure 2. Linkage disequilibrium (LD) map comparing All AS patients and controls.** Darker color indicates higher linkage disequilibrium (LD), lighter color indicates less LD. Numbers in the squares indicate correlation coefficient (R²) value. The left part of the picture contains 5 SNPs (from rs9438876 to rs11249215). They are from *RUNX3*. The middle part of the picture contains 2 SNPs (rs8070463 and rs4439799). They are from *TBKBP1*. The right part of the picture contains 4 SNPs (from rs7379457 to rs32579). They are from *PPARGC1B*. Haplotypes are constructed from the darker blocks (high linkage disequilibrium). They are TG, GT and GG.

can lead to a marked improvement in OXPHOS defects caused by mutations in mitochondrial DNA (mtDNA) or nuclear DNA (nDNA) [32]. Kiyo-aki found PGC-1β accelerated osteoclastic bone resorption through the coordination of mitochondrial biogenesis and the cell-differentiation program [33]. Our data shows that rs7379457 SNP which localizes to the promoter of *PPARGC1B* is related to the susceptibility to AS and severity of AS. As a result, the functions of osteoclasts are inhibited due to decreased oxidative phosphorylation. With the imbalance between osteoblasts and osteoclasts, ossification predominates and thus leads to osteophyte formation and even ankylosis.

The *RUNX3* gene (Runt-related transcription factor 3) encodes for RUNX3, and it localizes to chromosome 1p36.11. RUNX3 is a downstream target of the transforming growth factor-β (TGF-β) pathway, which is considered a tumor suppressor pathway, as components are frequently altered in cancers, especially those of the gastrointestinal tract [34]. *RUNX3* is inactivated in gastric cancer by hemizygous deletion, promoter hypermethylation, histone modification, and protein mislocalization, suggesting a tumor-suppressive role of RUNX3 in this malignancy [35–37]. Since the discovery of the potential role of RUNX3 in the initiation and the progression of gastric cancer, RUNX3 has been found to be involved in the development of a variety of cancers, including colon, liver, lung and breast cancer [38–41]. *RUNX3* knockout mice spontaneously develop inflammatory bowel disease characterized by leukocyte infiltration, mucosal hyperplasia, formation of lymphoid clusters, and increased production of IgA. RUNX3 belongs to the runt domain family of transcription factors, which are key regulators of lineage-specific gene expression and more recently are found to be linked to human autoimmunity [42]. When RUNX3 is suppressed in human T cells, either through gene inactivation or with small interference

**Table 4.** Haplotype analysis in block 1.

| | rs109077 | rs32582 | Case Ratio | Control Ratio | Chi Square | p value |
|---|---|---|---|---|---|---|
| All AS patients vs. controls | T | G | 529:263 | 536:272 | 0.037 | 0.847 |
| | G | T | 136:656 | 141:667 | 0.022 | 0.883 |
| | G | G | 123:669 | 130:678 | 0.094 | 0.759 |
| Severe AS patients vs. controls | T | G | 114:50 | 537:271 | 0.574 | 0.449 |
| | G | T | 28:136 | 142:666 | 0.024 | 0.878 |
| | G | G | 22:142 | 130:678 | 0.739 | 0.390 |
| Normal AS patients vs. controls | T | G | 415:213 | 536:272 | 0.010 | 0.920 |
| | G | T | 108:520 | 141:667 | 0.016 | 0.900 |
| | G | G | 101:527 | 130:678 | 1.04E-5 | 0.997 |

Haplotypes are constructed. Case ratio means in the case group, the frequency of this kind of haplotype vs. other kinds of haplotype; control ratio means in the control group, the frequency of this kind of haplotype vs. other kinds of haplotype. None of the constructed haplotype has significant difference between cases and controls.

RNA, Foxp3 expression is reduced, which in turn disrupts the recognition of regulatory T cells. As with other autoimmune diseases, AS patients exhibit an imbalance of CCR4+CCR6+ helper T cells and regulatory T cells [43] [44]. RUNX3 is highly expressed in dendritic cells (DC), where it functions as a component of the transforming growth factor (TGF-β) signaling cascade [45]. It is obvious that RUNX3 is not only a tumor suppressor but also plays an important role in autoimmune diseases and inflammations. In our data, the rs1395621 and rs9438876 SNP show significant relationship to severity of AS. We conclude the RUNX3 can influence the AS severity due to its effect on the inflammatory process.

TBKBP1 (tumor necrosis factor family member-associated NF-κB activator binding kinase 1 binding protein) is an adaptor protein that binds to TBK1, also known as sintbad. The precise function of TBKBP1 in the process of TBK1 activation has not been defined fully, but there is evidence that the adaptor proteins link the kinases to the upstream signaling pathways, possibly by its interaction with TRAF3 [46]. Ken performed bone-marrow transfer experiments which revealed that TBK1-mediated signaling in hematopoietic cells is critical for the induction of antigen specific B and CD4+ T cells, whereas in non-hematopoietic cells TBK1 is required for CD8+ T-cell induction. These data suggest that TBK1 is a key signaling molecule for DNA-vaccine-induced immunogenicity, in addition to being part of the classic NF-κB inflammatory pathway [47]. Acute or chronic inflammation is an important feature of AS, with degree of inflammation correlated to severity of disease [48]. Appropriately, our data shows that rs8070463 SNP of TBKBP1 is related to the severity of AS.

In conclusion, PPARGC1B is associated with the susceptibility to AS; PPARGC1B, RUNX3 and TBKBP1 are associated with the severity of AS in the Chinese Han population. These findings support the GWAS results that these three genes are related to AS. Our findings can provide context for better understanding of the genetic and molecular pathogenesis of AS. The specific SNPs in these genes can be used to guide genetic analysis and counseling, medical and surgical treatment options, and ultimate prognosis. Further studies are needed to elucidate the molecular roles these genes play in AS.

## Supporting Information

**Figure S1 Linkage disequilibrium map comparing severe AS patients and controls.** The distribution and position of SNPs are the same as Figure 2. Haplotypes are constructed from the darker blocks (high linkage disequilibrium). They are TG, GT and GG.

**Figure S2 Linkage disequilibrium map comparing normal AS patients and controls.** The distribution and position of SNPs are the same as Figure 2. Haplotypes are constructed from the darker blocks (high linkage disequilibrium). They are TG, GT and GG.

**Table S1** Genotype and allele frequencies of PPARGC1B SNPs among all AS patients, severe AS patients, normal AS patients versus controls. SNPs in PPARGC1B are compared between all AS patients, severe AS patients, and normal AS patients versus the

control subjects. P-value for each SNP is shown, and p-value for individual genotypes are shown only if significant at 0.05 level. # indicates p-value is less than 0.05 but cannot pass Bonferroni correction which shows marginal significant difference. *indicates p-value is less than 0.01 which shows significant difference after Bonferroni correction. OR and 95% CI are adjusted by age and sex. The rs7379457 SNP shows significant difference when comparing all AS patients to controls, TT genotype carrier frequency is higher than controls (p = 0.005*). This SNP also shows significant difference in comparing normal AS patients to controls, TT genotype carrier frequency is higher than controls (p = 0.002*); CC genotype carrier frequency is lower than controls (p = 0.006*).

**Table S2** Genotype and allele frequencies of RUNX3 SNPs among all AS patients, severe AS patients, normal AS patients versus controls. SNPs in RUNX3 are compared between all AS patients, severe AS patients, and normal AS patients versus the control subjects. # indicates p-value is less than 0.05 but cannot pass Bonferroni correction which shows marginal significant difference. *indicates p-value is less than 0.01 which shows significant difference after Bonferroni correction. After Bonferroni correction, the rs1395621 SNP shows significant difference when comparing severe AS patients to controls, AA genotype carrier frequency is lower than controls (p = 0.007*) and A allele carrier frequency is lower than controls (p = 0.003*). The rs9438876 SNP shows significant difference when comparing normal AS patients to controls, the AA genotype is lower than controls (p = 0.007*).

**Table S3** Genotype and allele frequencies of TBKBP1 SNPs among all AS patients, severe AS patients, normal AS patients versus controls. SNPs in TBKBP1 are compared between all AS patients, severe AS patients, and normal AS patients versus the control subjects. # indicates p-value is less than 0.05 but cannot pass Bonferroni correction which shows marginal significant difference. *indicates p-value shows significant difference after Bonferroni correction. After Bonferroni correction the rs8070463 SNP shows significant difference in genotype distribution when comparing severe AS patients to controls, CC genotype carrier frequency is lower than controls (p = 0.003*). This SNP also shows significant difference in C allele distribution when comparing severe AS patients to controls, C allele carrier frequency is lower than controls (p = 0.004*). The rs8070463 SNP is related to the severity of AS.

## Acknowledgments

The authors wish to thank all the patients and families that participated in this study, and all clinical doctors helped us in Chinese PLA general hospital.

## Author Contributions

Constructed the haplotype: JL. Collected the blood samples: CC ZL. Conceived and designed the experiments: ZL YW. Performed the experiments: ZL WC. Analyzed the data: ZL WC. Contributed reagents/materials/analysis tools: CC. Wrote the paper: ZL LS YW.

## References

1. Brown MA, Wordsworth BP, Reveille JD (2002) Genetics of ankylosing spondylitis. Clin Exp Rheumatol 20: S43–9.
2. Braun J, Sieper J (2007) Ankylosing spondylitis. Lancet; 369: 1379–90.
3. Carette S, Graham D, Little H, Rubenstein J, Rosen P (1983) The natural disease course of ankylosing spondylitis. Arthritis Rheum 26: 186–90.
4. Gran JT, Skomsvoll JF (1997) The outcome of ankylosing spondylitis: a study of 100 patients. Br J Rheumatol 36: 766–71.

5. Wanders A, Landewé R, Spoorenberg A, de Vlam K, Mielants H, et al. (2004) Scoring of radiographic progression in randomised clinical trials in ankylosing spondylitis: a preference for paired reading order. Ann Rheum Dis. Dec;63(12): 1601–4. Epub Aug 5.

6. Hamersma J, Cardon LR, Bradbury L, Brophy S, van der Horst-Bruinsma I, et al. (2001) Is disease severity in ankylosing spondylitis genetically determined?

7. The Australo-Anglo-American Spondyloarthritis Consortium (TASC) & the Wellcome Trust Case Control Consortium (WTCCC) (2007) Association scan of 14,500 nsSNPs in four common diseases identifies variants involved in autoimmunity. Nat Genet. 39(11): 1329–1337.

8. The Australo-Anglo-American Spondyloarthritis Consortium (TASC) & the Wellcome Trust Case Control Consortium (WTCCC) (2011) Interaction between ERAP1 and HLA-B27 in ankylosing spondylitis implicates peptide handling in the mechanism for HLA-B27 in disease susceptibility. Nature Genetics volume 43 number 8 August.

9. Sirota M, Schaub MA, Batzoglou S, Robinson WH, Butte AJ (2009) Autoimmune Disease Classification by Inverse Association with SNP Alleles PLoS Genet. Dec; 5(12): e1000792.

10. Lehne B, Lewis CM, Schlitt T (2011) From SNPs to genes: disease association at the gene level. PLoS ONE June, Volume 6, Issue 6, e20133.

11. van der Linden S, Valkenburg HA, Cats A (1984) Evaluation of diagnostic criteria for ankylosing spondylitis. A proposal for modification of the New York criteria. Arthritis Rheum. 27: 361–368.

12. Calin A, Garrett S, Whitelock H, Kennedy LG, O'Hea J, Mallorie P, et al. (1994) A new approach to defining functional ability in ankylosing spondylitis: the development of Bath ankylosing spondylitis disease functional index (BASFI). J Rheumatol 21: 2281–2285.

13. Garrett S, Jenkinson TR, Whitelock HC, Kennedy LG, Gaisford P, et al. (1994) A new approach to defining disease status in AS: the Bath ankylosing spondylitis disease activity index (BASDAI). J Rheumatol 21: 2286–2291.

14. Baraliakos X, Listing J, von der Recke A, Braun J (2009) The natural course of radiographic progression in ankylosing spondylitis–evidence for major individual variations in a large proportion of patients. J Rheumatol 36: 997–1002.

15. Creemers MC, Franssen MJ, van't Hof MA, Gribnau FW, van de Putte LB, et al. (2005) Assessment of outcome in ankylosing spondylitis: an extended radiographic scoring system. Ann Rheum Dis 64: 127–9.

16. Sieper J, Rudwaleit M, Baraliakos X, Brandt J, Braun J, et al. (2009) The Assessment of SpondyloArthritis international Society (ASAS) handbook: a guide to assess spondyloarthritis. Ann Rheum Dis 68(Suppl II): 1–44.

17. Amor B, Santos RS, Nahal R, Listrat V, Dougados M (1994) Predictive factors for the longterm outcome of spondyloarthropathies. J Rheumatol 21: 1883–87.

18. Kiaer T, Gehrchen M (2010) Transpedicular closed wedge osteotomy in ankylosing spondylitis: results of surgical treatment and prospective outcome analysis. Eur Spine J 19: 57–64.

19. Tost J, Gut IG (2005) Genotyping single nucleotide polymorphisms by MALDI mass spectrometry in clinical applications. Clinical Biochemistry 38: 335–350.

20. Reveille JD, Ball EJ, Khan MA (2001) HLA-B27 and genetic predisposing factors in spondyloarthropathies. Curr.Opin. Rheumatol. 13: 265–272.

21. Taylor AL, Balakrishnan C, Calin A (1998) Reference centile charts for measures of disease activity, functional impairment, and metrology in ankylosing spongdylitis. Arthritis & Rheumatism Vol 41. No 6. June. 1119–1125.

22. Braun J, van der Heijde D, Dougados M, Emery P, Khan MA, et al. (2002) Staging of patients with ankylosing spondylitis: a preliminary proposal. Ann Rheum Dis Dec;61 Suppl 3:iii9–23.

23. Sirota M, Schaub MA, Batzoglou S, Robinson WH, Butte AJ (2009) Autoimmune disease classification by Inverse association with SNP alleles. PLoS genetics December, Volume 5, Issue 12, e1000792.

24. Vionnet N, Hani EH, Dupont S, Gallina S, Francke S, et al. (2000) Genome wide search for type 2 diabetes-susceptibility genes in French whites: evidence for a novel susceptibility locus for early-onset diabetes on chromosome 3q27-qter and independent replication of the type 2-diabetes locus on chromosome 1q21-q24. Am J Hum Genet 67: 1470–80.

25. Wirtenberger M, Tchatchou S, Hemminki K, Schmutzhard J, Sutter C, et al. (2006) Associations of genetic variants in the estrogen receptor coactivators PPARGC1A, PPARGC1B and EP300 with familial breast cancer. Carcinogenesis, 27: 2201–2208.

26. Puigserver P, Wu Z, Park CW, Graves R, Wright M, et al. (1998) A cold-inducible coactivator of nuclear receptors linked to adaptive thermogenesis, Cell 92: 829–839.

27. Lehman JJ, Barger PM, Kovacs A, Saffitz JE, Medeiros DM, et al. (2000) Peroxisome proliferator-activated receptor coactivator-1 promotes cardiac mitochondrial biogenesis, J. Clin. Invest. 106: 847–856.

28. Yoon JC, Puigserver P, Chen G, Donovan J, Wu Z, et al. (2001) Spiegelman, Control of hepatic gluconeogenesis through the transcriptional coactivator PGC-1, Nature 413: 131–138.

29. Herzig S, Long F, Jhala US, Hedrick S, Quinn R, et al. (2001) CREB regulates hepatic gluconeogenesis through the coactivator PGC-1, Nature 413: 179–183.

30. Vega RB, Huss JM, Kelly DP (2000) The coactivator PGC-1 cooperates with peroxisome proliferator-activated receptor a in transcriptional control of nuclear genes encoding mitochondrial fatty acid oxidation enzymes, Mol. Cell. Biol. 20: 1868–1876.

31. Dimauro S, Schon EA (2008) Mitochondrial disorders in the nervous system. Annu. Rev. Neurosci. 31: 91–123.

32. Srivastava S, Diaz F, Iommarini L, Aure K, Lombes A, et al. (2009) PGC-1 1alpha/beta induced expression partially compensates for respiratory chain defects in cells from patients with mitochondrial disorders. Human Molecular Genetics, Vol. 18, 10: 1805–1812.

33. Ishii KA, Fumoto T, Iwai K, Takeshita S, Ito M, et al. (2009) Coordination of PGC-1beta and iron uptake in mitochondrial biogenesis and osteoclast activation. Nat Med. Mar;15(3): 259–66. Epub 2009 Mar 1.

34. Derynck R, Akhurst RJ, Balmain A (2001) TGF-beta signaling in tumor suppression and cancer progression. Nat Genet 29: 117–29.

35. Li QL, Ito K, Sakakura C (2002) Causal relationship between the loss of RUNX3 expression and gastric cancer. Cell 109: 113–24.

36. Li QL, Ito K, Sakakura C, Fukamachi H, Inoue K, et al. (2005) RUNX3, a novel tumor suppressor, is frequently inactivated in gastric cancer by protein mislocalization. Cancer Res 65: 7743–50.

37. Fujii S, Ito K, Ito Y, Ochiai A (2008) Enhancer of zeste homologue 2 (EZH2) down-regulates RUNX3 by increasing histone H3 methylation. J Biol Chem 283: 17324–32.

38. Subramaniam MM, Chan JY, Yeoh KG, Quek T, Ito K, et al. (2009). Molecular pathology of RUNX3 in human carcinogenesis. Biochim Biophys Acta 1796: 315–331.

39. Goel A, Arnold CN, Tassone P, Chang DK, Niedzwiecki D, et al. (2004) Epigenetic inactivation of RUNX3 in microsatellite unstable sporadic colon cancers. Int J Cancer 112: 754–9.

40. Li QL, Kim HR, Kim WJ, Choi JK, Lee YH, et al. (2004) Transcriptional silencing of the RUNX3 gene by CpG hypermethylation is associated with lung cancer. Biochem Biophys Res Commun 314: 223–8.

41. Lau QC, Raja E, Salto-Tellez M, Liu Q, Ito K, et al. (2006) RUNX3 is frequently inactivated by dual mechanisms of protein mislocalization and promoter hypermethylation in breast cancer. Cancer Res 66: 6512–20.

42. Alarcón-Riquelme ME (2004) Role of RUNX in autoimmune diseases linking rheumatoid arthritis, psoriasis and lupus. Arthritis Res. Ther. 6: 169–173.

43. Klunker S, Chong MM, Mantel PY, Palomares O, Bassin C, et al. (2009) Transcription factors RUNX1 and RUNX3 in the induction and suppressive function of Foxp3+ inducible regulatory T cells. J Exp Med 206(12): 2701–2715.

44. Wu Y, Ren M, Yang R, Liang X, Ma Y, et al. (2011) Reduced immunomodulation potential of bone marrow-derived mesenchymal stem cells induced CCR4+CCR6+Th/Treg cell subset imbalance in ankylosing spondylitis. Arthritis Res Ther 13(1): R29.

45. Fainaru O, Woolf E, Lotem J, Yarmus M, Brenner O, et al. (2004) Runx3 regulates mouse TGF-beta-mediated dendritic cell function and its absence results in airway inflammation. EMBO J. 23: 969–979.

46. Unterholzner L, Sumner RP, Baran M, Ren H, Mansur DS, et al. (2011) Vaccinia Virus Protein C6 Is a Virulence Factor that Binds TBK-1 Adaptor Proteins and Inhibits Activation of IRF3 and IRF7 PLoS pathogens Sep;7(9): e1002247. Epub 2011 Sep 8.

47. Ishii KJ, Kawagoe T, Koyama S, Matsui K, Kumar H, et al. (2008) TANK-binding kinase-1 delineates innate and adaptive immune responses to DNA vaccines. Nature. Feb 7;451(7179): 725–9.

48. Reveille JD, Ball EJ, Khan MA (2001) HLA-B27 and genetic predisposing factors in spondyloarthropathies. Curr.Opin. Rheumatol. 13: 265–272.

# 11

# Interaction Pattern of Arg 62 in the A-Pocket of Differentially Disease-Associated HLA-B27 Subtypes Suggests Distinct TCR Binding Modes

**Elisa Nurzia[1]⊚, Daniele Narzi[2]⊚, Alberto Cauli[3], Alessandro Mathieu[3], Valentina Tedeschi[1], Silvana Caristi[1], Rosa Sorrentino[4], Rainer A. Böckmann[2]\*, Maria Teresa Fiorillo[1]\***

1 Department of Biology and Biotechnology "C. Darwin", Sapienza University, Rome, Italy, 2 Computational Biology, Department of Biology, University of Erlangen-Nürnberg, Erlangen, Germany, 3 2nd Chair of Rheumatology, Department of Medical Sciences, University of Cagliari, Cagliari, Italy, 4 Istituto Pasteur-Fondazione Cenci Bolognetti, Department of Biology and Biotechnology "C. Darwin", Sapienza University, Rome, Italy

## Abstract

The single amino acid replacement Asp116His distinguishes the two subtypes HLA-B\*2705 and HLA-B\*2709 which are, respectively, associated and non-associated with Ankylosing Spondylitis, an autoimmune chronic inflammatory disease. The reason for this differential association is so far poorly understood and might be related to subtype-specific HLA:peptide conformations as well as to subtype/peptide-dependent dynamical properties on the nanoscale. Here, we combine functional experiments with extensive molecular dynamics simulations to investigate the molecular dynamics and function of the conserved Arg62 of the α1-helix for both B27 subtypes in complex with the self-peptides pVIPR (RRKWRRWHL) and TIS (RRLPIFSRL), and the viral peptides pLMP2 (RRRWRRLTV) and NPflu (SRYWAIRTR). Simulations of HLA:peptide systems suggest that peptide-stabilizing interactions of the Arg62 residue observed in crystal structures are metastable for both B27 subtypes under physiological conditions, rendering this arginine solvent-exposed and, probably, a key residue for TCR interaction more than peptide-binding. This view is supported by functional experiments with conservative (R62K) and non-conservative (R62A) B\*2705 and B\*2709 mutants that showed an overall reduction in their capability to present peptides to CD8+ T cells. Moreover, major subtype-dependent differences in the peptide recognition suggest distinct TCR binding modes for the B\*2705 versus the B\*2709 subtype.

**Editor:** Clive M. Gray, University of Cape Town, South Africa

**Funding:** This work was supported by VolkswagenStiftung (Grant I/82735 to MTF and Grant I/82733 to DN and RAB) http://www.volkswagen-stiftung.de/ and by Fondazione Pasteur-Cenci Bolognetti to RS. http://www.istitutopasteur.it/. The funders had no role in study design, data collection and analysis, decision to publish, or preparation of the manuscript.

**Competing Interests:** The authors have declared that no competing interests exist.

\* E-mail: mariateresa.fiorillo@uniroma1.it (MTF); rainer.boeckmann@biologie.uni-erlangen.de (RAB)

⊚ These authors contributed equally to this work.

## Introduction

Major histocompatibility complex (MHC) class I molecules are highly polymorphic glycoproteins involved in the presentation of foreign peptides to cytotoxic CD8+ T lymphocytes. In this process, which is pivotal for immune surveillance of intracellular pathogens, a key step is the recognition of the MHC class I complex (heavy chain (HC), $\beta_2$-microglobulin ($\beta_2$m) and peptide, see Fig. 1A) by a T-cell receptor (TCR). Peptides, typically 8–10 amino acid residues long, are produced during intracellular protein degradation [1]. A detailed knowledge of the rules governing peptide binding arose from crystallographic studies and peptide elution analysis from purified MHC molecules [2–7]. Less is known about the dynamic properties of the MHC class I complex [8] and whether or how the peptide or the heavy chain binding groove may adapt their conformation in the process of recognition by TCR, either by induced fit or by conformational selection [9–12].

HLA-B27 is one of the most investigated human MHC class I antigens given the strong association with Ankylosing Spondylitis (AS), a rheumatic autoimmune disorder [13,14]. Nevertheless, HLA-B27 confers to carriers some immunological benefits such as effective cytotoxic T cell (CTL) responses by presenting epitopes from many infectious agents such as influenza virus (flu), Epstein-Barr virus (EBV), hepatitis C virus (HCV) and human immunodeficiency virus (HIV) [15–18].

The pathogenic role of HLA-B27 has not yet been fully elucidated. Notably, some HLA-B27 subtypes are not associated with AS [19–21]. This applies to the HLA-B\*2709 allele which occurs in up to 19% of B27 healthy carriers in Sardinia [22]. B\*2709 represents a good investigative tool in pairwise comparative studies with B\*2705, the most common B27 allele and strongly associated with AS in worldwide populations. Indeed, the two allelic products are distinguished only by a single substitution in the residue 116 (Asp in B\*2705 and His in B\*2709) located in the floor of pocket F where the peptide C-terminus accommodates [23]. Asp116His is a relevant polymorphism that gives rise to different repertoires of bound peptides and cytotoxic CD8+ T cells (CTL) [24–26]. As an example, pVIPR, a self-peptide derived from type I receptor of Vasoactive Intestinal Peptide evokes

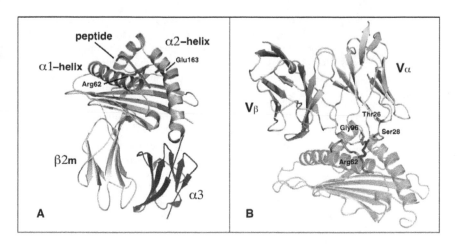

**Figure 1. MHC:peptide complex unbound (A) and bound (B) to a TCR.** A) Cartoon representation of HLA*B2705 presenting the pLMP2 peptide (PDB ID: 1UXS). The peptide-binding groove is shown in beige, the α3 domain in red, the β2-microglobulin in green and the bound LMP2 peptide in blue. Arg62 and Glu163 are emphasized in stick representation. B) Cartoon representation of the binding groove of HLA-B*0801 (in beige) in complex with an EBV derived nonapeptide (in purple) bound to the Vα and Vβ chains of the LC13 T-Cell receptor (in green, PDB ID: 1MI5). Arg62 of the MHC binding groove as well as the residues of the Vα chain making contacts with Arg62 (Thr26, Ser28 and Gly96) are shown in stick representation.

autoreactive CTL responses in B*2705 individuals, mostly patients with AS, but not in B*2709 healthy individuals [26,27]. This peptide exhibits a double conformation, canonical (pVIPR A) and non-canonical (pVIPR B) on B*2705, and only the canonical (pVIPR A) binding mode in complex with B*2709 [28]. This finding allows speculating on a cause-effect correlation between the double conformation of pVIPR and a defective negative thymic selection that prevents autoreactive CTLs to be deleted thus allowing them to gain access to the circulating T cell pool. pVIPR shares high sequence similarity with pLMP2, a viral peptide from EBV which is displayed in two drastically different conformations by B*2705 (non-canonical) and B*2709 molecules (canonical) [29]. The remarkable structural similarities between pLMP2 and pVIPR on B*2705 molecules are functionally mirrored by the occurrence of pLMP2/pVIPR cross-reactive CTL in B*2705 positive patients with AS [29]. Both these peptides have an Arg at position 1, a feature shared by a large portion of B27 bound peptides [30]. Crystallographic analysis revealed tight interactions of this residue bound in the A pocket to the three residues Glu163 (α2-helix), Trp167 (α2-helix), and Arg62 (α1-helix). Both van der Waals interactions as well as water-mediated salt bridges between these residues contribute significantly to the peptide binding [28,29,31,32].

Until now, no crystal structure of TCRs bound to B27:peptide complexes has been solved. Therefore, no information on conformational changes in these structures upon TCR engagement is available. However, several crystal structures of other MHC complexes bound to TCRs and sharing common key residues (Arg62, Gln65, Ala150) with the two B27 subtypes investigated here are available in the Protein Data Bank [33–35]. Notably, in all these structures and independently from the initial state, the Arg62 side chain adopts a conformation enabling the contact with the CDRα1 once the TCR engages the MHC:peptide (Fig. 1B). In the pLMP2:, pVIPR: and TIS:B*2705/09 crystal structures, the Arg62 side chain is always oriented towards the HLA binding groove and even engaged in a (water-mediated) salt bridge to Glu163 of the opposed α2-helix [28,29,32]. The salt bridge is formed across the N-terminal part of the peptide. In this conformation, the Arg62 side chain is hardly accessible for interactions to a TCR (see Fig. 1A).

The time evolution of conformations sampled by a biomolecular system (here MHC:peptide complexes) can be monitored at atomic resolution by performing molecular dynamics (MD) simulations [36]. MD simulations were already applied to the study of various HLA-B molecules in complex with different peptides [8,37–43].

In the present study, MD simulations of B*2705 and B*2709 molecules bound to peptides having an Arg (pVIPR, pLMP2 and TIS) [44] or a Ser (NPflu) [45] at position 1, document a TCR-independent but peptide-dependent conformational change of Arg62. The simulations show a predominant solvent-exposed conformation of the Arg62 side chain for B27:peptide complexes with an arginine in position 1 of the peptide.

The relevance of Arg62 for T-cell recognition was investigated by functional experiments in which self (pVIPR) or viral peptides (pLMP2, NPflu) are presented to specific CTLs in association with B*2705 or B*2709 mutants in which a Lys or an Ala replaces Arg62.

## Results

### MD simulations of HLA-B27:peptide systems

Crystal structures of B*2705 and B*2709 with bound peptides were resolved at 100 K [28,29,32]. Here, we investigated the conformational dynamics focusing on the Arg62 residue of seven different HLA:peptide systems at physiological temperature, by MD simulations of 400 ns length. The simulated systems were pLMP2, pVIPR, TIS associated with either B*2705 or B*2709 molecules, and NPflu in complex with B*2705 only (see Methods). TIS is part of TIS11B, a member of epidermal growth factor early response genes that has been eluted from both B*2705 and 09 molecules [24,46,47]. Thermodynamic and structural studies have demonstrated an almost total equivalence of B*2705:TIS and B*2709:TIS complexes [32,44] and therefore this peptide has been included in the MD simulations as reference. NPflu is an immunodominant, HLA-B27-restricted epitope derived from the nucleoprotein of Influenza A virus and the only investigated peptide here lacking Arg at P1 [45]. No simulation of B*2709:NPflu was undertaken given the instability of this complex caused by the presence of pArg9 (C-terminal anchor) which is disfavoured in the F pocket of B*2709 (His 116) [24,47].

## Arg62 conformational flexibility in B*2705 and B*2709 subtypes is peptide-dependent

In pLMP2 and pVIPR pArg1 forms a direct salt bridge with Glu163 in both B*2705 and B*2709 subtypes as shown by the x-ray crystal structures (left panels in Fig. 2A). As a measure of the Arg62 conformations sampled in the simulations, the minimum distance between Arg62 and Glu163 (see Fig. 1A) was calculated as a function of the simulation time for all systems. The distribution of distances was used to analyze the free energy profile along this degree of freedom, ($\Delta$G(dist)) [48]:

$$\Delta G(dist) = - RT \ln(\rho(dist)/\rho_{max})$$

$\rho$(dist) is the density of states at a given distance and $\rho_{max}$ the maximal density of the respective distribution [48]. The $\Delta$G profile as well as the time traces for the distance between Arg62 and Glu163 are shown in Figure 2B and C. The grey area indicates the distance range as observed in the crystal.

The side chain of Arg62 showed a large conformational flexibility for all systems involving peptides with a N-terminal Arg. In these systems, the water-mediated salt bridge between Arg62 and Glu163 present in the crystal structures was destabilized resulting in a global rearrangement of the A pocket. As shown in Figure 2A, the side chain of Arg62 adopted a completely solvent exposed conformation. This exposed confor-

mation resembles the one observed for the same side chain in the different reported MHC/TCR crystal structures (see Fig.1B) [34]. A local energy minimum corresponding to the bound conformation observed in crystal structures was found for both B*2705 and B*2709 subtypes presenting peptides with Arg in position 1 (pVIPR, pLMP2, TIS). In these systems, the free energy profile additionally shows the presence of stable exposed conformations of the Arg62 side chain (local/global energy minimum corresponding to Arg62-Glu163 distances >6.0 Å). For B*2705 in complex with pLMP2, distances between Arg62 and Glu163 of 15 Å and more were observed (Fig. 2B). This separation is due to a partial unfolding of the α1-helix resulting in an increased separation between the two helices [43]. The contact between Arg62 and Glu163 present in the starting structure and lost during the MD simulation is intermediately restored for HLA-B*2705 in complex with pVIPR in both A and B conformations (Fig. 2A top panel and 2C).

The breakage of the water-mediated salt-bridge between Arg62 and Glu163 is facilitated by the positive charges of the guanidinium group of pArg1 and of pArg3/pLys3. These can partially stabilize the negative charge of Glu163 after loss of contact with Arg62 by formation of transient, partially water-mediated, salt bridges to Glu163 (see Fig. 2D for distances between pArg3/pLys3 to Glu163). Additionally, the Glu163-Arg62 interaction may be replaced by a salt bridge to the positively charged N-terminal amine group instead of the guanidinium group of pArg1. This occurs in the B*2705:pLMP2, B*2709:pLMP2 and B*2709:pVIPR complexes.

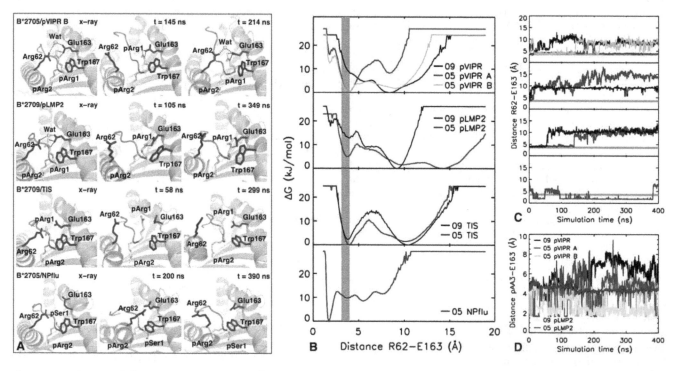

**Figure 2. Conformational variability of the Arg62 side chain.** A) Representation of the N-terminal binding pockets of HLA-B*2705 presenting pVIPR in non-canonical conformation (top row), of HLA-B*2709 presenting pLMP2 (2nd row) and TIS (3rd row), and of HLA-B*2705 presenting the NPflu peptide (bottom row). Residues of the binding groove (Arg62, Glu163 and Trp167, red sticks) and the first two N-terminal residues (pArg1 and pArg2) of the peptide (in blue) are highlighted. The x-ray structures of the respective systems are shown in the first column. For comparison, three representative snapshots taken at different times of the simulations are depicted. Water molecules involved in water mediated salt-bridge between Arg62 and Glu163 are shown if present (blue sphere). B) Free energy profiles as a function of the distance between Arg62 and Glu163 computed for all eight simulated systems. The gray area indicates the range of the distances found in the corresponding crystal structures. C) Time traces of the distance between Arg62 and Glu163 as obtained from the MD simulations (legends as in B). D) Time traces of the distance between Glu163 and pArg3 of pLMP2 and pLys3 of pVIPR, respectively.

Intriguingly, the only investigated system B*2705:NPflu with a peptide lacking pArg1 but having pSer1, an uncharged, albeit polar residue as well as pTyr3, showed a considerably different energetic profile when compared with the other systems. A significantly more stable salt bridge (not water-mediated) between Arg62 and Glu163 was observed in the simulations. Such an interaction is absent in the crystal structure of NPflu [45].

## R62K and R62A replacements in B*2705 and B*2709 subtypes do not alter the cell surface expression and molecular stability

In order to investigate the functional role of Arg62, we performed single amino acid substitutions in both B27 subtypes. In particular, we generated B*2705 and B*2709 mutants

substituting Arg62 by Lys (R62K) that conserves the positive charge and by Ala (R62A) in which a non-polar residue replaces the positively charged residue. For functional experiments, we stably transfected the cDNAs encoding the four B27 mutants in HeLa cells. Afterwards, HeLa transfectants have been cloned and several different clones analysed by flow cytometry to assess the expression of B27 mutants on the cell surface. One clone for each B27 mutant was chosen for further experiments. The B27 mutants expression profile has been analysed with either ME1, a mAb recognizing the properly folded B27 molecules (heavy chain/ $\beta$2m/peptide) or HC10 that reacts with the heavy chains dissociated from the $\beta$2m [49,50]. The staining with the conformational dependent antibody ME1 showed an expression level of the folded R62K and R62A B27 mutants slightly lower and higher, respectively, than wt (Fig. 3A and C). On the opposite,

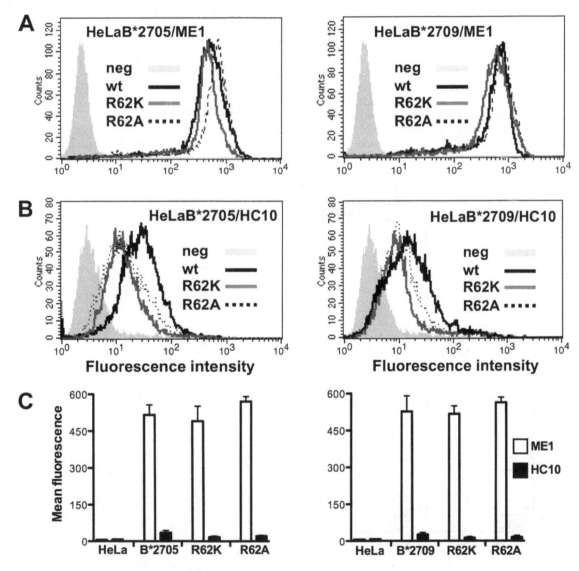

**Figure 3. Cell surface expression of R62A and R62K B*2705/09 mutants on Hela transfectants.** A) Surface expression of R62A and R62K mutants within B*2705 (left panel) and B*2709 context (right panel) compared to that of wt molecules. Cells were stained with ME1 mAb and analysed by flow cytometry analysis. B) Surface expression of free heavy chains of R62A and R62K B*2705 mutants (left panel) and R62A and R62K B*2709 mutants (left panel) versus wt molecules analysed with HC10 mAb. Grey histograms represent wt HeLa cells (neg) used as controls. Mouse IgG negative controls have not been shown. One representative experiment is shown here. C) Comparison of the surface expression of wt (B*2705 on left panel; B*2709 on right panel) molecules with the relative mutants as folded heterodimers (white bars) and $\beta$2m-free heavy chains (black bars). Untransfected HeLa cells (HeLa in the figure) do not expressed unfolded heavy chains. The results are expressed as mean fluorescence ± SD of five/six independent experiments.

the analysis with the HC10 mAb showed that both R62K and R62A mutants in the context of B*2709 and, even more, in that of B*2705 displayed an evident decreased amount of β2m-free heavy chains compared to wt molecules (Fig. 3B and C). The data suggest that these mutations do not induce dissociation of the three party complexes on the cell surface. No free heavy chains are detectable on the cell surface of untransfected HeLa cells (Fig. 3B).

## Arg 62 is relevant for TCR recognition of peptides with pArg1 associated with B*2705 and B*2709 molecules

HeLa transfectants expressing the B*2705 and B*2709 mutant forms have been used as target cells for specific HLA-B27-restricted CD8+ cytotoxic T cells to assess whether the substitution of Arg62 by a conservative (Lys) or non-conservative (Ala) amino acid could affect the T cell recognition of pVIPR and pLMP2. The results shown in Figure 4 attest a distinct behaviour among three different pVIPR-specific CTL lines derived from two B*2705 positive patients with AS (EP and BAR). In the case of EP1 CTL line, the pVIPR:B*2705 mutant complexes were recognized even better as compared to the wt molecules. On the contrary, the same CTL line was less effective when the peptide was presented by either R62K or R62A B*2709 mutants compared to the wt molecules. As for EP4 from the same patient with AS, the TCR recognition appeared highly dependent on the presence of Arg62 since the recognition of pVIPR was totally abrogated on both R62K and R62A B*2705 mutants and on R62A B*2709 mutant and heavily reduced (up to 70% on R62K B*2709 mutant (Fig. 4).

The effector functions of BAR28 CTL line were tested only in the B*2705 context. It exhibited a clear lack of peptide recognition on the non-conservative mutant R62A, and a partial decrement on the R62K mutant compared to the wt (Fig. 4).

As for the recognition of pLMP2, we tested four CTL lines: two from a B*2705 patient with AS (PIC) and two from two different B*2709 individuals (DE and PMC). PIC3 and PIC5 CTL lines behaved similarly showing reduced lytic activity against both B*2705 and B*2709 mutant HeLa cells incubated with pLMP2 in comparison with the wt molecules (Fig. 5). Interestingly, pLMP2 was recognized slightly better when presented by the conservative mutant in B*2705 context vs the non-conservative one, while the opposite occurred in the B*2709 context. DE5 displayed only a negligible recognition of pLMP2 on mutant R62K B*2705 and the same trend of PIC3 and PIC5 with the B*2709 mutants. The CTL line PMC6 tested only in the B*2705 context, showed lack of reactivity towards pLMP2 on both mutants. No CTL line, either pVIPR- or pLMP2- specific, was able to lyse untransfected HeLa cells incubated with the relevant peptide (data not shown).

These results demonstrate that the Arg62, located in the A-pocket of HLA-B27 binding groove, could play an important role as TCR docking residue.

## Arg62 is crucial for TCR recognition also when the peptide possesses a p1 residue different from Arg

The effect of Arg62 substitutions in the B27 molecules was also investigated with a peptide not having Arg at position 1. In this

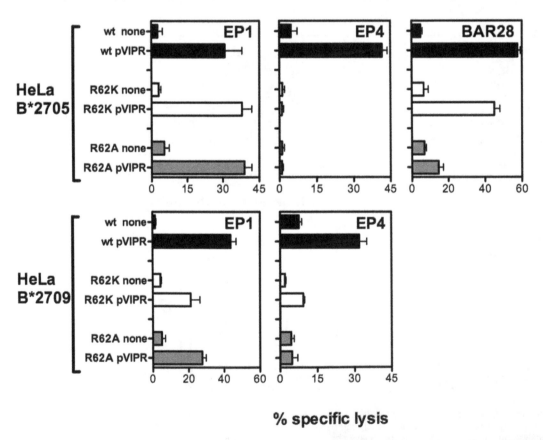

**% specific lysis**

**Figura 4. CTL recognition of pVIPR displayed by R62K and R62A B*2705/09 mutants and by wt subtypes.** 4 h standard [51]chromium-release assay showing the reactivity pattern of pVIPR responsive CTLs raised in B*2705 positive patients with AS (EP and BAR) against HeLa cells transfected with B*2705 and 09 molecules or expressing the indicated mutant forms. These cells used as targets have been pulsed ON with pVIPR (70 μM) or cultured in medium alone. Effector/target ratio was 15:1. Bars represent the mean percentage of lysis ± SD of three independent experiments.

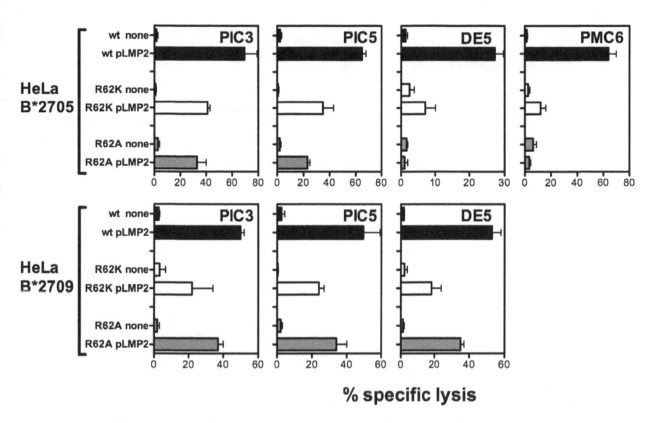

**% specific lysis**

**Figura 5. CTL reactivity against pLMP2 bound to R62K and R62A B*2705/09 mutants and wt molecules.** pLMP2-driven CTL lines derived from a B*2705 positive patients with AS (PIC) and two B*2709 positive individual (DE and PMC) have been tested in a 4 h standard [51]chromium-release assay using HeLa transfectants expressing wt or mutants of B*2705 and B*2709 subtypes as target cells after ON treatment with pLMP2 (70 μM) or in absence of peptide. Effector/target ratio was 15:1. Mean percentage of lysis ± SD of three separate experiments is shown here.

case, the constellation among Arg62, Glu163 and Trp167 that stabilizes peptides with pArg1 is different. To address this issue, we tested the recognition of NPflu by a specific CTL line (SER62) derived from a B*2705 positive individual. As expected, the B*2709 molecules were not able to present the peptide because of the Arg at the C-terminus (Fig. 6). In the B*2705 context, the non-conservative substitution R62A abrogated the peptide recognition while R62K mutant showed a 35% reduction of lytic activity compared to the wt molecules. This result obtained with a B27 epitope having Ser instead of Arg at P1, suggests a general relevance of Arg62 for TCR recognition of B27/peptide complexes that is only partially influenced by the amino acid specificities at P1 residue.

## Discussion

Subtype- and peptide-dependent structural and dynamical features of the HLA:peptide complexes dictate the conditions for T-cell recognition and are likely to be involved in the differential association of some HLA-B27 subtypes with AS. To investigate this matter, a combination of theoretical and experimental procedures was employed.

We focused on the interactions established by the Arg62 inside the A pocket that anchors the peptide N-terminus. This is a residue of the α1-helix, highly conserved in the alleles of the HLA-B locus (>95%) whose orientation could be strongly influenced by the P1 residue of the specific ligand [51,52]. In all resolved B27 crystal structures, this arginine is oriented towards the binding groove, frequently forming water-mediated salt bridges to Glu163 on the opposed α2-helix, thereby clamping the peptide in the binding groove. In contrast, available MHC:peptide:TCR structures suggest an engagement of Arg62 in TCR binding implying an exposed Arg62 conformation. Examples are given by the allogeneic H-2K[b] MHC class I molecule bound to an octapeptide and the KB5-C20 TCR (PDB ID: 1KJ2 2.71 Å) [33]; the HLA-B*0801 in association with a nonamer from EBNA3A of EBV bound to the LC13 TCR (PDB ID: 1MI5 2.50 Å) (Fig. 1B) [34] and the HLA-B*3501 in complex with the endecapeptide EPLP bound to ELS4 TCR (PDB ID: 2NX5 2.70 Å) [35]. In the HLA-B*3501 and HLA-B*0801 structures, four key aminoacids Arg62, Gln65, Ala150, Gln155 are engaged by specific residues of the respective bound TCRs. All these residues are shared by B*2705 and B*2709 subtypes. The same residues, with the exception of Gln155 replaced by Arg155, are involved in the contacts between H-2K[b] subtype and the KB5-C20 T-Cell receptor.

Accordingly, Webb and colleagues [53] predicted that the Arg62 in the H2-Kb e H2-Kbm8 would contact the CDR1α of the anti-HSV T lymphocytes and, serving as "electrostatic guide for TCR docking", would be pivotal for T-cell selection depending on its dynamics and positioning.

The tight Arg62-pArg1-Trp167 stacking interaction has been invoked as a possible explanation for the relative high frequency, in the B27 repertoire, of peptides with dibasic N-terminal motif pArg1-pArg2 [30], that, however, have an intrinsic resistance to cytosolic degradation. To this regard, it has been shown that mutations of Glu163 alone or both Glu163 and Trp167 had a limited effect on the B*2705 molecules for usage of peptides with basic P1 residues, thus indicating that the increased cytosolic stability is responsible for such a preferential binding [54]. However, B*2705 mutants substituted at Arg62 residue have

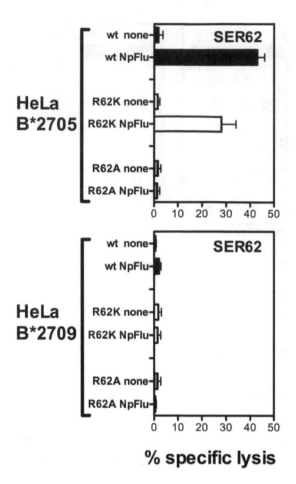

**Figure 6. Recognition of Npflu associated to R62K and R62A B*2705/09 mutants and wt molecules.** Cytotoxic activity of a specific CTL obtained from a B*2705 positive subject (SER) against HeLa cells transfected with wt and B*2705 and B*2709 mutants and incubated with NPflu peptide (70 µM) or in medium alone and used as targets. Effector/target ratio was 15:1. Bars represent the mean percentage of lysis ± SD of three independent experiments.

never been generated and assessed for their peptide binding repertoire.

Here, we have investigated the structure and dynamics of the Arg62-Glu163 peptide clamp pair in MD simulations of the HLA-B*2705/09 subtypes bound to peptides with arginine (pVIPR, pLMP2, TIS) and serine (NPflu) at the N-terminal peptide position, under physiological conditions. In our computational setting, all MD simulations of B*2705 and B*2709 subtypes bound to peptides with pArg1 (pVIPR, pLMP2 and TIS) revealed a very large conformational flexibility of the Arg62 side chain. Notably, during the 400 ns simulation, the contact between Arg62 and Glu163 present in the respective crystal structures was lost (examples are shown in Figure 2A) and the side chain of Arg62 adopts a flexible exposed conformation, similar to that displayed in the MHC-peptide/TCR complexes reported above (see also Fig. 1B). This conformational change with the exposed Arg62 was stable in the majority of simulated systems except for B*2705 bound to pVIPR both in the canonical and non-canonical conformations. Here, the Arg62-Glu163 bond is intermediately re-established. The Arg62 reorientation is accompanied by a partial rearrangement of the A pocket. The Arg62 re-orientation was favourable when Arg1 could interact with Glu163 or when

other positively charged residues such as pArg3 in pLMP2 or pLys3 in pVIPR could form a transient or stable salt bridge with Glu163. In contrast, with a polar residue present at P1 as Ser in NPflu, the system showed a marked different energetic profile with a tightened Arg62-Glu163 clamp across the peptide, although not present in the crystal [45]. Thus, the peptide sequence dictates the conformation of TCR-accessible heavy chain amino acids. Several MHC:peptide:TCR crystal structures reported in the literature as well as our molecular dynamics simulations suggested a key role for Arg62. For a deeper comprehension of its relevance to the B*2705 and B*2709 molecular stability and, more importantly, to the antigen presentation to TCR, we generated HeLa cells stably expressing R62A and R62K B27 mutant forms. Both conservative and non-conservative substitutions did not significantly change the cell surface expression level of B27 mutants as inferred by comparison with wt B*2705 and B*2709 alleles (Fig. 3). This was observed by flow cytometry analysis with ME1 [49], a mAb recognizing the properly folded B27 molecules or with HC10 [50] that reacts against the free heavy chains. Therefore, a change in the expression level and/or molecular stability of the mutants did not bias T-cell data.

A comparison of T-cell results for pVIPR and pLMP2 presented by the wt molecules and by the R62A and R62K B27 mutants suggests a relevance of R62 for TCR interaction. For all but one CTL line (EP1), the mutations in Arg62 led to a significant decrease or even total abrogation of lytic activity with respect to pVIPR presentation by wt B27 molecules. Interestingly, the EP1 CTL line displayed a full activation by R62K and R62A B*2705 mutants but not by the same mutants in the B*2709 context. We do not expect that mutations of Arg62 lead to a different distribution of pVIPR conformations observed in crystal structures in complex with B*2705 and thereby to a modified T-cell response. The crystal structures of both conformations show a similar interaction pattern in this region of the binding groove.

For pLMP2 presentation in the disease-associated B*2705 context, both mutants are less effective than wt in activating the CTL lytic activity with the non-conservative R62A mutant working slightly worse than the conservative R62K mutant. This order is reversed in the case of peptide presentation by the non-disease associated B*2709 (Fig. 5) suggesting different TCR binding modes to B*2709 as compared to B*2705. DE5 CTL provides a striking example: it failed to react against pLMP2 when presented by R62A B*2705 mutant while it was activated by the same mutant in the B*2709 context. All together, these data strongly suggest that R62 mutations in the A pocket could be differently buffered in respect to TCR recognition by the His-Asp polymorphism at 116 in the F pocket. Also T cell recognition of NPflu, the only peptide analysed here having Ser at P1, appeared to be influenced by mutations at R62 in the B*2705 context while, as already mentioned, it is not presented by the B*2709 subtype. As for the cases of B*2705 presenting pLMP2 or pVIPR, CTL activity required a positively charged residue at position 62 (R or K). This result is consistent with previous T-cell recognition data showing that the side chain of pSer1 was not directly involved in interactions with the TCR but rather the region around P1 represents a docking site for the TCR. Accordingly, the replacement of pSer1 by amino acids with bulky side chains (R, K or Y) induced a marked reduction of T-cell recognition due to the steric interference with TCR binding [45,55].

This combined experimental and theoretical study would suggest a differential contribution of Arg62 to the TCR recognition of B*2705/09:peptide complexes. MD simulations of the wt B27:peptide systems revealed the meta-stability of the Arg62-Glu163 peptide clamp frequently observed in crystal structures, and the preference of Arg62 to adopt a solvent-exposed, TCR oriented side-chain conformation. Functional experiments showed that the positive charge of Arg62 is preferred for the TCR recognition of disease-associated B*2705 complexes. Differently, a small amino acid such as Ala is favourable over Lys in the non-disease-associated B*2709 subtype. In conclusion, this study gives a strong indication for a B27 subtype-dependent functional role of Arg 62 in the antigen recognition by TCR.

## Materials and Methods

### Ethics Statement

This study has been approved by the Ethics Committee of the University of Cagliari where blood samples of patients with AS and healthy controls have been collected (365/09/CE). All participants involved in this study gave their written informed consent.

### MD simulations

The starting structures of the HLA-B*2709 and HLA-B*2705 proteins presenting the peptides studied here were taken from the Protein Data Bank (PDB entries: 1UXW: B*2709 with pLMP2 at 1.71 Å [29], 61UXS: B*2705 with pLMP2 at 1.55 Å [29], 1OF2: B*2709 with pVIPR at 2.20 Å [28], 1OGT: B*2705 with pVIPR in canonical (VIPR A) and non-canonical (VIPR B) conformation at 1.47 Å [28], 1W0W: B*2709 with TIS at 2.11 Å [32], 1W0V: B*2705 with TIS at 2.27 Å [32]. Additionally the HLA-B*2705-peptide complex with the immunodominant viral peptide from influenza nucleoprotein (NPflu) NP383–391 was also investigated (PDB ID: 2BST) at 2.10 Å [45].

Protonation states of the titratable groups present in the investigated proteins [56] were chosen according to results of pKa calculations performed on the studied systems using the WHATIF package [57].

The GROMACS software package [58] (version 4.0.4) with the OPLS-AA/L all-atom force field [59] was used to carry out the MD simulations. The proteins were solvated in a dodecahedron box, imposing a minimum distance between the protein and the box of 1.4 nm. Almost 27,000 TIP4 water molecules were added to the different systems [60]. $Na^+$ and $Cl^-$ ions were added to the systems in order to reproduce the physiological ionic concentration (0.15 M). An excess of $Na^+$ was added to compensate for the net negative charge of the MHC complexes. The long-range electrostatic interactions (distances >1.0 nm) were computed by the Particle Mesh Ewald (PME) method [61]. The short-range electrostatic interactions were treated explicitly with a non-bonded pairlist cut off of 1.0 nm. The bond lengths of the hydrogen atoms were constrained by applying the Lincs algorithm thus permitting the use of a time step of 2 fs for numerical integration of the equations of motion [62]. The temperature was kept constant by coupling the system to an external thermal bath (310 K) with a coupling time constant $\tau_T = 0.1$ ps [63]. The systems were weakly coupled to a pressure bath (1 Bar) [63] with a coupling time constant $\tau_p = 1.0$ ps. 200 steps of energy minimization (steepest descent algorithm), followed by 100 ps of MD simulation with harmonic position restraints (force constant 1000 kJ mol$^{-1}$ nm$^{-2}$) on the heavy atoms of the protein preceded the production runs. All MD simulations were run for 400 ns ($2 \times 10^8$ integration steps), adding up to a total simulated time of 3.2 μs.

### Synthetic peptides

The following peptides have been used in this study: pVIPR (RRKWRRWHL, 400–408) from human vasoactive intestinal peptide type 1 receptor [26]; pLMP2 (RRRWRRLTV, 236–244)

[16] from Epstein-Barr virus latent membrane protein 2; NPflu (SRYWAIRTR, 383–391) [15,45] from influenza A virus nucleoprotein; TIS (RRLPIFSRL, 325–333) [24] from TIS11B, member of epidermal growth factor early response genes. Peptides were purchased from PRIMM GmbH (Dubendorf, Zuerich, CH), dissolved in 100% DMSO and their concentration estimated by BCA test according to the manufacturer's protocol (Pierce, Thermo scientific, IL, USA).

### B27 mutants and cDNA cloning

cDNAs encoding for B*2705 and B*2709 had been cloned in pCEP4 mammalian expression vector (Invitrogen, Carlsbad, CA, USA) as reported previously [23]. The mutated constructs were generated by PCR-based cassette mutagenesis of the B*2705 and B*2709 wt cDNAs by using the following primers: (forward) 5'-GCCCGGTACCGGACTCAGAATCTCCTCAG-3' and (reverse) 5'-CAATACTCCGGACCCTCCTGCTCTATCC-3' that amplify part of HLA-B27 cDNA upstream to the codon encoding for R62. This 240 bp fragment that included part of 5'-UTR of HLA-B27, introduced a KpnI site (underlined) at 5'-end and a Kpn2I site (underlined) at 3'-end. A second PCR was performed to introduce the specific mutation R62A and R62K using as primers: forward for R62A substitution 5'-GAGGGTCCGGAGTAT TGGGAC**GCG**GAGACAC-3' (in bold the codon introducing the mutation) and forward for R62K substitution 5'-GAGGGTCCGGAGTATTGGGAC**AAG**GAGACA-3' (in bold the codon introducing the mutation) and reverse, 5'-CCGCAAGCTTCTGGGGAGGAAACACAGGTCAGCGGAAC-3' (the same for all mutants). These primers amplified a fragment of 900 bp and introduced a Kpn2I site at 5'-end (underlined) and a HindIII site (underlined) at 3'-end. The PCRs were conducted in a standard buffer with 2.5 mM $MgSO_4$, 10 pmol of each primers, 0,2 mM of dNTP mix, 1,25 U of Pfu Taq Polymerase (Fermentas, Thermo scientific, IL, USA) and $H_2O$ to a final volume of 50 μl. After a first step at 94°C (30 s), annealing at 62°C (30 s), and extension at 72°C (30 s) for 5 cycles, other 27 cycles were run at 94°C (30 s), 66°C (30 s), 72°C (30 s), before a final extension at 72°C (7 min) in a GeneAmp PCR system 9700 Thermal cycler (Applied Biosystems, Carlsbad, CA, USA). The PCR products were sequentially digested with KpnI (Fermentas, Thermo scientific, IL, USA) and Kpn2I (Fermentas, Thermo scientific, IL, USA) as for the fragment of 240 bp and with Kpn2I and HindIII (Fermentas, Thermo scientific, IL, USA) as for the fragment of 900 bp and then purified from agarose gel by using GFX$^{TM}$ PCR DNA and Gel Band Purification Kit (GE Healthcare Europe GmbH, MI, Italy). Afterwards, the 240 bp and the 900 bp fragments of the respective B27 subtypes were mixed at ratio of 5:5:1 with pCEP4 vector cut with KpnI and HindIII and gel purified using the same kit as above. The ligations were conducted overnight at 16°C with T4 DNA ligase (New England Biolabs, Beverly, MA). XL1-Blue *Escherichia coli* electrocompetent cells (Stratagene; Agilent Technologies, Italy) were transformed by the products of ligations and several colonies for each subtypes were screened by B27-specific PCR and the positive ones checked by automated DNA sequencing.

### Transfection of HeLa cells

HeLa cells (ATCC number CCL2$^{TM}$; www.atcc.com/) were transfected with pCEP4 constructs containing cDNAs for wt B*2705 and B*2709 and R62A and R62K mutants using Lipofectamine 2000 Reagent (Invitrogen, Carlsbad, CA, USA) according to the manufacturer's instructions. After transfection, cells were diluted in DMEM supplemented with 10% heat-inactivated fetal bovine serum, 2 mM L-glutamine, 100 U/mL penicillin and 100 μg/mL streptomycin at $1 \times 10^6$ cells/mL.

Selection for hygromycin B-resistant cells was initiated 48 h post-transfection with 200 μg/mL hygromycin B (PAA, Pasching, Austria). After two weeks of culture, cells were diluted at one cell/well in 96-well flat-bottom microplates and clones, stably expressing B27 molecules, were selected and used to perform subsequent experiments.

## mAbs and immunofluorescence

For immunofluorescence experiments, cells were stained with ME1 (a conformational dependent IgG1mAb, recognizing HLA-B27, -B7, -B42, -B67, -B73 and Bw22) [49] and HC10 (a IgG2a mAb, reacting with a determinant on β2-microglobulin free heavy chains of HLA-B, -C and some HLA-A alleles) [50] and then by F(ab')2 of rabbit anti-mouse FITC (Jackson ImmunoResearch Europe Ltd., Suffolk, UK). Isotype matched mouse Igs were used as negative controls to define background staining. Flow cytometry analysis was made immediately after staining, without fixation, by using a FACSCalibur (BD Biosciences). For each sample, 10.000 events were acquired using forward/side light scatter characteristics and analyzed using Cell Quest software (Becton Dickinson).

## Cell lines

Autologous B lymphoblastoid cell lines (B-LCLs) from B27 positive subjects were generated by *in vitro* immortalization of B cells using the standard type 1 Epstein-Barr virus isolate B95.8 [23] and cultured in RPMI (Lonza, Basel Switzerland) supplemented with 10% fetal calf serum, 2 mM L-glutamine, 100 units/ml penicillin, 100 μg/ml streptomycin. wt and transfected HeLa cells, described above, were cultured in DMEM (Lonza, Basel Switzerland) supplemented with 10% fetal bovine serum, 2 mM L-glutamine, 100 units/ml penicillin, 100 μg/ml streptomycin. HeLa transfectants were cultured in presence of 200 μg/ml hygromycin B (PAA, Pasching, Austria) to maintain the expression of B27 molecules.

## Generation of antigen-specific CTL lines

Peripheral blood mononuclear cells from B*2705 positive patients with AS and healthy donors, either B*2705 or B*2709 positive, were isolated by density gradient centrifugation with Lymphoprep and depleted of the CD4+ T cells by Dynabeads M-450 CD4+ (Dynal ASA, Oslo, Norway). Cell cultures were seeded at $1 \times 10^4$ cells/well in 96-well flat-bottom microplates and stimulated by autologous B-LCLs at 0.5:1 antigen-presenting cells/responder ratio. The antigen-presenting cells had been pulsed overnight with pVIPR (70 μM), pLMP2 (50 μM) or NPflu (50 μM) peptides before being γ-irradiated (200 Gy). CTL lines were grown in RPMI 1640 medium supplemented with 10% heat-inactivated pooled human serum, 2 mM L-glutamine, 100 U/mL penicillin and 100 μg/mL streptomycin. 20 units/ml human rIL-2 (Roche Applied Science) was added to each well after 3 days. CTL lines were then re-stimulated on day 10–12. One week later, the specificity of CTL lines was tested by a standard $^{51}$Cr release assay using as targets peptide-pulsed autologous B-LCL and T2B*2705 transfectants [64]. Phenotypic analysis of peptide-specific CTL lines was performed by immunostaining using the following monoclonal antibodies: OKT3, OKT4, and OKT8 (Orthodiagnostics, Stanford, CA). CTL lines were maintained in culture by weekly stimulation with γ-irradiated autologous B-LCL in complete RPMI medium (see above) and human rIL-2 (20–100 units/ml), and were used for functional assays 8–10 days after stimulation. The study has been approved by the Institutional Review Board of the University of Cagliari were blood samples have been collected.

## $^{51}$Cr-Release Assay

Specific reactivity of CTL lines towards pVIPR, pLMP2 and NPflu was tested by a standard 4-h $^{51}$Cr-release assay. Target cells (HeLa transfectants either expressing wt B*2705 and B*2709 molecules or R62A and R62K mutated forms) were incubated overnight with the different peptides at indicated concentrations or cultured in medium alone. One day later, target cells were labeled with sodium $^{51}$chromate, washed and plated ($3 \times 10^3$ target cells/well) with effector T cells at 15:1 effector/target ratio, in absence of free peptide.

## Acknowledgments

We would like to thank B27 donors and patients with AS for participation in this study and Federica Lucantoni for excellent technical assistance. We are grateful to Andreas Ziegler for a critical reading of the manuscript. Computer time was provided by the Computer Center of the University of Erlangen-Nürnberg (RRZE).

## Author Contributions

Conceived and designed the experiments: MTF RAB RS AM. Performed the experiments: EN DN AC VT SC. Analyzed the data: MTF RAB EN DN AM AC RS. Contributed reagents/materials/analysis tools: AC AM RS. Wrote the paper: MTF RAB RS EN DN.

## References

1. Yedwell JW (2007) Plumbing the sources of endogenous MHC class I peptide ligands. Curr Opin Immunol 19: 79–86.
2. Madden DR, Gorga JC, Strominger JL, Wiley DC (1991) The structure of HLA-B27 reveals nonamer self-peptides bound in an extended conformation. Nature 353: 321–325.
3. Madden DR, Gorga JC, Strominger JL, Wiley DC (1992) The three-dimensional structure of HLA-B27 at 2.1 Å resolution suggests a general mechanism for tight peptide binding to MHC. Cell 70: 1035–1048.
4. Li XC, Raghavan M (2010) Structure and function of major histocompatibility complex class I antigens. Curr Opin Organ Transplant 15: 499–504.
5. Rammensee H, Bachmann J, Emmerich NP, Bachor OA, Stevanović S (1999) SYFPEITHI: database for MHC ligands and peptide motifs. Immunogenetics 50: 213–219.
6. Sathiamurthy M, Hickman HD, Cavett JW, Zahoor A, Prilliman K, et al. (2003) Population of the HLA ligand database. Tissue Antigens 61: 12–19.
7. Sidney J, Peters B, Frahm N, Brander C, Sette A (2008) HLA class I supertypes: a revised and updated classification. BMC Immunol 9: 1.
8. Pöhlmann T, Böckmann RA, Grubmüller H, Uchanska-Ziegler B, Ziegler A, et al. (2004) Differential peptide dynamics is linked to major histocompatibility complex polymorphism. J Biol Chem 279: 28197–28201.
9. Lange OF, Lakomek NA, Fares C, Schröder GF, Walter KFA, et al. (2008) Recognition dynamics up to microseconds revealed from an RDC-derived ubiquitin ensemble in solution. Science 320: 1471–1475.
10. Koshland DE (1958) Application of a theory of enzyme specificity to protein synthesis. Proc Natl Acad Sci USA 44: 98–104.
11. Rudolph MG, Stanfield RL, Wilson IA (2006) How TCRs bind MHCs, peptides, and coreceptors. Annu Rev Immunol 24: 419–466.
12. Gakamsky DM, Luescher IF, Pecht I (2004) T cell receptor-ligand interactions: a conformational preequilibrium or an induced fit. Proc Natl Acad Sci USA 101: 9063–9066.
13. Brewerton DA, Hart FD, Nicholls A, Caffrey M, James DC (1973) Ankylosing spondylitis and HL-A 27. Lancet 1: 904–907.
14. Schlossstein L, Terasaki PI, Bluestone R, Pearson CM (1973) High association of an HL-A antigen, W27, with ankylosing spondylitis. N Engl J Med 288: 704–706.
15. Bowness P, Moss PA, Rowland-Jones S, Bell JI, McMichael AJ (1993) Conservation of T cell receptor usage by HLA B27-restricted influenza-specific cytotoxic T lymphocytes suggests a general pattern for antigen-specific major histocompatibility complex class I-restricted responses. Eur J Immunol 23: 1417–1421.

16. Brooks JM, Murray RJ, Thomas WA, Kurilla MG, Rickinson AB (1993) Different HLA-B27 subtypes present the same immunodominant Epstein-Barr virus peptide. J Exp Med 178: 879–887.

17. Neumann-Haefelin C, McKiernan S, Ward S, Viazov S, Spangenberg HC, et al. (2006) Dominant influence of an HLA-B27 restricted CD8+ T cell response in mediating HCV clearance and evolution. Hepatology 43: 563–572.

18. Wilson JD, Ogg GS, Allen RL, Davis C, Shaunak S, et al. (2000) Direct visualization of HIV-1-specific cytotoxic T lymphocytes during primary infection. AIDS 14: 225–233.

19. Gonzalez-Roces S, Alvarez MV, Gonzalez S, Dieye A, Makni H, et al. (1997) HLA-B27 polymorphism and worldwide susceptibility to ankylosing spondylitis. Tissue Antigens 49: 116–123.

20. Khan MA, Mathieu A, Sorrentino R, Akkoc N (2007) The pathogenetic role of HLA-B27 and its subtypes. Autoimmun Rev 6: 183–189.

21. Reveille JD, Maganti RM (2009) Subtypes of HLA-B27: history and implications in the pathogenesis of ankylosing spondylitis. Adv Exp Med Biol 649: 159–176.

22. Paladini F, Taccari E, Fiorillo MT, Cauli A, Passiu G, et al. (2005) Distribution of HLA-B27 subtypes in Sardinia and continental Italy and their association with spondylarthropathies. Arthritis Rheum 52: 3319–3321.

23. Del Porto P, D'Amato M, Fiorillo MT, Tuosto L, Piccolella E, et al. (1994) Identification of a novel HLA-B27 subtype by restriction analysis of a cytotoxic γδ T cell clone. J Immunol 153: 3093–3100.

24. Fiorillo MT, Meadows L, D'Amato M, Shabanowitz J, Hunt DE, et al. (1997) Susceptibility to ankylosing spondylitis correlates with the C-terminal residue of peptides presented by various HLA-B27 subtypes. Eur J Immunol 27: 368–373.

25. Fiorillo MT, Greco G, Maragno M, Potolicchio I, Monizio A, et al. (1998) The naturally occurring polymorphism $Asp^{116}$-$His^{116}$ differentiating the ankylosing spondylitis associated HLA-B*2705 from the non-associated HLA-B*2709 subtype influences peptide-specific CD8 T cells recognition. Eur J Immunol 28: 2508–2516.

26. Fiorillo, MT, Maragno M, Butler R, Dupuis ML, Sorrentino R (2000) CD8+ T cell autoreactivity to an HLA-B27-restricted self-epitope correlates with ankylosing spondylitis. J Clin Invest 106: 47–53.

27. Fiorillo MT, Sorrentino R (2009) T cell responses against viral and self-epitopes and HLA-B27 subtypes differently associated with Ankylosing Spondylitis. Adv Exp Med Biol 649: 255–262.

28. Hulsmeyer M, Fiorillo MT, Bettosini F, Sorrentino R, Saenger W, et al. (2004) Dual, HLA-B27 subtype-dependent conformation of a self-peptide. J Exp Med 199: 271–281.

29. Fiorillo MT, Ruckert C, Hulsmeyer M, Sorrentino R, Saenger W, et al. (2005) Allele-dependent similarity between viral and self-peptide presentation by HLA-B27 subtypes. J Biol Chem 280: 2962–2971.

30. Lopez de Castro JA, Alvarez I, Marcilla M, Paradela A, Ramos M, et al. (2004) HLA-B27: a registry of constitutive peptide ligands. Tissue Antigens 63: 424–445.

31. Hillig RC, Hulsmeyer M, Saenger W, Welfle K, Misselwitz R, et al. (2004) Thermodynamic and structural analysis of peptide- and allele-dependent properties of two HLA-B27 subtypes exhibiting differential disease association. J Biol Chem 279: 652–666.

32. Hülsmeyer M, Welfle K, Pöhlmann T, Misselwitz R, Alexiev U, et al. (2005) Thermodynamic and structural equivalence of two HLA-B27 subtypes complexed with a self-peptide. J Mol Biol 346: 1367–1379.

33. Reiser JB, Grégoire C, Darnault C, Mosser T, Guimezanes A, et al. (2002) A T cell receptor CDR3β loop undergoes conformational changes of unprecedented magnitude upon binding to a peptide/MHC class I complex. Immunity 216: 345–354.

34. Kjer-Nielsen L, Clements CS, Purcell AW, Brooks AG, Whisstock JC, et al. (2003) A structural basis for the selection of dominant alphabeta T cell receptors in antiviral immunity. Immunity 18: 53–64.

35. Tynan FE, Reid HH, Kjer-Nielsen L, Miles JJ, Wilce MC, et al. (2007) A T cell receptor flattens a bulged antigenic peptide presented by a major histocompatibility complex class I molecule. Nat Immunol 8: 268–276.

36. Karplus M, Petsko GA (1990) Molecular-Dynamics simulations in biology. Nature 347: 631–639.

37. Rognan D, Scapozza L, Folkers G, Daser A (1994) Molecular Dynamics simulation of MHC-Peptide complexes as a tool for predicting potential T Cell epitopes. Biochemistry 33: 11476–11485.

38. Rognan D, Krebs S, Kuonen O, Lamas JR, Lopez de Castro JA, et al. (1997) Fine specificity of antigen binding to two class I major histocompatibility proteins (B*2705 and B*2703) differing in a single amino acid residue. J Comput Aided Mol Des 11: 463–478.

39. Sieker F, Springer S, Zacharias M (2007) Comparative molecular dynamics analysis of tapasin-dependent and -independent MHC class I alleles. Protein Sci 16: 299–308.

40. Sieker F, Straatsma TP, Springer S, Zacharias M (2008) Differential tapasin dependence of MHC class I molecules correlates with conformational changes upon peptide dissociation: A molecular dynamics simulation study. Mol Immunol 45: 3714–3722.

41. Fabian H, Huser H, Narzi D, Misselwitz R, Loll B, et al. (2008) HLA-B27 subtypes differentially associated with disease exhibit conformational differences in solution. J Mol Biol 376: 798–810.

42. Omasits U, Knapp B, Neumann M, Steinhauser O, Stockinger H, et al. (2008) Analysis of key parameters for molecular dynamics of pMHC molecules. Mol Simul 34: 781–793.

43. Narzi D, Becker CM, Fiorillo MT, Uchanska-Ziegler B, Ziegler A, et al. (2012) Dynamical characterization of two differentially disease associated MHC Class I proteins in complex with viral and self-peptides. J Mol Biol 415: 429–442.

44. Ziegler A, Loll B, Misselwitz R, Uchanska-Ziegler B (2009) Implications of structural and thermodynamic studies of HLA-B27 subtypes exhibiting differential association with ankylosing spondylitis. Adv Exp Med Biol 649: 177–195.

45. Stewart-Jones GB, di Gleria K, Kollnberger S, McMichael AJ, Jones EY, et al. (2005) Crystal structures and KIR3DL1 recognition of three immunodominant viral peptides complexed to HLA-B*2705. Eur J Immunol 35: 341–351.

46. Rotzschke O, Falk K, Stefanovic S, Gnau V, Jung G, et al. (1994) Dominant aromatic/aliphatic C-terminal anchor in HLA-B*2702 and B*2705 peptide motifs. Immunogenetics 39: 74–77.

47. Ramos M, Paradela A, Vazquez M, Marina A, Vazquez J, et al. (2002) Differential association of HLA-B*2705 and B*2709 to ankylosing spondylitis correlates with limited peptide subsets but not with altered cell surface stability. J Biol Chem 277: 28749–28756.

48. van Gunsteren WF, Daura X, Mark AE (2002) Computation of Free Energy. Helv Chim Acta 85: 3113–3129.

49. Ellis SA, Taylor C, McMichael A (1982) Recognition of HLA-B27 and related antigen by a monoclonal antibody. Hum Immunol 5: 49–59.

50. Stam NJ, Spits H, Ploegh HL (1986) Monoclonal antibodies raised against denatured HLA-B locus heavy chain permit biochemical characterization of certain HLA-C locus products. J Immunol 137: 2299–2306.

51. Kjer-Nielsen L, Clements CS, Brooks AG, Purcell AW, Fontes MR, et al. (2002) The structure of HLA-B8 complexed to an immunodominant viral determinant: peptide-induced conformational changes and a mode of MHC class I dimerization. J Immunol 169: 5153–5160.

52. Reid SW, McAdam S, Smith KJ, Klenerman P, O'Callaghan CA, et al. (1996) Antagonist HIV-1 Gag peptides induce structural changes in HLA B8. J Exp Med 184: 2279–2286.

53. Webb AI, Borg NA, Dunstone MA, Kjer-Nielsen L, Beddoe T, et al. (2004) The structure of H-2K(b) and K(bm8) complexed to a herpes simplex virus determinant: evidence for a conformational switch that governs T cell repertoire selection and viral resistance. J Immunol 173: 402–409.

54. Gomez P, Mavian C, Galocha B, Garcia-Medel N, López de Castro JA (2009) Presentation of cytosolically stable peptides by HLA-B27 is not dependent on the canonic interactions of N-terminal basic residues in the A pocket. J Immunol 182: 446–455.

55. Bowness P, Allen R, McMichael AJ (1994) Identification of T cell receptor recognition residues for a viral peptide presented by HLA B27. Eur J Immunol 24: 2357–2363.

56. Narzi D, Winkler K, Saidowsky J, Misselwitz R, Ziegler A, et al. (2008) Molecular determinants of major histocompatibility complex class I complex stability. J Biol Chem 283: 23093–23103.

57. Vriend G (1990) WHAT IF: A molecular modeling and drug design program. J Mol Graph 8: 52–56.

58. Hess B, Kutzner C, van der Spoel D, Lindahl E (2008) GROMACS 4: Algorithms for highly efficient, load-balanced, and scalable molecular simulation. J Chem Theory Comput 4: 435–447.

59. Kaminski GA, Friesner RA, Tirado-Rives J, Jorgensen WL (2001) Evaluation and reparametrization of the OPLS-AA force field for proteins via comparison with accurate quantum chemical calculations on peptides. J Phys Chem B 105: 6474–6487.

60. Jorgensen WL, Chandrasekhar J, Madura JD, Impey RW, Klein ML (1983) Comparison of simple potential functions for simulating liquid water. J Chem Phys 79: 926–935.

61. Darden TA, York DM, Pedersen LG (1993) Particle mesh Ewald: "An N log(N) method for Ewald sums in large systems". J Chem Phys 98: 10089–10092.

62. Hess B, Bekker H, Berendsen HJC, Fraaije JGEM (1997) LINCS: a linear constraint solver for molecular simulations. J Comp Chem 18: 1463–1472.

63. Berendsen HJC, Postma JPM, van Gunsteren W, Di Nola A, Haak JR (1984) Molecular dynamics with coupling to an external bath. J Chem Phys 81: 3684–3690.

64. Nurzia E, Panimolle F, Cauli A, Mathieu A, Magnacca A, et al. (2010) CD8+ T-cell mediated self–reactivity in HLA-B27 context as a consequence of dual peptide conformation. Clin Immunol 135: 476–482.

# 12

# Unplanned Reoperation within 30 Days of Fusion Surgery for Spinal Deformity

**Zheng Li, Jianxiong Shen\*, Guixing Qiu, Haiquan Yu, Yipeng Wang, Jianguo Zhang, Hong Zhao, Yu Zhao, Shugang Li, Xisheng Weng, Jinqian Liang, Lijuan Zhao**

Department of Orthopaedic Surgery, Peking Union Medical College Hospital, Chinese Academy of Medical Sciences & Peking Union Medical College, Beijing, China

## Abstract

No recent studies have analyzed the rates of or reasons for unanticipated revision surgery within 30 days of primary surgery in spinal deformity patients. Our aim was to examine the incidence, characteristics, reasons, and risk factors for unplanned revision surgery in spinal deformity patients treated at one institution. All patients with a diagnosis of spinal deformity presenting for primary instrumented spinal fusion at a single institution from 1998 to 2012 were reviewed. All unplanned reoperations performed within 30 days after primary surgery were analyzed in terms of demographics, surgical data, and complications. Statistical analyses were performed to obtain correlations and risk factors for anticipated revision. Of 2758 patients [aged 16.07 years (range, 2–71), 69.8% female] who underwent spinal fusion surgery, 59 (2.1%) required reoperation within 30 days after primary surgery. The length of follow up for each patient was more than 30 days. Of those that required reoperation, 87.0% had posterior surgery only, 5.7% had anterior surgery, and 7.3% underwent an anteroposterior approach. The reasons for reoperation included implant failure (n = 20), wound infection (n = 12), neurologic deficit (n = 9), pulmonary complications (n = 17), and coronal plane imbalance (n = 1). The risk factors for reoperation were age, diagnosis, and surgical procedure with osteotomy.

**Editor:** Laxmaiah Manchikanti, University of Louisville, United States of America

**Funding:** This work was supported by National Natural Science Foundation of P.R. China (Grant Number: 81272053 and 81330044; http://www.nsfc.gov.cn/Portal0/default152.htm). The funders had no role in study design, data collection and analysis, decision to publish, or preparation of the manuscript.

**Competing Interests:** The authors have declared that no competing interests exist.

\* E-mail: shenjianxiong@medmail.com.cn

## Introduction

Patients with spinal deformity usually present with symptoms such as visible deformity, pain, progression of deformity, sagittal or coronal imbalance, and/or neural compromise [1]. Fusion surgery for spinal deformity is intended to be the final therapeutic intervention in the management of this condition [2]. The goals of surgical treatment are to obtain a stable and solid fusion after a safe and optimal 3-dimensional correction of the spinal deformity [3]. Achieving these goals should also improve the patients' quality of life in the long term, compared to those who did not undergo surgical treatment [4]. Optimal management of spinal deformity continues to challenge both patients and surgeons. Despite recent improvements in the efficacy and safety of spinal fusion, complications following surgical correction of scoliosis deformity remain a reality [5], and various potential problems requiring further surgical intervention may develop in the immediate postoperative period or over time [6].

Unplanned reoperation within 30 days of primary surgery has recently been suggested as a useful quality marker in hospitals performing spinal surgery [7]. Reoperation is associated with poor clinical outcomes, including higher risk of complications and implant failures [6,8]. In addition, the costs and the time associated with hospitalization for unplanned reoperation patients have been increasing [9]. A previous study reported that 7.5% of 452 cases of idiopathic scoliosis correction required reoperation [10,11]. Another study documented a 3.9% overall reoperation rate [12]. In cases of adult spinal deformity, the cumulative reoperation rate has been found to be 25.8% [13]. The reasons for reoperation include infection, pseudarthrosis, adjacent segment problems, implant failure, neurologic complications, and curve progression [11]. To our knowledge, however, the rate and causes of unplanned reoperation within 30 days after primary surgery have not been reported.

The objective of this study was, therefore, to determine the incidence and factors contributing to unplanned reoperation within 30 days of fusion surgery for spinal deformity in our department.

## Results

Between 1998 and 2012, a total of 2758 consecutive patients underwent spinal fusion for spinal deformity at our institution. The mean age at the time of initial surgery was 16.07±8.3 years (range, 2–71 years). Females made up 69.8% of the cases (n = 1925), and males made up 30.2% of the cases (n = 833). The majority of patients (n = 2400, 87.0%) were treated using a posterior approach and instrumented spinal fusion. A total of 202 (7.3%) patients underwent a combined anterior and posterior spinal fusion, and 156 (5.7%) had an instrumented anterior spinal fusion. There was no overall difference between the revision and non-revision groups with respect to age and gender (Table 1).

**Table 1.** Patient Characteristics of Cohort.

| | Reoperation (n = 59) | No operation (n = 2699) | p |
|---|---|---|---|
| Age (range) | 17.86±9.0 (2–55) | 16.07±8.2 (2–71) | p>0.05 |
| Sex | | | p>0.05 |
| Female | 33 | 1870 | |
| Male | 26 | 829 | |
| Max cobb | 69°±16° | 68°±1.9° | p>0.05 |
| Mean levels fused | 11.3±2.9 | 11.3±3.9 | p>0.05 |

## Reasons for Reoperation

Of the 2758 patients identified as having primary surgery for spinal deformity, 59 patients (2.1%) underwent reoperation within 30 days of primary surgery for scoliosis. Table 2 illustrates the percentages of patients in the reoperation group and the cohort as a whole with respect to the reason for revision.

Twenty repeat operations were performed due to implant-related failures. Of these, 6 (30%) were due to pullout of the hooks, 6 were because of improper implant location, 6 were due to loosening of pedicle screws, and 2 were due to screw cap loosening (Fig. 1, 2, and 3).

Infection was only noted in patients who underwent posterior spinal instrumentation and fusion as the index procedure; no infections occurred after anterior spinal instrumentation. This difference was significant (p<0.001). In all, 59 reoperations due to infections were performed in 12 patients. Eight of these 12 cases were due to deep wound infections, and four were due to superficial wound infections. The implants were not removed in any of these patients following the reoperation.

Nine revisions were performed because of the patient's neurologic deficit, 6 revisions were due to paraplegia, and 3 revisions were due to nerve root injury. Of the 6 patients who presented with paraplegia, 4 presented with complete paralysis of the lower extremity, and 2 presented with incomplete paralysis of the lower extremity.

Reoperations were performed in 17 patients due to pulmonary complications. Eight of these patients returned to the operating room for hydrothorax, 5 for hemothorax, 2 for pneumothorax and 2 for chylothorax.

One revision was performed for coronal plane imbalance.

## Sex, Age, Diagnosis and Surgical Approach

The breakdown of the primary diagnoses is as follows: 1255 (45.5%) IS, 1039 (37.8%) congenital scoliosis, 182 (6.6%)

**Table 2.** Reoperation Reasons.

| Reason for Reoperation | Reoperations (%) | Total patients (%) |
|---|---|---|
| implant failure | 20/59 (33.9%) | 20/2758 (0.73%) |
| infection | 12/59 (20.3%) | 12/2758 (0.44%) |
| neurologic deficit | 9/59 (15.3%) | 9/2758 (0.37%) |
| pulmonary complications | 17/59 (28.9%) | 17/2758 (0.62%) |
| coronal plane imbalance | 1/59 (1.7%) | 1/2758 (0.04%) |
| Total | 59/59 (100%) | 59/2758 (2.1%) |

neuromuscular scoliosis, 79 (2.9%) neurofibromatosis scoliosis, 101 (3.7%) degenerative scoliosis, 51 (1.8%) Marfan syndrome with scoliosis and 51 (1.8%) other (syndrome-related scoliosis, ankylosing spondylitis, achondroplasia with scoliosis). Patients with Marfan syndrome with scoliosis had a much higher rate of reoperation (7.84%) and had a significantly higher rate of reoperation when compared with the idiopathic scoliosis group (p = 0.0001) and the neuromuscular scoliosis group (p = 0.007). Patients with congenital scoliosis had a much higher rate of reoperation when compared with the idiopathic scoliosis group (P = 0.0001) (Table 3 and Figure 4).

We found a significant difference in the rates of reoperation based on gender. The reoperation rate was 3.0% (26/833) for males and 1.71% (33/1925) for females (P = 0.019). Patients were divided into two age groups: ≤19 years and >19 years. We found significantly fewer reoperations in the ≤19-year-old group compared with the >19-year-old group (p = 0.006) (Table 4).

The reoperation rate by surgical approach is listed in Table 4. There was a non-statistically significant increase in reoperation rates for patients having combined anteroposterior segmental fusion when compared with anterior or posterior fusion alone (p = 0.634). When patients were group according to whether osteotomy was performed in the operation, osteoectomy group had a higher rate of reoperation compared to non-osteoectomy group (p = 0.01). The most common reasons for repeat surgery in patients who underwent posterior instrumentation and fusion were implant failure, pulmonary complications, and wound infection. For anterior surgery, the most common reason for repeat surgery was pulmonary complications. For combined anteroposterior surgery, the most common reason for reoperation was implant failure.

Analysis of the reasons for neural complications indicated that patients with Marfan syndrome with scoliosis had the highest rate of neural complications and had a significantly higher rate when compared to the idiopathic scoliosis group (p = 0.01). The congenital scoliosis group also had a significantly higher rate when compared to the idiopathic scoliosis group (p = 0.03) (Table 5). When patients were group according to whether osteoectomy was performed during the operation, the osteoectomy group had a higher rate of reoperation for neural complications compared to non-osteoectomy group (p = 0.01) (Table 5).

## Discussion

Unplanned reoperations represent major events for patients and have considerable impacts on the healthcare system, especially when the reoperations occur within 30 days after the initial surgery [14–16]. Reoperation rate has been used as a criterion for evaluating surgical department practice and even overall hospital care [17]. Unplanned reoperations increase the burden on the healthcare system as they result in operating theatre occupation, affect surgical waiting lists and lead to longer hospital stays and therefore higher costs [18]. These procedures can have an impact on staff trust and self-confidence. Although several studies have analyzed the rates of long-term reoperation after primary surgery for spinal deformity, the incidence and factors contributing to unplanned reoperation within 30 days of fusion surgery for spinal deformity have not been previously reported. This retrospective study is the first to provide data on the incidence and factors contributing to unplanned reoperation within 30 days of fusion surgery for spinal deformity. The overall unplanned reoperation rate within 30 days of primary surgery for spinal deformity in our study was 2.1%. There was no difference in patients' characteristics regarding age, gender, maximum Cobb measurement, and

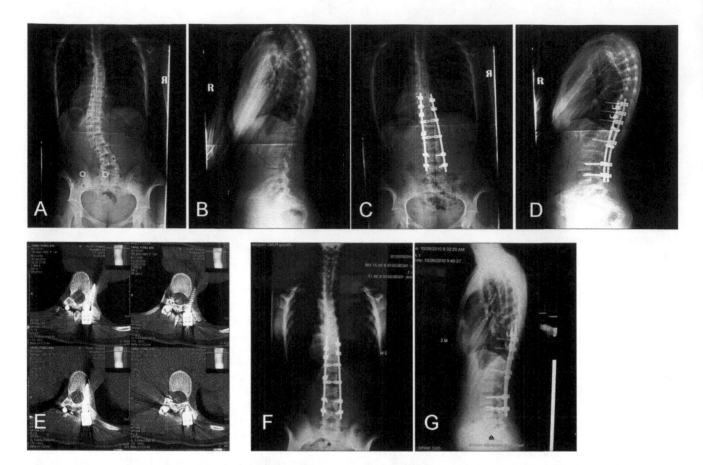

**Figure 1. Patient is a 15 year-old female with Marfan syndrome with scoliosis.** A and B, Standing preoperative anteroposterior and lateral radiographs. C and D, Standing anteroposterior and lateral radiographs 4 days after operation. E, Magnetic resonance images, showing improper implant location. F and G, Standing anteroposterior and lateral radiographs 4 days after reoperation.

mean number of levels fused. The most common reasons for repeat surgery within 30 days of initial surgery were implant-related failures, pulmonary complications, wound infection, and neurologic deficits. Age older than 18 years, congenital scoliosis, syndrome-related spine deformity and inclusion of osteoectomy in the operation were risk factors for unplanned reoperation within 30 days of fusion surgery for spinal deformity.

A number of studies have been published investigating the rate of surgical revisions after spinal deformity surgery. In a retrospective review of patients who underwent instrumented spinal fusion for primary adult spinal deformity, Pichelmann et al reported a revision rate of 9.0% with a mean time to revision of 4.0 years with 45% of the revisions occurring within the first 2 years [13]. The most common reason for revision was pseudarthrosis, with wound infection as the second most common reason. In our study, implant-related failure was the most common reason for revision. Implant failure remains a major surgical challenge in the correction of spinal deformity. Aside from technical error and improper instrumentation, poor quality of bone and its structure are the main causes of implant failure. In our series, the implant-related failure complications requiring reoperation included hook pull-out, improper implant location, pedicle screw loosening, and screw cap loosening.

Postoperative spine infection is a complication that may have a significant impact on clinical outcome and is an important consideration in surgical decision-making [19,20]. Therefore, optimal prevention and management of infection reflects not only

a well-coordinated multidisciplinary team and an experienced surgeon but also the quality of the entire institution. Many series report postoperative infections as the most prevalent indication for repeat surgery, with the prevalence of infection after scoliosis surgery being 4.7% [21,22]. Our series contained five superficial wound infections and 13 deep wound infections that required repeat surgery. In line with previous studies, all of the infections were observed in patients whose index procedure was posterior spinal instrumentation and fusion. No infections occurred following anterior spinal instrumentation.

Previous studies have reported that no reoperations were needed for neurologic complications [23]. In our series, however, 9 revisions were due to neurologic deficit: 6 of which were due to paraplegia and 3 were due to nerve root injury. Of the 6 patients who presented with paraplegia, 4 presented with complete paralysis of the lower extremity and 2 presented with incomplete paralysis of the lower extremity.

Pulmonary complication was the next most common reason for readmission [23,24]. This complication includes hydrothorax, hemothorax, pneumothorax and chylothorax. Surgical technique has a significant influence on postoperative pulmonary complications. Anderson et al. found that the incidence of postoperative pulmonary complications in patients who underwent anterior fusion was 3 times that in patients who underwent posterior fusion. In our study, however, we found no significant difference between the surgical approaches.

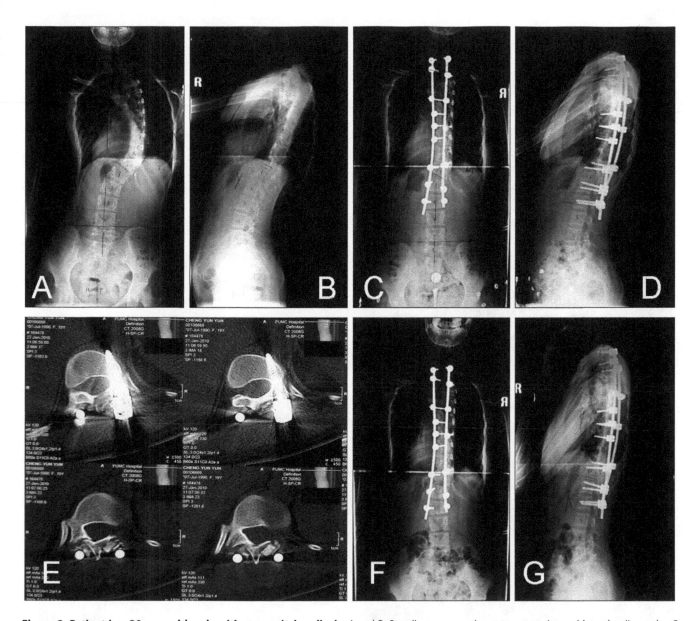

**Figure 2. Patient is a 20 year-old male with congenital scoliosis.** A and B, Standing preoperative anteroposterior and lateral radiographs. C and D, Standing anteroposterior and lateral radiographs 4 days after operation. E, Magnetic resonance images showing improper implant location. F and G, Standing anteroposterior and lateral radiographs 5 days after reoperation.

It is important to be able to identify the risk factors for developing complications that could require revision surgery within 30 days after initial surgery; the precise knowledge of reoperation risks is valuable information for both patients and surgeons. Previous studies have shown that older age, increased body mass index, and osteopenia are significant risk factors for developing a complication [14,25]. Mok et al [9] identified risk factors for infection (age, diabetes, hypothyroidism, and surgeon's experience) and adjacent segment decompensation (age, smoking, and cardiac comorbidity). The current study represents, to our knowledge, the first analysis of risk factors for readmission within 30 days after initial surgery for spinal deformity. In accordance with the data of previous authors [9], patient age over 18 years conferred a risk of developing a complication that required reoperation 1.8 times higher than those younger than 18. Congenital scoliosis and Marfan syndrome with scoliosis presented

a significantly higher revision rate than other spinal deformities. Furthermore, with regard to the reasons for neural complications, patients with congenital scoliosis and syndrome-related scoliosis also had a higher rate when compared to the other groups. Moreover, no statistically significant difference was found in the reoperation rate based on the surgical approach. Patients whose surgery included osteoectomy had a higher rate of reoperation compared to the non-osteoectomy group.

In conclusion, this is the first study to provide insight into the incidence and factors contributing to unplanned reoperation within 30 days of fusion surgery for spinal deformity. The rate of unanticipated revision surgery within 30 days after primary surgery is 2.1%. The reasons for reoperation included implant-related failures, pulmonary complications, infections, neurologic deficit and coronal plane imbalance. The importance of comorbidities often present in this patient population is highlighted by

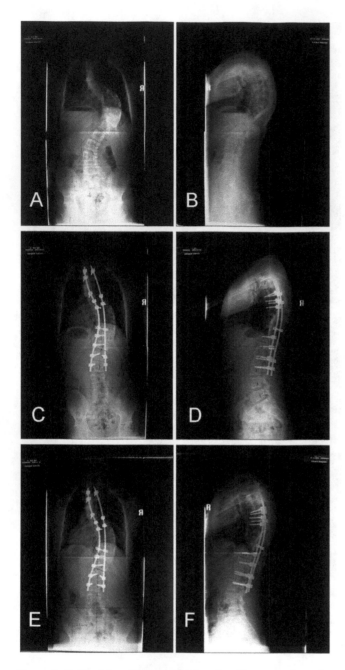

**Figure 3. Patient is a 16 year-old female with neuromuscular scoliosis.** A and B, Standing preoperative anteroposterior and lateral radiographs. C and D, Standing anteroposterior and lateral radiographs 4 days after operation showing pedicle screw loosening. E and F, Standing anteroposterior and lateral radiographs 5 days after reoperation.

the significantly elevated risks found with increasing age, congenital scoliosis and Marfan syndrome with scoliosis as well as inclusion of osteoectomy in the operation. The information contained in this report will assist surgeons with preoperative risk stratification and facilitate discussions with patients to make informed choices in surgical decision-making.

**Table 3.** Diagnosis and Reoperation Rates.

| Diagnosis | Reoperation | No Reoperation | Rate | Total |
|---|---|---|---|---|
| Congenital scoliosis | 34 | 1005 | 3.27% | 1039 |
| Idiopathic scoliosis | 14 | 1241 | 1.12% | 1255 |
| Neuromuscular scoliosis | 2 | 180 | 1.10% | 182 |
| Neurofibromatosis with scoliosis | 2 | 77 | 2.53% | 79 |
| Degenerative scoliosis | 2 | 99 | 1.98% | 101 |
| Marfan syndrome with scoliosis | 4 | 47 | 7.84% | 51 |
| Others | 1 | 50 | 1.96% | 51 |
| Total | 59 | 2699 | 2.14% | 2758 |

Others include syndrome-related scoliosis, ankylosing spondylitis, achondroplasia with scoliosis.

## Materials and Methods

### Ethics statement

All of these protocols were approved by the Clinical Research Ethics Committee of the Peking Union Medical College Hospital. Data were obtained from surgical patients after obtaining approval from the Clinical Research Ethics Committee of the Peking Union Medical College Hospital and fully informed written consent from the patients or patients' parents.

### Patient Population

We retrospectively reviewed a prospectively collected database at our institution to identify patients who underwent a definitive spinal fusion between 1998 and 2012 for a diagnosis of spinal

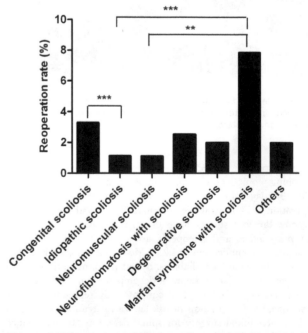

**Figure 4. Diagnosis and Reoperation Rates.** The statistically significant differences compared with the control are noted as *p<0.05, **p<0.01 and ***p<0.001. Others include syndrome-related scoliosis, ankylosing spondylitis, achondroplasia with scoliosis.

**Table 4.** Risk factors for reoperation.

| | Reoperation within 30 days | No reoperation | Total | Reoperation rate (%) | P |
|---|---|---|---|---|---|
| Sex | | | | | 0.019 |
| Male | 26 | 807 | 833 | 3.12 | |
| Female | 33 | 1892 | 1925 | 1.71 | |
| Age | | | | | 0.006 |
| ≤19years | 42 | 2279 | 2321 | 1.81 | |
| >19 years | 17 | 420 | 437 | 3.89 | |
| Procedure | | | | | 0.006 |
| Osteotomy | 21 | 562 | 583 | 3.74 | |
| No Osteotomy | 38 | 2137 | 2175 | 1.78 | |
| Kyphosis | | | | | 0.613 |
| Kyphosis | 2 | 64 | 66 | 3.13 | |
| Without kyphosis | 57 | 2635 | 2692 | 2.16 | |
| surgical approach | | | | | 0.634 |
| Anterior | 4 | 152 | 156 | 2.56 | |
| Posterior | 49 | 2351 | 2400 | 2.04 | |
| Combined | 6 | 196 | 202 | 2.90 | |

deformity. Spinal deformity was defined as any major coronal, sagittal, or combined deformity requiring instrumented fusion. We excluded patients who underwent spinal deformity surgery for other etiologies, such as acute vertebral fracture, spinal tumor, active infection, paraplegia, and those who had previously undergone primary surgery. The length of follow up for each patient was more than 30 days. A revision or reoperation surgery within 30 days of fusion surgery was defined as any unanticipated return to the operating room after the index procedure. All surgeries were performed by the senior author.

## Data Collection

Patients' names, dates of birth, genders, medical record numbers, diagnoses, dates of surgery, ages at surgery, approaches (anterior, posterior, or combined), and types of implants were recorded in the surgical logs. All subsequent reoperations at our institution were also recorded, and chart reviews were performed to ensure that no patients had undergone a known reoperation at another institution. The primary reason for the reoperation was recorded. If, for some reason, there appeared to be two or more possible factors responsible for further surgery, the predominant factor was chosen as the reason for reoperation and used in subsequent analyses. The reasons for reoperation were categorized into one of the following groups: (1) implant failure, (2) wound infection, (3) neurologic deficit (4) pulmonary complications, or (5) coronal plane imbalance. The decision to reoperate was based on the clinical judgment of the treating surgeon.

**Table 5.** Risk factors for reoperation for neurologic deficit.

| | Reoperation for neurologic deficit within 30 days | Reoperation within 30 days | No reoperation | Total | Reoperation rate (%) | P |
|---|---|---|---|---|---|---|
| Procedure | | | | | | 0.01 |
| Osteotomy | 6 | 21 | 562 | 583 | 1.03 | |
| No Osteotomy | 3 | 38 | 2137 | 2175 | 0.14 | |
| Diagnosis | | | | | | 0.09 |
| Congenital scoliosis | 6 | 34 | 1005 | 1039 | 0.58 | 0.03* |
| Idiopathic scoliosis | 1 | 14 | 1241 | 1255 | 0.14 | |
| Neuromuscular scoliosis | 0 | 2 | 180 | 182 | 0 | |
| Neurofibromatosis with scoliosis | 0 | 2 | 77 | 79 | 0 | |
| Degenerative scoliosis | 1 | 2 | 99 | 101 | 0.99 | |
| Marfan syndrome with scoliosis | 1 | 4 | 47 | 51 | 1.96 | 0.01* |
| Others | 0 | 1 | 50 | 51 | 0 | |

*When compared to idiopathic scoliosis group.

## Statistical Analysis

Statistical analyses were performed using Student's $t$-test for continuous variables and the Fisher exact test and $X^2$ test for categorical variables. A P-value of <0.05 defined significance.

## References

1. Wiggns GC, Rauzzino MJ, Bartkowski HM, Nockels RP, Shaffrey CI (2001) Management of complex pediatric and adolescent spinal deformity. J Neurosurg 95: 17–24.
2. Lykissas MG, Jain VV, Nathan ST, Pawar V, Eismann EA, et al. (2013) Mid- to long-term outcomes in adolescent idiopathic scoliosis after instrumented posterior spinal fusion: a meta-analysis. Spine (Phila Pa 1976) 38: E113–119.
3. Csernatony Z, Kiss L, Mano S, Hunya Z (2013) Our experience and early results with a complementary implant for the correction of major thoracic curves. Eur Spine J.
4. Liang CZ, Li FC, Li H, Tao Y, Zhou X, et al. (2012) Surgery is an effective and reasonable treatment for degenerative scoliosis: a systematic review. J Int Med Res 40: 399–405.
5. Charosky S, Guigui P, Blamoutier A, Roussouly P, Chopin D (2012) Complications and risk factors of primary adult scoliosis surgery: a multicenter study of 306 patients. Spine (Phila Pa 1976) 37: 693–700.
6. Campos M, Dolan L, Weinstein S (2012) Unanticipated revision surgery in adolescent idiopathic scoliosis. Spine (Phila Pa 1976) 37: 1048–1053.
7. McSorley S, Lowndes C, Sharma P, Macdonald A (2013) Unplanned reoperation within 30 days of surgery for colorectal cancer in NHS Lanarkshire. Colorectal Dis 15: 689–694.
8. Lehman RA Jr (2011) Postoperative lymphocele after revision circumferential long-segment scoliosis construct for pseudarthrosis. Spine J 11: 684–685.
9. Mok JM, Cloyd JM, Bradford DS, Hu SS, Deviren V, et al. (2009) Reoperation after primary fusion for adult spinal deformity: rate, reason, and timing. Spine (Phila Pa 1976) 34: 832–839.
10. Ramo BA, Richards BS (2012) Repeat surgical interventions following "definitive" instrumentation and fusion for idiopathic scoliosis: five-year update on a previously published cohort. Spine (Phila Pa 1976) 37: 1211–1217.
11. Sponseller PD (2010) Pediatric revision spinal deformity surgery: issues and complications. Spine (Phila Pa 1976) 35: 2205–2210.
12. Richards BS, Hasley BP, Casey VF (2006) Repeat surgical interventions following "definitive" instrumentation and fusion for idiopathic scoliosis. Spine (Phila Pa 1976) 31: 3018–3026.
13. Pichelmann MA, Lenke LG, Bridwell KH, Good CR, O'Leary PT, et al. (2010) Revision rates following primary adult spinal deformity surgery: six hundred forty-three consecutive patients followed-up to twenty-two years postoperative. Spine (Phila Pa 1976) 35: 219–226.
14. Rama-Maceiras P, Rey-Rilo T, Moreno-Lopez E, Molins-Gauna N, Sanduende-Otero Y, et al. (2011) Unplanned surgical reoperations in a tertiary hospital: perioperative mortality and associated risk factors. Eur J Anaesthesiol 28: 10–15.
15. Mukerji N, Jenkins A, Nicholson C, Mitchell P (2012) Unplanned reoperation rates in pediatric neurosurgery: a single center experience and proposed use as a quality indicator. J Neurosurg Pediatr 9: 665–669.
16. Price JD, Romeiser JL, Gnerre JM, Shroyer AL, Rosengart TK (2013) Risk analysis for readmission after coronary artery bypass surgery: developing a strategy to reduce readmissions. J Am Coll Surg 216: 412–419.
17. Almoudaris AM, Burns EM, Bottle A, Aylin P, Darzi A, et al. (2013) Single measures of performance do not reflect overall institutional quality in colorectal cancer surgery. Gut 62: 423–429.
18. Froschl U, Sengstbratl M, Huber J, Fugger R (2006) Unplanned reoperations for infection complications: a survey for quality control. Surg Infect (Larchmt) 7: 263–268.
19. Muschik M, Luck W, Schlenzka D (2004) Implant removal for late-developing infection after instrumented posterior spinal fusion for scoliosis: reinstrumentation reduces loss of correction. A retrospective analysis of 45 cases. Eur Spine J 13: 645–651.
20. Mok JM, Guillaume TJ, Talu U, Berven SH, Deviren V, et al. (2009) Clinical outcome of deep wound infection after instrumented posterior spinal fusion: a matched cohort analysis. Spine (Phila Pa 1976) 34: 578–583.
21. Sponseller PD, Shah SA, Abel MF, Newton PO, Letko L, et al. (2010) Infection rate after spine surgery in cerebral palsy is high and impairs results: multicenter analysis of risk factors and treatment. Clin Orthop Relat Res 468: 711–716.
22. Theiss SM, Lonstein JE, Winter RB (1996) Wound infections in reconstructive spine surgery. Orthop Clin North Am 27: 105–110.
23. Carreon LY, Puno RM, Lenke LG, Richards BS, Sucato DJ, et al. (2007) Non-neurologic complications following surgery for adolescent idiopathic scoliosis. J Bone Joint Surg Am 89: 2427–2432.
24. Davis MA (2009) Posterior spinal fusion versus anterior/posterior spinal fusion for adolescent idiopathic scoliosis: a decision analysis. Spine (Phila Pa 1976) 34: 2318–2323.
25. Pateder DB, Park YS, Kebaish KM, Cascio BM, Buchowski JM, et al. (2006) Spinal fusion after revision surgery for pseudarthrosis in adult scoliosis. Spine (Phila Pa 1976) 31: E314–319.

## Author Contributions

Conceived and designed the experiments: ZL JS. Performed the experiments: ZL JS GQ YW JZ HZ YZ SL XW JL LZ HY. Analyzed the data: ZL LZ. Contributed reagents/materials/analysis tools: ZL JS. Wrote the paper: ZL JS.

# 13

# IL23R Gene Confers Susceptibility to Ankylosing Spondylitis Concomitant with Uveitis in a Han Chinese Population

**Hongtao Dong[1]\*, Qiuming Li[1], Ying Zhang[2], Wei Tan[2]\*, Zhengxuan Jiang[3]\***

1 Department of Ophthalmology, the First Affiliated Hospital of Zhengzhou University, Zhengzhou, China, 2 Department of Ophthalmology, The First People's Hospital of Zunyi, The Third Affiliated Hospital of Zunyi Medical University, Zunyi, China, 3 Department of Ophthalmology, the Second Affiliated Hospital of Anhui Medical University, Hefei, China

## Abstract

**Purpose:** The interleukin-23 receptor (IL-23R) has been shown to be associated with ankylosing spondylitis (AS) in many different populations. This study examined whether IL-23R polymorphisms were associated with susceptibility to this disease in a Chinese Han population.

**Methods:** Three single-nucleotide polymorphisms (SNP), rs7517847, rs11209032, and rs17375018, were genotyped in 291 AS patients and 312 age-, sex-, and ethnically matched healthy controls using a polymerase chain reaction (PCR) restriction fragment length polymorphism (RFLP) assay.

**Results:** The genotype and allele frequencies of rs17375018, rs7517847, and rs11209032 were not different between the patients with AS and the healthy controls. On the one hand, stratification analysis indicated that the rs17375018 GG genotype and the G allele were increased in AS patients who were HLA-B27 positive (corrected $p = 0.024$, odds ratio [OR] 2.35, 95% CI 1.30–4.24; $p_c = 0.006$, OR 1.98, 95% CI 1.28–3.07, respectively). On the other hand, the analysis according to clinical characteristics showed a significantly increased prevalence of the homozygous rs17375018 GG genotype and the G allele in patients with AS and uveitis compared with the controls ($p_c = 0.024$ and $p_c = 0.024$, respectively). In addition, haplotype analysis performed with the SHEsis platform revealed no significant difference concerning the haplotypes between AS patients and healthy controls.

**Conclusions:** In this study, the results suggested that the rs17375018 of IL23R was positively associated with HLA-B27-positive AS and that the rs17375018 GG of IL-23R was associated with AS concomitant with uveitis. We found no evidence for an association between the other two SNPs of IL-23R and AS.

**Editor:** James T. Rosenbaum, Oregon Health & Science University, United States of America

**Funding:** This work was supported by the Foundation for health science and technology innovative talents of Henan province, china (4107); the Governor Foundation of Special Research of Clinical Application in Guizhou Province, 2012(131); the Key project of Natural Science Foundation of Higher Educational Bureau of Anhui Province (KJ2013A), the Foundation of Anhui Medical University (2012xkj053). The funders had no role in study design, data collection and analysis, decision to publish, or preparation of the manuscript.

**Competing Interests:** The authors have declared that no competing interests exist.

\* E-mail: jzx1287@163.com (ZJ); dhtkidy@126.com (HD); tanwei950118@sina.com (WT)

## Introduction

Ankylosing spondylitis (AS) is a chronic inflammatory disease characterized by a diverse spectrum of clinical manifestations, including the alteration of joint architecture, joint fusions, and functional impairment in the sacroiliac and spine joint [1,2]. The exact pathogenesis and the etiology of AS are not fully understood. Many studies have suggested that genetic factors and certain environmental factors are involved in its development [3,4,5]. The idea that genetic factors are strongly implicated in the pathogenesis of this disease is supported by twins having a much higher risk of developing AS [5]. Previous studies revealed that AS was strongly associated with the human leukocyte antigen B-27 allele (HLA-B27) in different populations [6,7]. However, HLA-B27 only partly accounts for the genetic predisposition to AS. Another study revealed that non-HLA genes may be involved in the development of AS [7]. Therefore, studies have been initiated to search for non-HLA genes. Studies found that immune-related genes such as endoplasmic reticulum aminopeptidase [8,9], interleukin-23 receptor (IL23R) [10,11], and interleukin-1 (IL-1) [12] were associated with AS in different populations. These results have provided useful information on the genetic predisposition to AS.

As both innate and adaptive immune responses and inflammatory mediators are involved in the pathogenesis of AS [7], molecules involved in the regulation of autoimmunity and inflammation are thought to represent good candidate genes. The interleukin-23 receptor (IL23R) gene is located on chromosome 1p31 and highly expressed in dendritic cells [13,14]. IL23R and its ligand, IL-23, are key components of the immune-regulatory pathway. Recently, studies have shown that some single nucleotide polymorphisms (SNPs) of the *IL23R* gene are strongly associated with several autoimmune diseases, such as Crohn's disease [15], rheumatoid arthritis [16], AS, and Behcet's disease. Therefore, we wanted to test whether *IL23R* gene polymorphisms are associated with AS in a Chinese Han population.

This case-control study was designed to test the association between specific variants of *IL23R* and the risk for AS. Three SNPs, rs17375018, rs11209032, and rs7517847, were investigated.

## Patients and Healthy Controls

### Study Population

A total of 291 AS patients and 312 healthy controls were recruited from The Third Affiliated Hospital of Zunyi Medical University. Both the patients and the controls were from a Chinese Han population. The control population consisted of unrelated healthy individuals from the same geographical regions as where the AS patients came from, and they were age-, sex-, and ethnically matched with the patients. The patients with AS were diagnosed according to the New York modified criteria [17]. The clinical characteristics of the AS patients were assessed at the time of diagnosis and summarized in Table 1. The study was approved by the local institutional ethics committee of The Third Affiliated Hospital of Zunyi Medical University. All procedures followed the tenets of the Declaration of Helsinki. Written informed consent was obtained from all the subjects. After obtaining the written informed consent, we took 5 ml of peripheral blood from each participant.

### SNP Selection and Genotyping

Blood samples were collected in EDTA tubes and kept at −70°C until use. Genomic DNA was extracted from the peripheral blood by the QIAamp DNA Blood Mini Kit (Qiagen, Hilden, Germany). We selected rs17375018 in this study because this SNP was found to be associated with Behcet's disease in Chinese and Japanese populations [18,19]. The rs7517847 and rs11209032 SNPs were chosen because they have been shown to be associated with certain immune-related diseases [15,20]. Amplification of the target DNA was performed by polymerase chain reaction (PCR). The PCR primers and restriction enzymes used in the present study were as described in a recent study [18]. The primers used in this study are presented in Table 2. A 5 μl reaction mixture, which consisted of 2.5 μl Premix Taq (Ex Taq Version; TaKaRa Biotechnology Co. Ltd., Dalian, China), 20 pmoles primers, and 0.2 μg of genomic DNA, was amplified by PCR. The conditions were as follows: initial denaturation at 95°C

for 5 min, followed by 38 cycles of denaturation at 94°C for 30 s, annealing at different temperatures (61°C for rs11209032, 55°C for 17375018, and 58°C for 7517847) for 30 s, extension at 72°C for 30 s, and a final extension at 72°C for 5 min. These SNPs were genotyped by PCR restriction fragment length polymorphism (RFLP) analysis. The PCR products of the rs11209032, rs17375018, and rs7517847 polymorphisms were digested with 4 U of XspI (TaKaRa, Dalian, China), BsurI (New England Biolabs, Inc, Ontario, Canada), and Ec0147I (New England Biolabs, Inc, Ontario, Canada) restriction enzymes (Table 2) in a 10 μl reaction volume overnight. The digestion products were visualized on a 3.5% agarose gel and stained with GoldView™ (SBS Genetech, Beijing, China). Direct sequencing was also performed by the Invitrogen Biotechnology Company using randomly selected subjects (20% of all samples) to validate the method used in this study.

### Statistical Analysis

The Hardy–Weinberg equilibrium (HWE) was tested using the $\chi^2$ test. The genotype frequencies were estimated by direct counting. The allele and the genotype frequencies were compared between the patients and the controls by the $\chi^2$ test using SPSS (version 10.0; SPSS Inc., Chicago, IL). Haplotype analysis was performed with the SHEsis platform [21]. The P values were corrected ($p_c$) with the Bonferroni correction by multiplying the P value with the number of analyses performed. $p_c < 0.05$ was considered significant.

### Results

The AS patient cohort included 291consecutive subjects (165 male, 126 female), all of whom were from a Chinese Han population. The average age of the patients was 34.6±8.2 years. The healthy control group consisted of 312 subjects (169 male, 143 female), with an average age of 37.9±8.4 years. There was no statistical difference between the AS patients and the controls concerning age and gender. The clinical features of the investigated AS patients and the controls are shown in Table 1.

The results showed that the distribution of the tested *IL23R* SNP genotypes and the alleles did not deviate from the Hardy–Weinberg equilibrium. The genotype and the allele frequencies of the tested *IL23R* SNPs are shown in Table 3. The results revealed that there were no significant differences between the AS patients and the controls concerning the genotype and the allele frequencies of the tested SNPs. As many studies have demonstrated that *HLA-B27* is strongly associated with AS in many different populations, *HLA-B27* may influence the association between the *IL23R* polymorphisms and AS in this study. Therefore, the

**Table 1.** Clinical features of the investigated AS patients and controls.

| Clinical features | AS patients | | Healthy controls | |
|---|---|---|---|---|
| | Total (*n*=291)% | | Total (*n*=312) % | |
| Age at onset (years±S.D) | 34.6±8.2 | | 37.9±8.4 | |
| Male | 165 | 56.7 | 169 | 54.2 |
| Female | 126 | 43.3 | 143 | 45.8 |
| HLA-B27 | 216 | 69.2 | 58 | 16.0 |
| Uveitis | 163 | 56.3 | 0 | |
| Arthritis | 291 | 100 | 0 | |

**Table 2.** Primers and restriction enzymes used for RFLP analysis of the IL23R gene.

| SNP | Primers | Restriction enzyme |
|---|---|---|
| rs7517847 | 5'- CCTTTCACCTATTCCCAAGGCC -3' | ECO147I |
| | 5'- GGGCCTAGGAGACAGCCCATAA -3' | |
| rs11209032 | 5'- CTCCCTACATCACCCTCTTTGCACT -3' | XSPI |
| | 5'- TGATAAGGCAATCCGGTGGTTC -3' | |
| rs17375018 | 5'- TTTTTCCCATCTTCTTTCTTAA -3' | BSURI |
| | 5'- CGCCCAGCCCTCTTCTCTAATT -3' | |

patients were divided into *HLA-B27*-positive and negative groups. The frequencies of the alleles and the genotypes of the *IL23R* polymorphism in the *HLA-B27*-positive AS patients and the controls are shown in Table 4. The results showed that the frequencies of the rs17375018 GG genotype and the G allele in the AS patients who were *HLA-B27* positive were significantly increased compared to *HLA-B27*-positive controls ($p_c$ = 0.024, OR 2.35, 95% CI 1.30–4.24; $p_c$ = 0.006, OR 1.98, 95% CI 1.28–3.07, respectively). Stratification analysis did not show any association of the examined *IL23R* SNPs with the *HLA-B27*-negative patients (data not shown). Haplotype analysis was performed with the SHEsis platform, and no significant difference concerning the haplotypes between AS patients and healthy controls. (data not shown).

We further investigated whether the *IL23R* SNPs were associated with certain clinical features of AS. The analysis showed that the frequencies of the rs17375018 GG genotype and the G allele were significantly higher in AS patients with uveitis compared to the controls ($p_c$ = 0.024 and $p_c$ = 0.024, respectively). The results are shown in Table 5. The results did not show any association between the other two tested *IL23R* SNPs and uveitis.

## Discussion

Recently, many candidate gene-association studies have been carried out to identify non-*HLA* genes involved in susceptibility to AS. This study investigated whether polymorphisms of *IL23R* contributed to AS in a Chinese Han population. Although there were no significant differences between the AS patients and the controls concerning the genotype and allele frequencies of the tested SNPs, the results showed that rs17375018 in *IL23R* was associated with *HLA-B27*-positive AS. We further investigated whether the *IL23R* SNPs were associated with certain clinical characteristics of AS. The results revealed that rs17375018 was associated with AS concomitant with uveitis.

AS is one of a number of common inflammatory diseases, which result in severe occupational disability as the disease progresses [1].

The development of AS is associated with complex interactions between environmental factors and immune responses [3,6]. It is clear that genetic factors influence the immune responses and the progression of AS. IL23 is one of the master regulators of immunity. Studies have shown that IL23 promotes inflammatory responses by inducing the production of IL17, IL6, IL8, and tumor necrosis factor-α and that it regulates the amplification and the stability of Th17 lymphocytes [14,22], which are associated with strong pro-inflammatory responses and severe autoimmunity. Therefore, the IL23 pathway may be involved in the pathogenesis of AS. We selected the *IL23R* gene as a candidate gene mainly based on the following facts: First, *IL23R* is an important component of the IL23 pathway, and the interaction of *IL23R* with its ligand, IL23, can promote the production of IL17, which is known to be involved in many chronic inflammatory diseases [14,23]. Second, the association between *IL23R* and inflammatory diseases has been extensively studied in recent years [9,10,15]. The results of these studies in different populations are controversial and do not specify clearly whether the *IL23R* polymorphism is a risk factor or a protective factor for AS [8,9,10,24]. Third, there is little information on the relationship between the *IL23R* polymorphic variant and the risk of AS in this population. These data prompted us to investigate the association of IL23R polymorphisms and AS in a Chinese Han population.

There are many SNPs in the IL23R gene, and a few are involved in the development of the disease. The rs17375018 SNP was chosen based on a previous study, which showed that this SNP was associated with Behcet's disease, another common uveitis entity observed in China [18]. The rs7517847 and rs11209032 SNPs were selected as the candidate SNPs mainly because their association with AS, Crohn's disease, and other autoimmune diseases in different populations has been studied previously [10,18,20]. In this study, the results showed that the GG genotype and the G allele of rs17375018 were associated with AS concomitant with uveitis. This result is consistent with that reported in Behcet's disease in a Chinese Han population and a Japanese population [18,19]. However, the rs17375018 of IL23R

**Table 3.** Frequencies of alleles and genotypes of *IL23R* polymorphisms in AS patients and controls.

| SNP | Genotype Allele | AS (N=291) | Controls (N=312) | $\chi^2$ | P value | pc | OR (95% CI) |
|---|---|---|---|---|---|---|---|
| rs17375018 | AA | 18(6.2%) | 26(8.3%) | 1.027 | 0.311 | NS | 0.73(0.39–1.35) |
| | AG | 108(37.1%) | 136(43.6%) | 2.621 | 0.105 | NS | 0.76(0.55–1.06) |
| | GG | 165(56.7%) | 150(48.1%) | 4.488 | 0.034 | NS | 1.41(1.03–1.95) |
| | A | 144(24.7%) | 188(30.1%) | 4.379 | 0.036 | NS | 0.76(0.59–0.98) |
| | G | 438(75.3%) | 436(69.9%) | 4.379 | 0.036 | NS | 1.31(1.02–1.69) |
| rs7517847 | TT | 104(35.7%) | 98(31.4%) | 1.266 | 0.260 | NS | 1.21(0.87–1.70) |
| | GT | 146(50.2%) | 153(49.0%) | 0.077 | 0.781 | NS | 1.05(0.76–1.44) |
| | GG | 41(14.1%) | 61(19.6%) | 3.196 | 0.074 | NS | 0.68(0.44–1.04) |
| | G | 228(39.2%) | 275(44.1%) | 2.968 | 0.085 | NS | 0.82(0.65–1.03) |
| | T | 354(60.8%) | 349(55.9%) | 2.968 | 0.085 | NS | 1.22 (0.97–1.54) |
| rs11209032 | GG | 53(18.2%) | 59(18.9%) | 0.048 | 0.826 | NS | 0.96(0.63–1.44) |
| | AG | 150(51.5%) | 167(53.5%) | 0.237 | 0.627 | NS | 0.92(0.67–1.27) |
| | AA | 88(30.3%) | 86(27.6%) | 0.525 | 0.469 | NS | 1.14(0.80–1.62) |
| | A | 326 (56.0%) | 339(54.3%) | 0.346 | 0.556 | NS | 1.07(0.85–1.34) |
| | G | 256(44.0%) | 285(45.7%) | 0.346 | 0.556 | NS | 0.93(0.74–1.17) |

OR = odds ratio; 95% CI = 95% confidence interval; pc = Bonferroni corrected *P*; NS = not significant.

**Table 4.** Frequencies of alleles and genotypes of *IL23R* polymorphism in *HLA-B27*-positive AS patients and controls.

| SNP | Genotype | *HLA-B27+* | *HLA-B27+* | $\chi^2$ | *P* | $p_c$ | OR |
|---|---|---|---|---|---|---|---|
|  | Allele | Patients | controls |  | value |  | (95%CI) |
| rs17375018 | AA | 14(6.5%) | 8(13.8%) | 3.310 | 0.069 | NS | 0.43(0.17–1.09) |
|  | AG | 71(32.9%) | 27(46.6%) | 3.725 | 0.054 | NS | 0.56(0.31–1.01) |
|  | GG | 131(60.6%) | 23(39.7%) | 8.186 | 0.004 | 0.024 | 2.35(1.30–4.24) |
|  | A | 99(22.9%) | 43(37.1%) | 9.540 | 0.002 | 0.006 | 0.51(0.33–0.78) |
|  | G | 333(77.1%) | 73(62.9%) | 9.540 | 0.002 | 0.006 | 1.98(1.28–3.07) |
| rs7517847 | TT | 81(37.5%) | 22(37.9%) | 0.004 | 0.952 | NS | 0.98(0.54–1.79) |
|  | GT | 105(48.6%) | 30(51.7%) | 0.177 | 0.674 | NS | 0.88(0.49–1.58) |
|  | GG | 30(13.9%) | 6(10.3%) | 0.503 | 0.478 | NS | 1.40(0.55–3.54) |
|  | G | 165(38.2%) | 42(36.2%) | 0.154 | 0.695 | NS | 1.09(0.71–1.67) |
|  | T | 267(61.8%) | 74(63.8%) | 0.154 | 0.695 | NS | 0.92 (0.60–1.41) |
| rs11209032 | GG | 34(15.7%) | 11(18.9%) | 0.346 | 0.556 | NS | 0.80(0.38–1.69) |
|  | AG | 124(57.4%) | 32(55.2%) | 0.093 | 0.760 | NS | 1.10(0.61–1.96) |
|  | AA | 58(26.9%) | 15(25.9%) | 0.023 | 0.880 | NS | 1.05(0.54–2.04) |
|  | A | 240(55.6%) | 62(53.4%) | 0.164 | 0.685 | NS | 1.09(0.72–1.64) |
|  | G | 192(44.4%) | 54(46.6%) | 0.164 | 0.685 | NS | 0.92(0.61–1.39) |

OR = odds ratio; 95% CI = 95% confidence interval;
$p_c$ = Bonferroni corrected *P*; NS = not significant.

was not associated with Vogt-Koyanagi-Harada syndrome (VKH) in a Chinese population [25]. This study failed to find any association between rs7517847, rs11209032, and AS. Similarly, another study found no association between these SNPs and Crohn's disease in a Japanese population [26] and no association

**Table 5.** Frequencies of alleles and genotypes of *IL23R* polymorphism in AS patients with uveitis, without uveitis, and controls.

| SNP | Genotype | AS patients | AS patients | Controls | $p_c$ |
|---|---|---|---|---|---|
|  | allele | with uveitis | without uveitis |  |  |
| rs17375018 | AA | 10(6.1%) | 8(6.3%) | 26(8.3%) |  |
|  | AG | 52(31.9%) | 56(43.7%) | 136(43.6%) |  |
|  | GG | 101(61.0%) | 64(50.0%) | 150(48.1%) | 0.024 |
|  | A | 72(22.1%) | 72(28.1%) | 188(30.1%) |  |
|  | G | 254(77.9%) | 184(71.9%) | 436(69.9%) | 0.024 |
| rs7517847 | TT | 62(38.0%) | 42(32.8%) | 98(31.4%) |  |
|  | GT | 77(47.2%) | 69(53.9%) | 153(49.0%) |  |
|  | GG | 24(14.7%) | 17(13.3%) | 61(19.6%) |  |
|  | G | 125(39.2%) | 103(40.2%) | 275(44.1%) |  |
|  | T | 201(60.8%) | 153(59.8%) | 349(55.9%) |  |
| rs11209032 | GG | 32(19.6%) | 21(16.4%) | 59(18.9%) |  |
|  | AG | 81(49.7%) | 69(53.9%) | 167(53.5%) |  |
|  | AA | 50(30.7%) | 38(29.7%) | 86(27.6%) |  |
|  | A | 181 (55.5%) | 145(56.6%) | 339(54.3%) |  |
|  | G | 145(44.5%) | 111(43.4%) | 285(45.7%) |  |

$p_c$, AS patients with uveitis vs. healthy controls; $p_c$ = Bonferroni corrected *P*.

with VKH and Fuchs' syndrome in a Chinese population [25,27]. In contrast, the rs7517847 and rs11209032 SNPs have been reported to be associated with AS in a Spanish population and with Crohn's disease in a Caucasian population [15,20]. In common with our findings, a previous study showed that the *IL23R* gene was not associated with AS in a Chinese Han population [8]. Interestingly, when the patients were divided into two groups according to whether they were *HLA-B27* positive or negative, the rs17375018 of *IL23R* was associated with *HLA-B27*-positive AS. This result suggests that *IL23R* may play an important role in the pathogenesis of AS through *HLA-B27*. Further analysis of the clinical features and the *IL23R* polymorphisms suggested that rs17375018 was strongly associated with AS concomitant with uveitis which is an autoimmune disease. It reported that *HLA-B27* is associated with acute anterior uveitis [28,29,30]. Taken together, these data suggest that AS concomitant with uveitis and acute anterior uveitis may share a common genetic factor in this population.

Although the current study found an association between *IL23R* polymorphisms and AS concomitant with uveitis, some limitations need to be considered. First, the sample size influenced the power to detect disease susceptibility genes. Second, in addition to the relatively small size, all the subjects came from a Chinese Han population. The results of this study need to be confirmed using large sample sizes and multi-ethnic populations. Extensive studies are needed to clarify the functional role of the *IL23R* gene in the pathogenesis of AS. Additionally, this study only selected three SNPs. Other SNPs of the *IL23R* gene need to be tested in further research.

In summary, our study showed that the rs17375018 of *IL23R* was positively associated with *HLA-B27*-positive AS and that the rs17375018 GG of *IL23R* was associated with AS concomitant with uveitis. We did not find any association between the other two SNPs and AS in this Chinese Han population.

## Acknowledgments

Thanks to all donors enrolled in the present study.

## Author Contributions

Conceived and designed the experiments: ZJ HD WT. Performed the experiments: HD ZJ QL. Analyzed the data: WT YZ QL. Contributed reagents/materials/analysis tools: HD WT ZJ. Wrote the paper: HD ZJ.

## References

1. Braun J, Sieper J (2007) Ankylosing spondylitis. Lancet 369: 1379–1390.
2. Lories RJ, Luyten FP, de Vlam K (2009) Progress in spondylarthritis. Mechanisms of new bone formation in spondyloarthritis. Arthritis Res Ther 11: 221.
3. Tam LS, Gu J, Yu D (2010) Pathogenesis of ankylosing spondylitis. Nat Rev Rheumatol 6: 399–405.
4. Brown MA (2009) Genetics and the pathogenesis of ankylosing spondylitis. Curr Opin Rheumatol 21: 318–323.
5. Brown MA, Kennedy LG, MacGregor AJ, Darke C, Duncan E, et al. (1997) Susceptibility to ankylosing spondylitis in twins: the role of genes, HLA, and the environment. Arthritis Rheum 40: 1823–1828.
6. Reveille JD (2011) The genetic basis of spondyloarthritis. Ann Rheum Dis 70 Suppl 1: i44–50.
7. Brown MA (2006) Non-major-histocompatibility-complex genetics of ankylosing spondylitis. Best Pract Res Clin Rheumatol 20: 611–621.
8. Davidson SI, Wu X, Liu Y, Wei M, Danoy PA, et al. (2009) Association of ERAP1, but not IL23R, with ankylosing spondylitis in a Han Chinese population. Arthritis Rheum 60: 3263–3268.
9. Burton PR, Clayton DG, Cardon LR, Craddock N, Deloukas P, et al. (2007) Association scan of 14,500 nonsynonymous SNPs in four diseases identifies autoimmunity variants. Nat Genet 39: 1329–1337.
10. Sung IH, Kim TH, Bang SY, Kim TJ, Lee B, et al. (2009) IL-23R polymorphisms in patients with ankylosing spondylitis in Korea. J Rheumatol 36: 1003–1005.
11. Reveille JD, Sims AM, Danoy P, Evans DM, Leo P, et al. (2010) Genome-wide association study of ankylosing spondylitis identifies non-MHC susceptibility loci. Nat Genet 42: 123–127.
12. Cui X, Rouhani FN, Hawari F, Levine SJ (2003) Shedding of the type II IL-1 decoy receptor requires a multifunctional aminopeptidase, aminopeptidase regulator of TNF receptor type 1 shedding. J Immunol 171: 6814–6819.
13. Parham C, Chirica M, Timans J, Vaisberg E, Travis M, et al. (2002) A receptor for the heterodimeric cytokine IL-23 is composed of IL-12Rbeta1 and a novel cytokine receptor subunit, IL-23R. J Immunol 168: 5699–5708.
14. Trinchieri G, Pflanz S, Kastelein RA (2003) The IL-12 family of heterodimeric cytokines: new players in the regulation of T cell responses. Immunity 19: 641–644.
15. Duerr RH, Taylor KD, Brant SR, Rioux JD, Silverberg MS, et al. (2006) A genome-wide association study identifies IL23R as an inflammatory bowel disease gene. Science 314: 1461–1463.
16. Hollis-Moffatt JE, Merriman ME, Rodger RA, Rowley KA, Chapman PT, et al. (2009) Evidence for association of an interleukin 23 receptor variant independent of the R381Q variant with rheumatoid arthritis. Ann Rheum Dis 68: 1340–1344.
17. van der Linden S, Valkenburg HA, Cats A (1984) Evaluation of diagnostic criteria for ankylosing spondylitis. A proposal for modification of the New York criteria. Arthritis Rheum 27: 361–368.
18. Jiang Z, Yang P, Hou S, Du L, Xie L, et al. (2010) IL-23R gene confers susceptibility to Behcet's disease in a Chinese Han population. Ann Rheum Dis 69: 1325–1328.
19. Mizuki N, Meguro A, Ota M, Ohno S, Shiota T, et al. (2010) Genome-wide association studies identify IL23R-IL12RB2 and IL10 as Behcet's disease susceptibility loci. Nat Genet 42: 703–706.
20. Karaderi T, Harvey D, Farrar C, Appleton LH, Stone MA, et al. (2009) Association between the interleukin 23 receptor and ankylosing spondylitis is confirmed by a new UK case-control study and meta-analysis of published series. Rheumatology (Oxford) 48: 386–389.
21. Shi YY, He L (2005) SHEsis, a powerful software platform for analyses of linkage disequilibrium, haplotype construction, and genetic association at polymorphism loci. Cell Res 15: 97–98.
22. McGeachy MJ, Chen Y, Tato CM, Laurence A, Joyce-Shaikh B, et al. (2009) The interleukin 23 receptor is essential for the terminal differentiation of interleukin 17-producing effector T helper cells in vivo. Nat Immunol 10: 314–324.
23. Bettelli E, Oukka M, Kuchroo VK (2007) T(H)-17 cells in the circle of immunity and autoimmunity. Nat Immunol 8: 345–350.
24. Rueda B, Orozco G, Raya E, Fernandez-Sueiro JL, Mulero J, et al. (2008) The IL23R Arg381Gln non-synonymous polymorphism confers susceptibility to ankylosing spondylitis. Ann Rheum Dis 67: 1451–1454.
25. Jiang Z, Yang P, Hou S, Li F, Zhou H (2010) Polymorphisms of IL23R and Vogt-Koyanagi-Harada syndrome in a Chinese Han population. Hum Immunol 71: 414–417.
26. Yamazaki K, Onouchi Y, Takazoe M, Kubo M, Nakamura Y, et al. (2007) Association analysis of genetic variants in IL23R, ATG16L1 and 5p13.1 loci with Crohn's disease in Japanese patients. J Hum Genet 52: 575–583.
27. Zhou H, Jiang Z, Yang P, Hou S, Li F, et al. (2010) Polymorphisms of IL23R and Fuchs' syndrome in a Chinese Han population. Mol Vis 16: 2585–2589.
28. Balaskas K, Ballabeni P, Guex-Crosier Y (2012) Retinal thickening in HLA-B27-associated acute anterior uveitis: evolution with time and association with severity of inflammatory activity. Invest Ophthalmol Vis Sci 53: 6171–6177.
29. Rosenbaum JT (1992) Acute anterior uveitis and spondyloarthropathies. Rheum Dis Clin North Am 18: 143–151.
30. Martin TM, Rosenbaum JT (2011) An update on the genetics of HLA B27-associated acute anterior uveitis. Ocul Immunol Inflamm 19: 108–114.

# 14

# Increased Risk of Ischemic Heart Disease in Young Patients with Newly Diagnosed Ankylosing Spondylitis – A Population-Based Longitudinal Follow-Up Study

**Ya-Ping Huang[1], Yen-Ho Wang[2,3], Shin-Liang Pan[2,3]\***

**1** Department of Physical Medicine and Rehabilitation, National Taiwan University Hospital Yun-Lin Branch, Yunlin, Taiwan, **2** Department of Physical Medicine and Rehabilitation, National Taiwan University Hospital, Taipei, Taiwan, **3** Department of Physical Medicine and Rehabilitation, National Taiwan University College of Medicine, Taipei, Taiwan

## Abstract

*Background:* Prospective data is sparse on the association between ischemic heart disease (IHD) and ankylosing spondylitis (AS) in the young. The purpose of this population-based, age- and sex- matched follow-up study was to investigate the risk of IHD in young patients with newly diagnosed AS.

*Methods:* A total of 4794 persons aged 18 to 45 years with at least two ambulatory visits in 2001 with the principal diagnosis of AS were enrolled in the AS group. The non-AS group consisted of 23970 age- and sex-matched, randomly sampled subjects without AS. The three-year IHD-free survival rate and cumulative incidence of IHD were calculated using the Kaplan-Meier method. The Cox proportional hazards regression model was used to estimate the hazard ratio of IHD after controlling for demographic and cardiovascular co-morbidities.

*Results:* During follow-up, 70 patients in the AS group and 253 subjects in the non-AS group developed IHD. The cumulative incidence rate of IHD over time was higher in the AS group than the non-AS group. The crude hazard ratio of IHD for the AS group was 1.47 (95% CI, 1.13 to 1.92; p = 0.0043) and the adjusted hazard ratio after controlling for demographic characteristics and comorbid medical disorders was 1.47 (95% CI, 1.13 to 1.92; p = 0.0045).

*Conclusions:* This study showed an increased risk of developing IHD in young patients with newly diagnosed AS.

**Editor:** Masataka Kuwana, Keio University School of Medicine, Japan

**Funding:** This work was supported by grants DOH93-TD-M-113-030, DOH94-TD-M-113-004, and DOH95-TD-M-113-002 from the Department of Health, Executive Yuan, Republic of China, and grant NSC 101-2314-B-002-088 from the National Science Council, Executive Yuan, Republic of China. The funders had no role in study design, data collection and analysis, decision to publish, or preparation of the manuscript.

**Competing Interests:** The authors have declared that no competing interests exist.

\* E-mail: panslcb@gmail.com

## Introduction

Ankylosing spondylitis (AS), characterized by enthesitis of the axial skeleton, is an autoimmune disease with systemic chronic inflammation. [1] AS predominantly affects young subjects, with a peak age of onset between 20- and 30-years-old, and is more prevalent in males. [2–4] Cardiovascular manifestations, such as aortic insufficiency, conduction disturbances of the atrioventricular node, and myocardial involvement, are important extra-articular manifestations of this disease. [5,6] It has been suggested that the cardiovascular manifestations seen in AS patients may result from systemic inflammation and immune-mediated atherogenesis. [7–9] However, whether AS patients have an increased risk of developing ischemic heart disease (IHD) is unclear. Several observational studies have shown an increased risk of IHD in AS patients, [10–15] but Mathieu et al. [16] and Brophy et al. [17] failed to find a higher rate of myocardial infarction in AS patients. Moreover, most studies evaluating cardiovascular risk were carried out on prevalent AS patients in middle or old age, [11,12] and little is known about IHD risk in young newly

diagnosed AS patients. The aim of this population-based, age- and sex-matched longitudinal follow-up study was therefore to evaluate the risk of developing IHD in young subjects (aged 45 or less) with newly diagnosed AS.

## Materials and Methods

### Data Source

The data used in this study were obtained from the complete National Health Insurance (NHI) claim database in Taiwan for the period 2000 to 2003. The NHI program has been implemented in Taiwan since 1995, and the coverage rate was 96% of the whole population at the end of 2000 and 97% at the end of 2003. It should be noted that the rationale for using the NHI database after 2000 is that, from Jan 1, 2000, according to the rules of the Bureau of NHI, the NHI claim data have been encoded using the standardized International Classification of Disease, 9th Revision, Clinical Modification (ICD-9-CM). To keep individual information confidential in order to satisfy regulations on personal privacy in Taiwan, all personal identification numbers in the data were encrypted by converting them into scrambled numbers before data processing. Because the database used consisted of de-identified secondary data released for research purposes, the study met the requirements of the "Personal Information Protection Act" in Taiwan and was exempt from full review by the National Taiwan University Hospital Research Ethics Committee. The data were analyzed anonymously and the need for informed consent was waived.

## Study Design and Subjects

We used an age- and sex-matched cohort design to study the effect of AS on the risk of developing IHD. The study population included an AS group and a non-AS group, both selected from Taiwanese residents in the complete NHI claim database for 2001, in which more than 21.6 million persons were registered. The Bureau of NHI has formed audit committees to randomly sample the claims data and review charts on a regular basis to verify the diagnostic validity and quality of care.

The AS group consisted of subjects who had received a principal diagnosis of AS (ICD-9-CM code 720 or 720.0) during ambulatory medical care visits between January 1, 2001 and December 31, 2001. The index visit was defined as the first ambulatory visit during which the principal diagnosis of AS was made. To maximize case ascertainment, only patients with at least two ambulatory visits (including the index visit) with a principal diagnosis of AS between January 1, 2001 and December 31, 2001 were considered for inclusion in the AS group (n = 18800). The exclusion criteria for the recruitment of subjects into the AS group were : (1) age less than 18 years (n = 545) or greater than 45 years (n = 6353) to restrict the research sample to the young adult population; (2) a previous diagnosis of AS during year 2000 (n = 6653) to increase the likelihood of identifying only AS cases newly diagnosed in 2001; (3) a diagnosis of any type of IHD (ICD-9-CM codes 410–414) (n = 227) before the index visit; and (4) a diagnosis of diffuse diseases of connective tissue (ICD-9-CM code 710, n = 271) or rheumatoid arthritis (ICD-9-CM code 714, n = 799) before the index visit, resulting in the exclusion of 14006 subjects because of one or more of these criteria. A total of 4794 subjects was therefore included in the final AS group.

The non-AS group was taken from the remaining subjects without a diagnosis of AS in the same 2001 NHI claim database. We assigned the first ambulatory visit during 2001 as the index visit. The exclusion criteria for recruiting subjects into the non-AS group were: (1) a diagnosis of AS before the index visit; (2) a diagnosis of IHD before the index visit; and (3) a diagnosis of diffuse diseases of connective tissue or rheumatoid arthritis before the index visit. We randomly sampled 5 age- and sex-matched persons for each subject in the AS group. A total of 23970 subjects was included in the non-AS group.

## Outcome and Follow-up

All the ambulatory medical care and inpatient records for each subject in the two groups were tracked from their index visit till the end of 2003 and the mortality data for the subjects who died during the follow-up were obtained from the national mortality registry. The date of the first principal diagnosis of IHD (ICD-9-CM codes 410–414) during the follow-up period was defined as the primary endpoint. All subjects were followed from the index visit to the first occurrence of IHD, death, or end of follow-up. We evaluated the effect of AS on IHD-free survival, adjusting for demographic features (age and sex) and the preexisting cardiovascular comorbidities of hypertension (ICD-9-CM code 401–405), diabetes (ICD-9-CM code 250), and hyperlipidemia (ICD-9-CM code 272). Information on comorbid medical disorders was

obtained by tracing all the ambulatory medical care and inpatients records in the NHI database in the year before the index visit.

## Statistical Analysis

The Chi-square test and Student's t test were used to compare differences in demographic characteristics and comorbid medical disorders between the AS and non-AS groups. Incidence rates of IHD were calculated as the number of incident IHD cases divided by IHD-free person-years. The IHD-free survival probabilities for the two groups were estimated using the Kaplan-Meier method. The cumulative incidence was then calculated as one minus the IHD-free survival probability, and differences in cumulative incidence rates between the two groups were tested using the log rank test. Cox proportional hazards regression analysis was used to estimate the effect of AS on occurrence of IHD after adjusting for medical comorbidities (diabetes, hypertension, and hyperlipidemia). Univariate analysis was initially performed for each variable, then the best subset selection method was used to obtain the final multiple regression model. An alpha level of 0.05 was considered statistically significant. The analyses were performed using SAS 9.2 software (SAS Institute, Cary, NC).

## Results

### Descriptive Findings

Table 1 shows the demographic characteristics and medical comorbidities for the AS and non-AS groups. The AS group had a higher prevalence of hyperlipidemia than the non-AS group (p = 0.0214). There was no significant difference between the two groups in the prevalence of diabetes mellitus (p = 0.6639) or hypertension (p = 0.8112).

### Cumulative Incidence of Ischemic Heart Disease

The median follow-up time was 31.9 months (inter-quantile range (IQR) = 6.6 months). Of the 4794 patients with AS, 70 developed IHD during 11961.5 person-years of follow-up, giving an incidence rate of 5.8 (95% confidence interval [CI], 4.6 to 7.4) per 1000 person-years. Of the 23970 subjects in the non-AS group, 253 developed IHD during 62337.0 person-years of follow-up, giving an incidence rate of 4.0 (95% CI, 3.6 to 4.6) per 1000 person-years. The cumulative incidence rate of IHD over time was higher in the AS group than the non-AS group (Figure 1, p = 0.0043).

**Table 1.** Demographic features and comorbid disorders of the AS and non-AS groups.

| Variable | Total study population, N = 28764 | | |
|---|---|---|---|
| | AS group, N = 4794 | Non-AS group, N = 23970 | p value |
| Men | 3539(73.8) | 17695 (73.8) | 1.0000 |
| Age, y | 31.2±7.6 | 31.1±7.6 | 0.2686 |
| Diabetes | 75(1.6) | 355(1.5) | 0.6639 |
| Hypertension | 103(2.2) | 502(2.1) | 0.8112 |
| Hyperlipidemia | 125(2.6) | 498(2.1) | 0.0214 |

Note: The values are the mean ± standard deviation or the number (%).

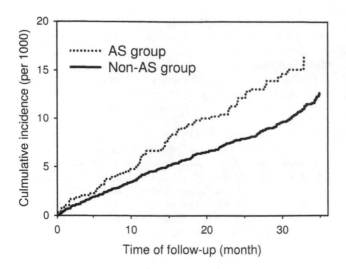

**Figure 1. Cumulative incidence of ischemic heart disease (IHD) in the ankylosing spondylitis group (dotted line) and non-AS group (solid line).**

## Cox Regression Analysis

The results of the Cox proportional hazards regression analysis are shown in Table 2. The left panel shows the crude hazard ratio (HR) for each variable based on the univariate analysis. The covariates with a p value less than 0.05 were age, AS, hypertension, diabetes, and hyperlipidemia. Compared to the non-AS group, the crude HR of IHD for the AS group was 1.47 (95% CI, 1.13 to 1.92; p = 0.0043). The middle panel shows the results using the full multivariate model. Age and sex were not included in the multiple regression analysis, since the AS and non-AS groups were matched for these variables. Using the best subset selection method, the final multiple regression model was obtained, as shown in the right panel. The variables included in the final model were AS, hypertension, and hyperlipidemia. The adjusted HR of developing IHD during the 3-year follow-up was 1.47 (95% CI, 1.13 to 1.92; p = 0.0045) for the AS group compared to the non-AS group. Hypertension was associated with a higher risk of IHD (adjusted HR 3.67; 95% CI, 2.39 to 5.64, p<0.0001). The adjusted HR of IHD for hyperlipidemia was 1.53 (95% CI, 0.90 to 2.62, p = 0.1201), which was not significant at an alpha level of 0.05.

### Sensitivity Analysis

Since ICD code 720 refers to AS and other spondylarthropathies, whereas ICD code 720.0 is specific for AS, we performed sensitivity analysis using a more restrictive case definition to include only subjects with ICD code 720.0 in the AS group. Of the 4794 subjects in the original AS group, the majority (4605, 96%) were diagnosed as ICD code 720.0. The estimated adjusted HR was 1.46 (95% CI, 1.12 to 1.92, p = 0.0058), very close to that obtained in the original analysis (Table 2, adjusted HR 1.47, 95% CI, 1.13 to 1.92, p = 0.0045). In addition, we used another restrictive case definition that included only AS patients who received two principal diagnoses of AS, with at least one being made by a rheumatologist, orthopedist, or physiatrist, and this resulted in an adjusted HR of 1.50 (95% CI, 1.12 to 2.00, p = 0.0058), again very close to the value obtained in the original analysis, suggesting that our findings will hold for different case definitions of AS.

In this study, we used a broad group of ICD-9-CM codes for case definition of hypertension, since physicians may use other ICD-9-CM codes for hypertension patients with a clinical presentation of hypertension-related systemic disease, such as ICD code 401 (essential hypertension), 402 (hypertensive heart disease), 403 (hypertensive renal disease), 404 (hypertensive heart and renal disease), or 405 (secondary hypertension). Since hypertension is a major risk factor of IHD, we investigated the impact of a different definition of hypertension on our findings by restricting the definition to include only ICD code 401 and found that the estimated adjusted hazard ratio of IHD for AS was almost unchanged (adjusted HR 1.47,95% CI, 1.12 to 1.91, p = 0.0047).

## Discussion

The present population-based follow-up study showed that young subjects with newly diagnosed AS were at a higher risk of developing IHD. The three-year cumulative incidence of IHD for the AS group was significantly higher than that for the non-AS group. These findings are consistent with the results from a population-based cohort study using the UK General Practice Research Database that found that men with AS had an increased risk of myocardial infraction compared to men in the general population (adjusted HR 1.44, 95% CI 1.15 to 1.81) [10].

The mechanism responsible for the higher IHD risk in AS patients is unclear, but evidence suggests that it may result from the chronic systemic inflammation seen in AS. [8,18,19] Early signs of atherosclerosis, such as increased carotid intra-media

**Table 2.** Crude and adjusted hazard ratio (HR) for the occurrence of ischemic heart disease during the three-year follow-up period in the AS and non-AS groups.

| Variable | Occurrence of ischemic heart disease | | | | | |
| | Univariate analysis | | Full multivariate model | | Best subset selected model | |
| | Crude HR (95% CI) | p value | Adjusted HR (95% CI) | p value | Adjusted HR (95% CI) | p value |
|---|---|---|---|---|---|---|
| Age (year) | 1.09 (1.07 to 1.11) | <.0001 | NA | NA | NA | NA |
| Sex (female vs. male) | 1.26 (1.00 to 1.60) | 0.0531 | NA | NA | NA | NA |
| AS (vs. non-AS) | 1.47 (1.13 to 1.92) | 0.0043 | 1.47 (1.13 to 1.92) | 0.0045 | 1.47 (1.13 to 1.92) | 0.0045 |
| Hypertension (yes vs. no) | 4.08 (2.73 to 6.09) | <.0001 | 3.56 (2.31 to 5.49) | <.0001 | 3.67 (2.39 to 5.64) | <.0001 |
| Diabetes mellitus (yes vs. no) | 2.30 (1.26 to 4.19) | 0.0068 | 1.40 (0.73 to 2.69) | 0.3149 | NA | NA |
| Hyperlipidemia (yes vs. no) | 2.35 (1.42 to 3.88) | 0.0009 | 1.42 (0.81 to 2.49) | 0.2225 | 1.53 (0.90 to 2.62) | 0.1201 |

Abbreviations: AS, ankylosing spondylitis; CI, confidence interval; NA, not applicable.

thickness, higher carotid pulse pressure, and impaired coronary flow reserve, are more prevalent in AS patients than healthy controls. [20–24] Elevated levels of inflammatory biomarkers, such as tumor necrosis factor alpha, C-reactive protein, and interleukin-6, have been found in AS patients. [8,25,26] Inflammation is considered to play an important role in endothelial dysfunction and the pathogenesis of arthrosclerosis, [27–30], and higher levels of these inflammatory markers have been correlated with an increased risk of atherosclerosis, coronary artery disease, and cardiovascular events. [23,24,31–33] Thus, AS-related systemic inflammation may be responsible for the higher IHD risk in young subjects with newly diagnosed AS seen in our study.

Previous studies have shown that AS patients have a higher prevalence of hypertension and diabetes mellitus, which may also contribute to the increased cardiovascular risk in AS. [19,34] However, in our study, there was no significant difference in the prevalence of diabetes or hypertension between the AS and non-AS groups (Table 1). This difference might be explained by the fact that only young subjects with newly diagnosed AS were recruited in our study, whereas most previous studies included all prevalent patients with AS and mainly older patients. Moreover, because the AS and non-AS groups had a similar prevalence of diabetes and hypertension, our findings suggest that AS independently contributes to an increased cardiovascular risk in the young.

In the present population insurance-based study, the estimated prevalence of AS was 0.12% using case definition that requires at least two ambulatory visits with a principal diagnosis of AS in 2001. This prevalence estimate is relatively lower than that obtained from a community-based survey on the prevalence of rheumatic disease in Taiwan [35] which used a 2 stage screening process in 1992. In that study, the estimated prevalence of AS in the adult Taiwanese population ranged from 0.19% to 0.54% [35].

Non-steroidal anti-inflammatory drugs (NSAIDs) are widely used for treating AS, [36,37] and, since their use has been associated with an increased cardiovascular risk, [38,39], this raises the possibility that the increased IHD risk in AS patients might result from a secondary effect of NSAID treatment. This was not taken into account in our study, since (i) observational studies on the effects of NSAID use on vascular risks are potentially confounded by indication, as patients with more severe rheumatic diseases are likely to receive higher NSAID doses and to have higher rheumatic disease-related vascular risk and (ii) NSAIDs are widely available as over the counter drugs, so NSAID use is not readily measurable using the insurance database. It is therefore difficult to separate potential adverse effects of NSAIDs from the biological effects of AS itself. Further studies are required to investigate this specific issue.

Since the present study was a large population insurance-based follow-up study and the temporal sequence between AS and IHD was ordered, the observed significant association seems unlikely to be due to selection bias or information bias (e.g. patients with AS would be more likely to be diagnosed as IHD than those without AS). A temporal relationship is essential for establishing a causal connection. Nevertheless, several limitations should be acknowledged. First, the diagnosis of AS, IHD, and medical comorbidities was determined by the ICD codes from the NHI claim database, and information about clinical history, physical examination, and radiographic findings was lacking. This is a major limitation of our study compared to studies using standardized protocols for the diagnosis of AS and there may be concern about the diagnostic accuracy of the database. However, the Bureau of NHI has formed different audit committees that make it a rule to randomly sample the claims data from every hospital and review charts on a regular basis to verify the diagnostic validity and quality of care. Accordingly, the NHI claim database is an established research database and independent studies have demonstrated the validity of the data. [40,41] Moreover, when restrictive definitions of AS were applied in the sensitivity analyses, the adjusted HR remained almost unchanged, indicating that our findings are likely to hold for various case definitions of AS. Second, although we excluded subjects with a previous diagnosis of AS during year 2000 to increase the likelihood of identifying AS patients newly diagnosed in 2001, it was possible that some prevalent AS cases with more longstanding AS, but coded for the first time in 2001, were included in the AS group. Third, the NHI database lacks some information about lifestyle factors, such as smoking, alcohol consumption, physical inactivity, and obesity, which may affect the interpretation of our results. Finally, since Taiwanese are mainly of Chinese ethnicity, it is uncertain whether our findings can be generalized to other ethnic groups.

## Conclusions

This population-based longitudinal follow-up study shows an increased risk of developing IHD in young patients with newly diagnosed AS and highlights the importance of early risk assessment for IHD in such patients.

## Author Contributions

Conceived and designed the experiments: YPH YHW SLP. Performed the experiments: YPH YHW SLP. Analyzed the data: YPH SLP. Contributed reagents/materials/analysis tools: YHW SLP. Wrote the paper: YPH YHW SLP.

## References

1. Braun J, Sieper J (2007) Ankylosing spondylitis. Lancet 369: 1379–1390.
2. Gran JT, Husby G, Hordvik M (1985 ) Prevalence of ankylosing spondylitis in males and females in a young middle-aged population of Tromso, northern Norway. Ann Rheum Dis 44: 359–367.
3. Feldtkeller E, Khan MA, van der Heijde D, van der Linden S, Braun J (2003) Age at disease onset and diagnosis delay in HLA-B27 negative vs. positive patients with ankylosing spondylitis. Rheumatol Int 23: 61–66.
4. Bakland G, Nossent HC, Gran JT (2005) Incidence and prevalence of ankylosing spondylitis in Northern Norway. Arthritis Rheum 53: 850–855.
5. Sukenik S, Pras A, Buskila D, Katz A, Snir Y, et al. (1987) Cardiovascular manifestations of ankylosing spondylitis. Clin Rheumatol 6: 588–592.
6. Lautermann D, Braun J (2002) Ankylosing spondylitis–cardiac manifestations. Clin Exp Rheumatol 20: S11–15.
7. Roman MJ, Salmon JE (2007) Cardiovascular Manifestations of Rheumatologic Diseases. Circulation 116: 2346–2355.
8. Divecha H, Sattar N, Rumley A, Cherry L, Lowe GD, et al. (2005) Cardiovascular risk parameters in men with ankylosing spondylitis in comparison with non-inflammatory control subjects: relevance of systemic inflammation. Clin Sci 109: 171–176.
9. Lehtinen K (1993) Mortality and causes of death in 398 patients admitted to hospital with ankylosing spondylitis. Ann Rheum Dis 52: 174–176.
10. Symmons DP, Goodson NJ, Cook MN, Watson DJ (2004) Men with ankylosing spondylitis have an increased risk of myocardial infarction Arthritis Rheum 50: Suppl: S477.
11. Han C, Robinson DW, Jr., Hackett MV, Paramore LC, Fraeman KH, et al. (2006) Cardiovascular disease and risk factors in patients with rheumatoid arthritis, psoriatic arthritis, and ankylosing spondylitis. J Rheumatol 33: 2167–2172.
12. Peters MJ, Visman I, Nielen MM, Van Dillen N, Verheij RA, et al. (2010) Ankylosing spondylitis: a risk factor for myocardial infarction?. Ann Rheum Dis 69: 579–581.
13. Bremander A, Petersson IF, Bergman S, Englund M (2011) Population-based estimates of common comorbidities and cardiovascular disease in ankylosing spondylitis. Arthritis Care Res (Hoboken) 63: 550–556.

14. Szabo SM, Levy AR, Rao SR, Kirbach SE, Lacaille D, et al. (2011) Increased risk of cardiovascular and cerebrovascular diseases in individuals with ankylosing spondylitis: a population-based study. Arthritis Rheum 63: 3294–3304.

15. Zöller B, Li X, Sundquist J, Sundquist K (2012) Risk of Subsequent Coronary Heart Disease in Patients Hospitalized for Immune-Mediated Diseases: A Nationwide Follow-Up Study from Sweden. PLoS ONE 7: e33442.

16. Mathieu S, Gossec L, Dougados M, Soubrier M (2011) Cardiovascular profile in ankylosing spondylitis: a systematic review and meta-analysis. Arthritis Care Res (Hoboken) 63: 557–563.

17. Brophy S, Cooksey R, Atkinson M, Zhou SM, Husain MJ, et al. (2012) No increased rate of acute myocardial infarction or stroke among patients with ankylosing spondylitis-a retrospective cohort study using routine data. Semin Arthritis Rheum 42: 140–145.

18. Grundtman C, Hollan I, Forre OT, Saatvedt K, Mikkelsen K, et al. (2010) Cardiovascular disease in patients with inflammatory rheumatic disease is associated with up-regulation of markers of inflammation in cardiac microvessels and cardiomyocytes. Arthritis Rheum 62: 667–673.

19. Mathieu S, Motreff P, Soubrier M (2010) Spondyloarthropathies: an independent cardiovascular risk factor? Joint Bone Spine 77: 542–545.

20. Gonzalez-Juanatey C, Vazquez-Rodriguez TR, Miranda-Filloy JA, Dierssen T, Vaqueiro I, et al. (2009) The High Prevalence of Subclinical Atherosclerosis in Patients With Ankylosing Spondylitis Without Clinically Evident Cardiovascular Disease. Medicine 88: 358–365.

21. Peters MJ, van Eijk IC, Smulders YM, Serne E, Dijkmans BA, et al. (2010) Signs of accelerated preclinical atherosclerosis in patients with ankylosing spondylitis. J Rheumatol 37: 161–166.

22. Bodnar N, Kerekes G, Seres I, Paragh G, Kappelmayer J, et al. (2011) Assessment of subclinical vascular disease associated with ankylosing spondylitis. J Rheumatol 38: 723–729.

23. Caliskan M, Erdogan D, Gullu H, Yilmaz S, Gursoy Y, et al. (2008) Impaired coronary microvascular and left ventricular diastolic functions in patients with ankylosing spondylitis. Atherosclerosis 196: 306–312.

24. Hamdi W, Chelli Bouaziz M, Zouch I, Ghannouchi MM, Haouel M, et al. (2012) Assessment of preclinical atherosclerosis in patients with ankylosing spondylitis. J Rheumatol 39: 322–326.

25. Braun J, Bollow M, Neure L, Seipelt E, Seyrekbasan F, et al. (1995) Use of immunohistologic and in situ hybridization techniques in the examination of sacroiliac joint biopsy specimens from patients with ankylosing spondylitis. Arthritis Rheum 38: 499–505.

26. Lange U, Teichmann J, Stracke H (2000) Correlation between plasma TNF-alpha, IGF-1, biochemical markers of bone metabolism, markers of inflammation/disease activity, and clinical manifestations in ankylosing spondylitis. Eur J Med Res 5: 507–511.

27. Ross R (1999) Atherosclerosis-an inflammatory disease. N Engl J Med 340: 115–126.

28. Libby P (2002) Inflammation in atherosclerosis. Nature 420: 868–874.

29. Libby P, Ridker PM, Maseri A (2002) Inflammation and atherosclerosis. Circulation 105: 1135–1143.

30. Hansson GK (2005) Inflammation, atherosclerosis, and coronary artery disease. N Engl J Med 352: 1685–1695.

31. Ridker PM, Hennekens CH, Buring JE, Rifai N (2000) C-reactive protein and other markers of inflammation in the prediction of cardiovascular disease in women. N Engl J Med 342: 836–843.

32. Ridker PM, Rifai N, Rose L, Buring JE, Cook NR (2002) Comparison of C-reactive protein and low-density lipoprotein cholesterol levels in the prediction of first cardiovascular events. N Engl J Med 347: 1557–1565.

33. Pearson TA, Mensah GA, Alexander RW, Anderson JL, Cannon RO, 3rd, et al. (2003) Markers of inflammation and cardiovascular disease: application to clinical and public health practice: A statement for healthcare professionals from the Centers for Disease Control and Prevention and the American Heart Association. Circulation 107: 499–511.

34. Peters MJ, van der Horst-Bruinsma IE, Dijkmans BA, Nurmohamed MT (2004) Cardiovascular risk profile of patients with spondylarthropathies, particularly ankylosing spondylitis and psoriatic arthritis. Semin Arthritis Rheum 34: 585–592.

35. Chou CT, Chen JM, Hsu CM, Chen SJ (2003) HLA-B27 and its subtypes in 4 Taiwanese Aborigine tribes: a comparison to Han Chinese patients with ankylosing spondylitis. J Rheumatol 30: 321–325.

36. Zochling J, van der Heijde D, Burgos-Vargas R, Collantes E, Davis JC Jr, et al. (2006) ASAS/EULAR recommendations for the management of ankylosing spondylitis. Ann Rheum Dis 65: 442–452.

37. van den Berg R, Baraliakos X, Braun J, van der Heijde D (2012) First update of the current evidence for the management of ankylosing spondylitis with non-pharmacological treatment and non-biologic drugs: a systematic literature review for the ASAS/EULAR management recommendations in ankylosing spondylitis. Rheumatology (Oxford).

38. Kearney PM, Baigent C, Godwin J, Halls H, Emberson JR, et al. (2006) Do selective cyclo-oxygenase-2 inhibitors and traditional non-steroidal anti-inflammatory drugs increase the risk of atherothrombosis? Meta-analysis of randomised trials. BMJ 332: 1302–1308.

39. Hermann M, Ruschitzka F (2007) Cardiovascular risk of cyclooxygenase-2 inhibitors and traditional non-steroidal anti-inflammatory drugs. Ann Med 39: 18–27.

40. Cheng CL, Kao-Yang YH, Lin SJ, Lee CH, Lai ML (2011) Validation of the national health insurance research database with ischemic stroke cases in Taiwan. Pharmacoepidemiol Drug Saf 20: 236–242.

41. Wu CH, Wang YH, Huang YP, Pan SL (2012) Does Adhesive Capsulitis of the Shoulder Increase the Risk of Stroke? A Population-Based Propensity Score-Matched Follow-Up Study. PLoS ONE 7: e49343.

# 15

# Physical Activity Assessment in Patients with Axial Spondyloarthritis Compared to Healthy Controls: A Technology-Based Approach

Thijs Willem Swinnen[1,2,3◑], Tineke Scheers[4,5◑], Johan Lefevre[4], Wim Dankaerts[3], Rene Westhovens[1,2], Kurt de Vlam[1,2]*

1 Rheumatology, University Hospitals Leuven, Leuven, Belgium, 2 Department of Development and Regeneration, KU Leuven, Leuven, Belgium, 3 Department of Rehabilitation Sciences, KU Leuven, Heverlee, Belgium, 4 Department of Kinesiology, KU Leuven, Heverlee, Belgium, 5 Research Foundation Flanders, Brussel, Belgium

## Abstract

*Introduction:* Traditionally, assessment in axial Spondyloarthritis (aSpA) includes the evaluation of the capacity to execute tasks, conceptualized as physical function. The role of physical activity, defined as movement-related energy expenditure, is largely unknown and almost exclusively studied using patient-reported outcome measures. The aims of this observational cross-sectional study are to compare physical activity between patients with aSpA and healthy controls (HC) and to evaluate the contribution of disease activity to physical activity differences between groups.

*Methods:* Forty patients with aSpA were matched by age, gender, period of data acquisition in terms of days and season to 40 HC. Physical activity was measured during five consecutive days (three weekdays and two weekend days) using ambulatory monitoring (SenseWear Armband). Self-reported disease activity was measured by the Bath Ankylosing Spondylitis Disease Activity Index (BASDAI). Differences in physical activity between patients with aSpA and HC were examined with Wilcoxon signed-rank tests and a mixed linear model. Difference scores between patients and HC were correlated with disease activity.

*Results:* Average weekly physical activity level (Med(IQR); HC:1.54(1.41–1.73); aSpA:1.45(1.31–1.67),MET) and energy expenditure (HC:36.40(33.43–41.01); aSpA:34.55(31.08–39.41),MET.hrs/day) were significantly lower in patients with aSpA. Analyses across intensity levels revealed no significant differences between groups for inactivity and time spent at light or moderate physical activities. In contrast, weekly averages of vigorous (HC:4.02(1.20–12.60); aSpA:0.00(0.00–1.20),min/d), very vigorous physical activities (HC0.00(0.00–1.08); aSpA:0.00(0.00–0.00),mind/d) and moderate/(very)vigorous combined (HC2.41(1.62–3.48); aSpA:1.63(1.20–2.82),hrs/d) were significantly lower in patients with aSpA. Disease activity did not interact with differences in physical activity between patients with aSpA and HC, evidenced by non-significant and very low correlations (range: −0.06–0.17) between BASDAI and HC-aSpA patients' difference scores.

*Conclusions:* Patients with aSpA exhibit lower physical activity compared to HC and these differences are independent of self-reported disease activity. Further research on PA in patients with aSpA should be prioritized.

**Editor:** Shervin Assassi, University of Texas Health Science Center at Houston, United States of America

**Funding:** Thijs Swinnen was funded by the Division of Rheumatology, University Hospitals Leuven (www.uzleuven.be) and Tineke Scheers was funded by the Research Foundation Flanders (F.W.O. Vlaanderen, www.fwo.be, 1134711N/1134709N). The funders had no role in study design, data collection and analysis, decision to publish, or preparation of the manuscript.

**Competing Interests:** The authors have declared that no competing interests exist. The SenseWear armbands were funded by the Division of Rheumatology, University Hospitals Leuven, nor was the manufacturer BodyMedia, Inc. involved in any part of this research.

* E-mail: kurt.devlam@uzleuven.be

◑ These authors contributed equally to this work.

## Introduction

The concept of spondyloarthritis embodies a family of rheumatic diseases characterized by distinct processes of tissue inflammation, destruction and/or pathological bone formation. Articular features typically occur at the synovio-entheseal complex [1,2], but also extra-articular features such as uveitis and psoriasis may complicate disease [3]. Clinically, a predominantly axial or peripheral articular presentation or a combination of both subtypes can be distinguished [4,5]. In axial spondyloarthritis

(aSpA), inflammatory back pain, stiffness and mobility impairment contribute to limitations in activities and restrictions in societal participation [4,6].

Physical activity (PA) can be defined as any bodily movement produced by contraction of skeletal muscle that substantially increases energy expenditure [7]. Community-based PA interventions for people with arthritis in general have shown to improve physical function, decrease pain, delay functional decline and reduce costs [8,9]. Despite this ample interest in PA in patients with arthritis in general, PA is a neglected construct in the aSpA literature [10]. The Assessment of SpondyloArthritis international Society (ASAS) expert group and the European League Against Rheumatism recommended exercise, a structured and planned form of PA [7], as a decisive part of the non-pharmacological treatment of ankylosing spondylitis (AS), [11]. Exercise programs for patients with AS, the hallmark aSpA condition, traditionally include flexibility exercises with only minor benefits on physical function, spinal mobility and patient global assessment at best [12,13]. Typically, these programs fail to deliver the optimal PA intensity according to the American College of Sports Medicine (ACSM) recommendations to develop health-related physical fitness in terms of cardio-respiratory endurance, muscular strength and body composition [12]. In contrast to other arthritis subgroups such as rheumatoid arthritis and osteoarthritis, the efficacy and safety of PA in relation to health outcomes is unknown for aSpA. Limited evidence from cross-sectional studies indicates a role for PA to improve fatigue [14], body composition [15] and quality of life [16], similar to findings in the healthy population. However, if patients exhibit less PA [15–17] and different i.e. disease-specific PA patterns compared to healthy controls is largely unknown. These data are needed to guide health policy and set research priorities.

PA assessment is currently not included in the ASAS minimal core set to monitor patients with aSpA in both clinical practice and research [18]. The key domain 'physical function' reflects difficulties in executing physical activities, not their amount or intensity, and is evaluated with the self-reported Bath Ankylosing Spondylitis Functional Index [19,20]. Since both expert rheumatologists and rehabilitation experts in the aSpA field increasingly recognize the need to establish the possible dose-dependent effects of PA [12,16,21], novel PA assessment strategies such as accelerometry are needed. Further, low correlations between PA and physical function measures in rheumatoid arthritis [22] or osteoarthritis [23] indicate that these related but distinct concepts should be assessed separately to optimally describe functioning. Taken together, establishing the role of PA in aSpA may lead to new perspectives on both the assessment of functioning and efficacy of PA on several clinical outcomes. This study investigated the role of self-reported disease activity in explaining PA differences.

To our best knowledge, this is the first study that aimed to identify differences in weekly PA between patients with aSpA and healthy controls using objective monitoring of PA in free-living conditions with a sophisticated multi-sensor device. Additionally, between and within group differences in PA will be explored for each timepoint (weekdays, Saturday and Sunday) to further detect different PA patterns. Lastly, this study aimed to unravel the role of disease activity in explaining the observed differences in PA between patients with aSpA and healthy controls.

## Materials and Methods

### Subjects

Forty patients with aSpA were consecutively recruited from our spondyloarthritis outpatient clinic at the University Hospitals Leuven. Axial SpA diagnosis was verified by an expert rheumatologist according to the European Spondylarthropathy Study Group criteria [5]. Exclusion criteria were: 1) history of spinal fractures or other fractures within 12 months, lower quadrant musculoskeletal injuries not related to SpA, discitis, pregnancy, spondylolisthesis, spondylolysis, 2) current symptoms of severe health conditions (eg. heart failure) that would influence the PA assessment according to the principal investigator, 3) not being able to stand or walk without an aid. An experienced physical

therapist ascertained exclusion criteria using the patient's medical record and the Self-administered Co-morbidity Questionnaire [24]. Forty healthy controls, matched by gender, age and period of data acquisition (season and monitoring days), were randomly selected from a large study on PA in Flemish adults [25]. A random number calculator (www.randomization.com) guided the selection procedure within strata of possible matches. All subjects provided written informed consent prior to participation. The study protocol was written in accordance to the Declaration of Helsinki and was approved by the Medical Ethics Committee of the University Hospitals Leuven (ML 5236).

### Measurements

**Disease activity.** The Bath Ankylosing Spondylitis Disease Activity Index (BASDAI), originally developed in patients with AS, is the widely accepted and ASAS endorsed disease-specific instrument to assess disease activity in aSpA [26]. The BASDAI questionnaire comprises six questions to evaluate the severity of fatigue, peripheral and axial pain, localized tenderness and morning stiffness during the last week. The psychometric properties of the BASDAI are well established [27–29].

**Physical activity.** The SenseWear Pro 3 Armband (Body-Media, Pittsburgh, USA) is a multi-sensor device containing a two-axial accelerometer and sensors measuring heat flux, galvanic skin response, skin temperature and near-body ambient temperature. The armband is positioned over the triceps muscle of the right arm. Algorithms provided by the manufacturer combine the sensor data with age, body weight, height, gender, smoking status and handedness to produce minute-by-minute estimates of energy expenditure (kcal), physical activity intensity (metabolic equivalent) and number of steps. Axial SpA patients and healthy controls were instructed to continuously wear the Armband for 5 and 7 consecutive days respectively, except during water-based activities which were reported in a non-wear log. A valid day was defined as a wear time of minimally 1296 minutes, which corresponds to 90% of a 24 hour period. To avoid bias, we selected the same weekdays in patients and healthy controls. Anthropometric measures were taken by the same observer at the moment of the outpatient visit, prior to the monitoring period. Height was measured with a stadiometer (Holtain Ltd, Dyfed, UK) to the nearest 0,1 cm and weight was measured with a digital scale (SECA, Birmingham, UK) to the nearest 0,1 kg. PA parameters were calculated for weekdays (average of three weekdays), Saturday and Sunday. Furthermore, a weekly average was estimated by the formula: $((\text{parameter}_{\text{average weekday}} * 5) + \text{parameter}_{\text{Saturday}} + \text{parameter}_{\text{Sunday}})/7$. Physical activity level (PAL) and energy expenditure (EE) both reflected the average daily energy expenditure, expressed as a multiple of the resting metabolic rate of 1 metabolic equivalent (1 MET = 1 kcal/kg/hr) and in MET.hrs/d, respectively. Time spent at different PA intensity levels was obtained using MET-values. MET-values ≤1.8 were considered to reflect inactivity, whereas MET-values >1.8 and <3 were defined as light activity [30]. MET-values ≥3 and <6 were classified as moderate activities. Vigorous activities were characterised by MET-values ≥6, but <9. MET-values ≥9 indicated very vigorous activities [31]. MET-values ≥3 reflected the overall health enhancing moderate and (very)vigorous physical activity (MVPA) estimate. The validity of the SenseWear in assessing these PA parameters is established in both healthy [32] and diseased persons [33].

### Data analysis

Continuous descriptive data of patients and healthy controls were contrasted using a paired t-test to account for the matched nature of the study and Chi-squared tests for proportions ($p < 0.05$). The *primary outcome analyses* involved: 1) the comparison of weekly average PA parameters between aSpA patients and controls using a Wilcoxon signed-rank test and 2) the verification of an interaction effect of disease activity on all PA comparisons between patients with aSpA and healthy controls. Difference scores within each matched pair (controls minus patients) were calculated and correlated with disease activity (BASDAI) with Spearman rank correlation coefficients. Because of the typical and large difference in work status between groups that may explain observed PA inequalities, we also correlated work status with PA difference scores using the point biserial correlation coefficient (spearman rank coefficient yielded the same results). A significant ($p < 0.05$) and moderate ($> 0.30$) coefficient was a priori set as the threshold for an interaction effect [34]. The *secondary outcome analyses* were exploratory comparisons (no a priori power calculations for this part) of PA parameters 1) between groups at any of the individual timepoints namely weekdays, Saturday and Sunday, 2) within each group across all timepoints and 3) between groups to detect different change patterns in PA estimates across all timepoints. All comparisons required longitudinal analyses whereby both the timepoints and groups were regarded as repeated measures. A general linear model which models covariances was employed using the MIXED procedure in SAS version 9.3 (SAS Institute, Cary, USA). For both timepoints and group, an unstructured covariance matrix was assumed. The model included fixed effects for time, group and their interaction. Model assumptions of constant variance and normality of the residuals were assessed by visual inspection of residual plots. Log-transformation was applied to PAL and EE to correct distorted residuals. However, log-transformation still yielded inappropriate residuals for time spent at light, moderate, vigorous, very vigorous and MVPA. For these parameters, the first and third types of comparison were made by means of a Friedman's test. To assess whether there was a difference between the groups at any time, a generalized estimating equations (GEE) model with identify link and normal distribution for the residuals was employed using sandwich estimators for the estimation of the (co)variances since it has been shown that this analysis yields consistent results, even if the model assumptions have not been satisfied. Post-hoc tests pairwise comparisons were made using Wilcoxon signed-rank tests. In order to attain a probability of 95%, p-values were Bonferroni corrected by multiplying them by 3.

## Results

Demographics and disease related characteristics are presented in Table 1 and indicate successful matching. During non-wear time, neither patients nor healthy controls reported additional PA. Full data are given in Table S1 available on the PLOS ONE website.

### Weekly physical activity between groups

Results of our primary outcome analysis are given in Table 2. Weekly PAL ($p = 0.048$) and EE ($p = 0.045$) were significantly lower in patients with aSpA (Table 2, Figure 1A). No differences between groups were found for weekly time spent at inactivity, light or moderate PA. For the latter, a trend for less moderate PA in patients was observed ($p = 0.07$). A lack of vigorous ($p < 0.001$) and very vigorous ($p < 0.001$) weekly PA in patients with aSpA versus controls was detected (Figure 1C, 1D, 3), in addition to reduced levels of MVPA combined ($p = 0.029$; Table 2, Figure 1B).

### Role of disease activity and work status

Disease activity did not interact with differences in weekly PA between patients and controls, evidenced by non-significant and very low correlations between BASDAI and difference scores ranging from $-0.06$ to $0.17$ (Table 3, Figure 2). Similarly low and non-significant correlations between work status and difference scores were observed ranging from $-0.11$ to $0.12$ (detailed data available from the corresponding author upon request).

### Differences between groups at time points

Concerning the secondary outcome analyses, significant differences between groups at any time point were found only for vigorous ($p < 0.001$), very vigorous PA ($p = 0.015$) and MVPA ($p = 0.028$) (see Table S1). Patients were spending less time at vigorous PA on weekdays ($p < 0.001$) and Saturday (Figure 3A, $p < 0.001$). Significantly less very vigorous PA on weekdays (Figure 3B, $p = 0.015$) and less MVPA on Saturday ($p = 0.021$) was found in patients. All plots have shown a pattern of less PA in aSpA patients at each time point (Figures not shown, additional figures available upon request from the corresponding author).

### Differences within groups at timepoints

Several significant effects within the aSpA group were detected (Table S1, EE: $p = 0.039$, light PA: $p = 0.049$; vigorous PA: $p = 0.009$). The visually clear lower EE on Sunday compared to Saturday ($p = 0.097$) and increased MVPA on Saturday ($p = 0.397$) did not reach significance. In contrast, patients with aSpA were showing significantly more time spent at light PA on weekdays compared to Sunday ($p = 0.021$). Also, patients were spending significantly more time at vigorous PA (Figure 3A) on weekdays compared to Saturday ($p = 0.027$), but not on Saturday compared to Sunday ($p = 0.128$). Significant effects within the healthy control group were identified for time spent inactive ($p = 0.013$) and at light PA ($p = 0.020$), with less inactive time on Saturday compared to Sunday ($p = 0.012$) and with more light PA on weekdays than Sunday ($p = 0.004$).

### Change profile across timepoints between groups

No significant differences in overall within group change patterns between patients with aSpA and controls were found ($p > 0.05$, Table S1). Visual inspection of all graphs (Figures not shown, but available on request from the corresponding author) has revealed quite stable PA estimates in aSpA patients across timepoints, while more variability on Saturday in the healthy control group was reflected both in the plots and quartile ranges (Table S1).

## Discussion

This is the first study demonstrating differences in PA between patients with aSpA and healthy controls using technology-based PA assessment. The lower weekly average estimates of PAL and EE observed indicate that total PA is reduced in patients with aSpA. To date, only three studies compared total PA between patients with aSpA and healthy controls. Marcora [17] studied disease-related cachexia in 19 patients with AS and 19 age-matched controls. To exclude PA behaviour as a non disease-related confounder of body composition, they compared self-reported PA levels between groups. With a p-value of 0.052 their analysis almost reached significance for lower PA levels in patients. From a Swedish registry study including self-reported PA, Haglund [16] concluded that patients with spondyloarthritis are slightly more likely to meet PA recommendations than healthy controls and both groups exhibit sufficient PA (about 70%) in general. Cultural differences and

**Table 1.** Demographics of healthy controls and patients with axial spondyloarthritis (aSpA).

| | | Healthy controls n = 40 | aSpA patients n = 40 | p-value |
|---|---|---|---|---|
| Gender | Men (n (%)) | 24 (60%) | 24 (60%) | NA |
| | Women (n (%)) | 16 (40%) | 16 (40%) | NA |
| Work status (n with job (%)) | | 39 (98%) | 25 (63%) | <.001[$] |
| Weight (kg) | | 75.69±13.31 | 76.36±17.12 | .847[¶] |
| Height (cm) | | 173.63±9.75 | 170.15±10.13 | .121[¶] |
| Body Mass Index (kg/m$^2$) | | 25.05±3.59 | 26.27±5.11 | .219[¶] |
| Age (years) | | 44.33±10.63 | 44.38±11.30 | .984[¶] |
| SWA wear-time (hrs/d) | | 23.71±0.17 | 23.67±0.03 | .501[¶] |
| Disease duration (years) | | NA | 11.40±9.50 | NA |
| BASDAI (0–10) | | NA | 3.69±2.59 | NA |
| Peripheral joints (0–10)* | | NA | 3.10±2.97 | NA |
| BASFI | | NA | 3.52±2.50 | NA |
| Cervical rotation (°)[#] | | NA | 62.41±14.61 | NA |
| Tragus to wall distance (cm)[#] | | NA | 13.23±3.73 | NA |
| Chest expansion (cm) | | NA | 4.06±1.98 | NA |
| Lumbar side flexion[#] | | NA | 11.23±4.09 | NA |
| Modified Schöber Index (cm)[#] | | NA | 3.59±1.00 | NA |
| Intermalleolar distance (cm)[#] | | NA | 97.43±20.00 | NA |
| BASMI (0–10) | | NA | 3.05±1.21 | NA |
| TSK-AA (11–44) | | NA | 13.83±3.28 | NA |
| NSAIDs (n (%)) | | NA | 21 (52,5%) | NA |
| Biologicals (n (%)) | | NA | 19 (47,5%) | NA |
| Analgesics (n (%)) | | NA | 14 (35%) | NA |
| DMARDs (n (%)) | | NA | 8 (20%) | NA |
| Corticosteroids (n (%)) | | NA | 0 (0%) | NA |
| Psychopharmaca (n (%)) | | NA | 3 (7,5%) | NA |

BASDAI, Bath Ankylosing Spondylitis Disease Activity Index; BASFI, Bath Ankylosing Spondylitis Functional Index; BASMI, Bath Ankylosing Spondylitis Metrology Index; NSAIDs, Non-Steroidal Anti-Inflammatory Drugs; DMARDs, Disease-Modifying AntiRheumatic Drugs; SWA, SenseWear Armband; TSK-AA, Tampa Scale for Kinesiophobia Activity Avoidance subscale;
*item 3 BASDAI;
[#]based on BASMI;
[¶]paired t-test (p<.05);
[$]chi-square test (p<.05);
NA, not applicable.

over-reporting of PA in survey research may explain these inconsistencies with other studies on PA around the globe [25,31]. Using a less sophisticated 3-axial accelerometer, Plasqui [15] found no differences in weekly PAL in a group of 25 patients with AS matched to healthy controls by gender, age and body mass. They observed a PAL (mean) between 1.70 and 1.99 indicating the selection of active or moderately active patients and controls, while our study sample can be classified as sedentary or light active with PAL values between 1.40 and 1.69 according to the World Health Organization guidelines on energy requirements [35]. In contrast to this work, the study of Plasqui [15] presented with a high risk of bias due to the small sample size (n = 25), the recruitment of first degree relatives as controls (about half the sample), no control for seasonal effects on PA and an inappropriate non-wear description (waking hours instead of 90% data of 24 hours period in this study). As we confirmed lower total PA with an objective methodology, we feel that research and maybe health policy on PA in aSpA should be prioritized.

This is the first study in the aSpA field that compared patients and controls across different PA intensity levels. We established a lack of weekly time spent at (very)vigorous PA and reduced MVPA, while only a trend for less moderate intensity PA between patients with aSpA and healthy controls was observed. The American College of Sports Medicine/American Heart association (ACSM/AHA) PA guideline recommends moderate intensity PA for a minimum of 30 min on five days each week or vigorous intensity PA for a minimum of 20 min on three days each week to maintain health [31]. Population surveys indicate that persons with self-reported doctor-diagnosed arthritis are less likely to meet PA guidelines for both moderate and vigorous activities (30 and 21%) compared to persons without arthritis (33 and 24%) [36]. We found that patients with aSpA and healthy controls spent on average 98 and 137 minutes (2.29 and 1.63 hrs) per day at moderate intensity and 0 and 4 minutes per day (0 and 0.07 hrs) at (very) vigorous PA. Both patients with aSpA and healthy controls appear to outperform the ACSM/AHA guideline for moderate, but not vigorous activities. Also, apparently sufficient levels but

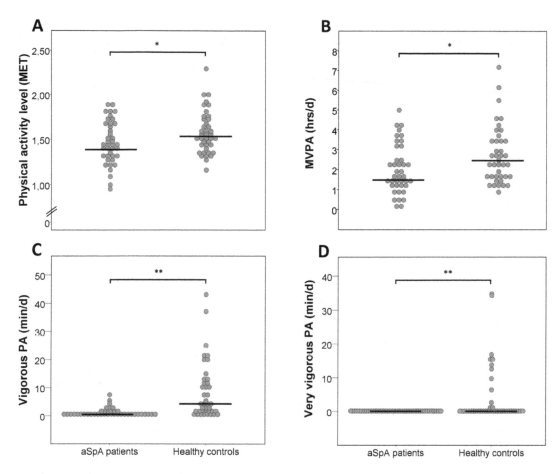

**Figure 1. Individual physical activity data between controls (n = 40) and patients with axial spondyloarthritis (n = 40): physical activity level expressed in metabolic equivalent (MET) (A), time spent at moderate and (very)vigorous physical activity (MVPA) in hrs/d (B), time spent at vigorous (C) and very vigorous (D) physical activities in min/d; *p<0.05, **p<0.01.**

**Table 2.** Comparison of physical activity parameters between healthy controls and patients with axial spondyloarthritis (aSpA).

| | | Healthy controls (n = 40)[#] | aSpA patients (n = 40)[#] | p-value[¶] |
|---|---|---|---|---|
| Weekly averages* | | | | |
| PAL | (MET) | 1.54 (1.41–1.73) | 1.45 (1.31–1.67) | **.048** |
| EE | (MET.hrs/d) | 36.40 (33.43–41.01) | 34.55 (31.08–39.41) | **.045** |
| Inactive | (hrs/d) | 17.85 (16.44–18.95) | 17.99 (16.83–19.17) | .450 |
| Light PA | (hrs/d) | 3.28 (2.73–4.10) | 3.87 (2.73–4.48) | .288 |
| Moderate PA | (hrs/d) | 2.29 (1.53–3.22) | 1.63 (1.20–2.80) | .070 |
| | (min/d)** | 137.40 (91.80–193.20) | 97.80 (72.00–168.00) | .070 |
| Vigorous PA | (hrs/d) | 0.07 (0.02–0.21) | 0.00 (0.00–0.02) | **<.001** |
| | (min/d)** | 4.02 (1.20–12.60) | 0.00 (0.00–1.20) | **<.001** |
| Very vigorous PA | (hrs/d) | 0.00 (0.00–0.03) | 0.00 (0.00–0.00) | **<.001** |
| | (min/d)** | 0.00 (0.00–1.08) | 0.00 (0.00–0.00) | **<.001** |
| MVPA | (hrs/d) | 2.41 (1.62–3.48) | 1.63 (1.20–2.82) | **.029** |
| | (min/d)** | 144.71 (96.98–208.05) | 98.19 (71.93–169.26) | **.029** |

[#]Data are presented as median (quartile range); PAL, physical activity level; EE, energy expenditure; PA, physical activity; MVPA, moderate/(very)vigorous physical activity combined;
*for a total week estimate, multiply values with seven;
**estimates transformed to minutes to facilitate interpretation;
[¶]Wilcoxon signed-rank tests, significant results in bold, p<0.05.

**Table 3.** Spearman correlation coefficients between disease activity (BASDAI*) and difference scores between healthy controls (HC) and patients with axial spondyloarthritis (aSpA) for all weekly average physical activity parameters (n = 40).

| | HC-aSpA patients difference scores[#] | R[¶] | p-value |
|---|---|---|---|
| Weekly averages** | | | |
| PAL (MET) | 0.14 (0.40) | 0.07 | .656 |
| EE (MET.hrs/d) | 3.15 (9.64) | 0.08 | .605 |
| Inactivity (hrs/d) | −0.25 (2.87) | −0.02 | .881 |
| Light PA (hrs/d) | −0.49 (2.32) | −0.06 | .710 |
| Moderate PA (hrs/d) | 0.43 (3.33) | 0.17 | .300 |
| Vigorous PA (hrs/d) | 0.07 (0.19) | −0.04 | .815 |
| Very vigorous PA (hrs/d) | 0.00 (0.03) | 0.06 | .706 |
| MVPA (hrs/d) | 0.66 (2.09) | 0.12 | .452 |

[#]Data are presented as median (quartile range);
*BASDAI, Bath Ankylosing Spondylitis Disease Activity Index; PA, physical activity; PAL, physical activity level; EE, energy expenditure; MVPA, moderate/(very)vigorous physical activity combined;
**for a total week estimate, multiply values with seven;
[¶]Correlation coefficients were neither significant nor relevant, no interaction was observed, p<0.05.

clinically relevant group differences in health enhancing MVPA were found (47 min less aSpA group). As this guideline only takes PA bouts of 10 minutes or more into account and allows combinations of moderate and vigorous activities to minimally accumulate 450 MET.min/week, direct comparison with our study data is impossible [31]. By including a control group, our study truthfully shows a disease-related loss of vigorous, very vigorous and moderate/(very)vigorous combined PA participation in patients with aSpA. Similarly, Farr [37] applied accelerometry in a sample of patients with osteoarthritis and observed a dramatic drop in patients who met the ACSM guideline for time spent at vigorous activities (men 2%, women 1%). In addition, the scarcity of time spent at vigorous and very vigorous intensity levels probably explains the differences in weekly average PAL and EE in patients versus controls. Last, although minimally clinically important difference estimates in aSpA do not exist for the PA estimates under study, the differences between groups exceeded

measurement error [38] and are similar to treatment effects in other populations [39].

To date, PA studies in aSpA have mainly focused on the role of PA on other outcomes. Da Costa [14] concluded that higher doses of leisure time PA determined by a structured interview were associated with less fatigue severity in aSpA patients with a normal mental status, while this effect was absent for patients reporting a poor mental status as measured with the SF-36 health survey's mental component subscore. Ward [40] has identified high PA intensities at work as a predictor of structural damage and activity limitations in AS. The latter finding points to the question whether the observed reduction of time spent in vigorous and very vigorous activity levels is adaptive (i.e. protective to the underlying disorder) or maladaptive (i.e. compromising the underlying disorder or other health outcomes) in the context of aSpA [2,41]. On one hand, a role for entheseal biomechanical stress in the development/maintenance of inflammation and/or damage in aSpA was recently proposed [2,42]. The observed stable and lower levels of

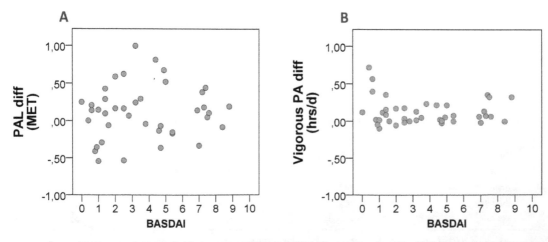

**Figure 2. Scatterplots of healthy control versus axial spondyloarthritis (aSpA) difference scores and disease activity as measured by the Bath Ankylosing Spondylitis Disease Activity Index (BASDAI): Physical activity level (PAL) A) and Vigorous PA (B); PA, physical activity; MET, metabolic equivalent; diff, difference score: for each matched pair (n = 40 pairs) healthy control value minus aSpA patient value.**

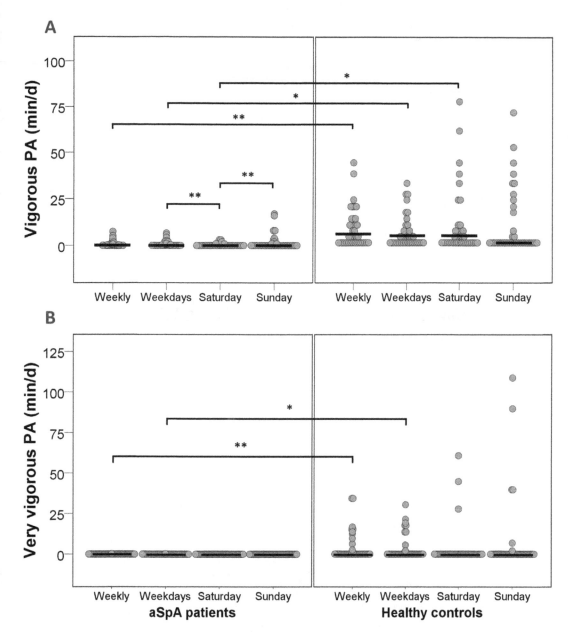

**Figure 3. Vigorous (A) and very vigorous (B) physical activities (PA) expressed in min/d for patients with axial spondyloarthritis (aSpA, n = 40) and matched healthy controls (n = 40). Horizontal lines represent median values for weekly average and time point estimates; *p<0.05, **p<0.01.**

PA in the aSpA group may be an effective strategy to alleviate aSpA disease processes. Indeed, the most frequently reported arthritis-specific coping strategy by patients is changing PA in terms of duration, frequency and intensity to complete an ongoing task [43]. On the other hand, a relationship between PA and cardiovascular health exists [31] and refraining from (very) vigorous activities may add to the increased cardiovascular risk of patients with aSpA [3]. Thus, increasing PA without vast entheseal biomechanical stress may be of uttermost importance to optimize health-related physical fitness in these patients. A large body of evidence from intervention studies supports only moderate effects of exercise to improve pain, stiffness, mobility impairment, patient's global assessment and activity limitations [13]. Ince et al. [38] targeted energy expenditure in line with the ACSM/AHA guidelines to develop cardio-respiratory endurance patients with

AS. Although core outcomes such as pain were not evaluated, the large effect sizes found for improvement in aerobic capacity point to rehabilitation opportunities in aSpA. Our finding that disease activity did not affect the observed differences between patients and healthy controls also suggests possibilities for PA intervention. Caution is however needed, because small but significant negative associations between total physical activity and both C-reactive protein [15] and BASDAI [16] were reported. In addition, no golden standard is available to assess disease activity and we only focused on self-reported disease activity. Future randomised studies including a wide spectrum of imaging, clinical (patient and physician perspective) and laboratory measures of disease activity may fully appreciate the role of disease activity. Also, as nor disease activity or work status, by intuition strong candidates to explain low PA, explained the PA differences observed, future research should focus on the identification of modifiable determinants of PA behaviour to promote health. For now, we interpret our finding as a non-recovery of reduced PA due to high disease activity, that needs a tailored rehabilitation approach beyond disease control.

The ASAS expert group recently embraced the World Health Organization's International Classification of Functioning, Disability and Health (WHO/ICF) framework to standardize the assessment of functioning in aSpA [44]. Unfortunately, the ASAS/WHO/ICF core sets [44–47] fail to recognize the crucial distinction between what a person can do in a standardized environment (activities) versus in a real-life situation (participation) [48]. More problematic is the continued use of self-reported outcome measures to appreciate functioning, possibly biased by psychological factors such as depression and anxiety [49]. This study adds to the optimal assessment of functioning in aSpA by quantifying the 'amount of' instead of 'difficulty with' movement-related participations and by introducing an unbiased objective measurement instrument in the patient's own environment.

The fact that our weekdays PA estimates were based on three instead of five weekdays may be considered as a limitation of this study. Because subjects were instructed to wear the SenseWear armband day and night, minimizing monitoring days based on a stability threshold established in healthy controls was needed to minimize patient burden without compromising validity [25,50]. To our opinion, high levels of compliance, matching days and season, and the participant's similar cultural background has resulted in accurate measures of habitual PA in both groups. Also, in our exploratory part, pairwise comparisons between groups at each time point and the observed higher variability of PA in healthy controls across timepoints that may relate to different change profiles between groups did not turn out significant, possibly indicating a lack of power. Only the primary outcomes comparing weekly PA between groups and evaluating the role of disease activity can be confidently interpreted.

## Conclusions

This is the first study establishing differences in PA between patients with aSpA and healthy controls using objective multi-sensor PA measures. Major findings were reduced weekly average energy expenditure and time spent at vigorous, very vigorous and moderate/(very)vigorous combined PA in patients with aSpA. Interestingly, disease activity did not affect the observed disparities in PA. Therefore, unraveling the relationship between PA and clinical outcomes in patients with aSpA should be a research and maybe health policy priority.

## Acknowledgments

The authors thank Ann Belmans (Leuven Biostatistics and Statistical Bioinformatics Centre, L-BioStat) for her statistical advice and all participants and all staff members who operationally contributed to this study.

## Author Contributions

Conceived and designed the experiments: TWS TS JL WD RW KDV. Performed the experiments: TWS TS. Analyzed the data: TWS TS JL WD RW KDV. Wrote the paper: TWS TS JL WD RW KDV.

## References

1. Luyten FP, Lories RJ, Verschueren P, de Vlam K, Westhovens R (2006) Contemporary concepts of inflammation, damage and repair in rheumatic diseases. Best Pract Res Clin Rheumatol 20: 829–848.

2. Benjamin M, McGonagle D (2009) The enthesis organ concept and its relevance to the spondyloarthropathies. Adv Exp Med Biol 649: 57–70.

3. Mathieu S, Gossec L, Dougados M, Soubrier M (2011) Cardiovascular profile in ankylosing spondylitis: a systematic review and meta-analysis. Arthritis Care Res (Hoboken) 63: 557–563.

4. Rudwaleit M, Khan MA, Sieper J (2005) The challenge of diagnosis and classification in early ankylosing spondylitis: do we need new criteria? Arthritis Rheum 52: 1000–1008.

5. Dougados M, van der Linden S, Juhlin R, Huitfeldt B, Amor B, et al. (1991) The European Spondylarthropathy Study Group preliminary criteria for the classification of spondylarthropathy. Arthritis Rheum 34: 1218–1227.

6. Dagfinrud H, Kjeken I, Mowinckel P, Hagen KB, Kvien TK (2005) Impact of functional impairment in ankylosing spondylitis: impairment, activity limitation, and participation restrictions. J Rheumatol 32: 516–523.

7. Caspersen CJ, Powell KE, Christenson GM (1985) Physical activity, exercise, and physical fitness: definitions and distinctions for health-related research. Public Health Rep 100: 126–131.

8. Brady TJ, Jernick SL, Hootman JM, Sniezek JE (2009) Public health interventions for arthritis: expanding the toolbox of evidence-based interventions. J Womens Health (Larchmt) 18: 1905–1917.

9. Baruth M, Wilcox S (2011) Effectiveness of two evidence-based programs in participants with arthritis: findings from the active for life initiative. Arthritis Care Res (Hoboken) 63: 1038–1047.

10. Conn VS, Hafdahl AR, Minor MA, Nielsen PJ (2008) Physical activity interventions among adults with arthritis: meta-analysis of outcomes. Semin Arthritis Rheum 37: 307–316.

11. Braun J, van den Berg R, Baraliakos X, Boehm H, Burgos-Vargas R, et al. (2011) 2010 update of the ASAS/EULAR recommendations for the management of ankylosing spondylitis. Ann Rheum Dis 70: 896–904.

12. Dagfinrud H, Halvorsen S, Vollestad NK, Niedermann K, Kvien TK, et al. (2011) Exercise programs in trials for patients with ankylosing spondylitis: do they really have the potential for effectiveness? Arthritis Care Res (Hoboken) 63: 597–603.

13. Dagfinrud H, Kvien TK, Hagen KB (2008) Physiotherapy interventions for ankylosing spondylitis. Cochrane Database Syst Rev: CD002822.

14. Da Costa D, Dritsa M, Ring A, Fitzcharles MA (2004) Mental health status and leisure-time physical activity contribute to fatigue intensity in patients with spondylarthropathy. Arthritis Rheum 51: 1004–1008.

15. Plasqui G, Boonen A, Geusens P, Kroot EJ, Starmans M, et al. (2012) Physical activity and body composition in patients with ankylosing spondylitis. Arthritis Care Res (Hoboken) 64: 101–107.

16. Haglund E, Bergman S, Petersson IF, Jacobsson LT, Strombeck B, et al. (2012) Differences in physical activity patterns in patients with spondyloarthritis. Arthritis Care Res (Hoboken).

17. Marcora S, Casanova F, Williams E, Jones J, Elamanchi R, et al. (2006) Preliminary evidence for cachexia in patients with well-established ankylosing spondylitis. Rheumatology (Oxford) 45: 1385–1388.

18. van der Heijde D, van der Linden S, Dougados M, Bellamy N, Russell AS, et al. (1999) Ankylosing spondylitis: plenary discussion and results of voting on selection of domains and some specific instruments. J Rheumatol 26: 1003–1005.

19. van der Heijde D, Calin A, Dougados M, Khan MA, van der Linden S, et al. (1999) Selection of instruments in the core set for DC-ART, SMARD, physical therapy, and clinical record keeping in ankylosing spondylitis. Progress report of the ASAS Working Group. Assessments in Ankylosing Spondylitis. J Rheumatol 26: 951–954.

20. Calin A, Garrett S, Whitelock H, Kennedy LG, O'Hea J, et al. (1994) A new approach to defining functional ability in ankylosing spondylitis: the development of the Bath Ankylosing Spondylitis Functional Index. J Rheumatol 21: 2281–2285.

21. Mihai B, van der Linden S, de Bie R, Stucki G (2005) Experts' beliefs on physiotherapy for patients with ankylosing spondylitis and assessment of their knowledge on published evidence in the field. Results of a questionnaire among international ASAS members. Eura Medicophys 41: 149–153.

22. Piva SR, Almeida GJ, Wasko MC (2010) Association of physical function and physical activity in women with rheumatoid arthritis. Arthritis Care Res (Hoboken) 62: 1144–1151.

23. Dunlop DD, Song J, Semanik PA, Sharma L, Chang RW (2011) Physical activity levels and functional performance in the osteoarthritis initiative: a graded relationship. Arthritis Rheum 63: 127–136.

24. Sangha O, Stucki G, Liang MH, Fossel AH, Katz JN (2003) The Self-Administered Comorbidity Questionnaire: a new method to assess comorbidity for clinical and health services research. Arthritis Rheum 49: 156–163.

25. Scheers T, Philippaerts R, Lefevre J (2011) Variability in physical activity patterns as measured by the SenseWear Armband: how many days are needed? Eur J Appl Physiol.

26. Sieper J, Rudwaleit M, Baraliakos X, Brandt J, Braun J, et al. (2009) The Assessment of SpondyloArthritis international Society (ASAS) handbook: a guide to assess spondyloarthritis [supplement]. Ann Rheum Dis (Suppl 2): ii1–44.

27. Jones SD, Calin A, Steiner A (1996) An update on the Bath Ankylosing Spondylitis Disease Activity and Functional Indices (BASDAI, BASFI): excellent Cronbach's alpha scores. J Rheumatol 23: 407.

28. Calin A, Nakache JP, Gueguen A, Zeidler H, Mielants H, et al. (1999) Defining disease activity in ankylosing spondylitis: is a combination of variables (Bath Ankylosing Spondylitis Disease Activity Index) an appropriate instrument? Rheumatology (Oxford) 38: 878–882.

29. Garrett S, Jenkinson T, Kennedy LG, Whitelock H, Gaisford P, et al. (1994) A new approach to defining disease status in ankylosing spondylitis: the Bath Ankylosing Spondylitis Disease Activity Index. J Rheumatol 21: 2286–2291.

30. Ainsworth BE, Haskell WL, Herrmann SD, Meckes N, Bassett DR Jr, et al. (2011) 2011 Compendium of Physical Activities: a second update of codes and MET values. Med Sci Sports Exerc 43: 1575–1581.

31. Haskell WL, Lee IM, Pate RR, Powell KE, Blair SN, et al. (2007) Physical activity and public health: updated recommendation for adults from the American College of Sports Medicine and the American Heart Association. Circulation 116: 1081–1093.

32. Langer D, Gosselink R, Sena R, Burtin C, Decramer M, et al. (2009) Validation of two activity monitors in patients with COPD. Thorax 64: 641–642.

33. Johannsen DL, Calabro MA, Stewart J, Franke W, Rood JC, et al. (2010) Accuracy of armband monitors for measuring daily energy expenditure in healthy adults. Med Sci Sports Exerc 42: 2134–2140.

34. Cohen J (1988) Statistical power analysis for the behavioural sciences. Hillsdale, NJ: Lawrence Erlbaum Associates.

35. Anonymous (2001) Human energy requirements. Report of a Joint FAO/WHO/UNU Expert Consultation. Rome.

36. Shih M, Hootman JM, Kruger J, Helmick CG (2006) Physical activity in men and women with arthritis National Health Interview Survey, 2002. Am J Prev Med 30: 385–393.

37. Farr JN, Going SB, Lohman TG, Rankin L, Kasle S, et al. (2008) Physical activity levels in patients with early knee osteoarthritis measured by accelerometry. Arthritis Rheum 59: 1229–1236.

38. Brazeau AS, Karelis AD, Mignault D, Lacroix MJ, Prud'homme D, et al. (2011) Test-retest reliability of a portable monitor to assess energy expenditure. Appl Physiol Nutr Metab 36: 339–343.

39. Scaglioni F, Marino M, Ciccia S, Procaccini A, Busacchi M, et al. (2012) Short-term multidisciplinary non-pharmacological intervention is effective in reducing liver fat content assessed non-invasively in patients with nonalcoholic fatty liver disease (NAFLD). Clin Res Hepatol Gastroenterol.

40. Ward MM, Reveille JD, Learch TJ, Davis JC Jr, Weisman MH (2008) Occupational physical activities and long-term functional and radiographic outcomes in patients with ankylosing spondylitis. Arthritis Rheum 59: 822–832.

41. Woolf CJ (2010) What is this thing called pain? J Clin Invest 120: 3742–3744.

42. D'Ambrosia P, King K, Davidson B, Zhou BH, Lu Y, et al. (2010) Pro-inflammatory cytokines expression increases following low- and high-magnitude cyclic loading of lumbar ligaments. Eur Spine J 19: 1330–1339.

43. Wilcox S, Der Ananian C, Abbott J, Vrazel J, Ramsey C, et al. (2006) Perceived exercise barriers, enablers, and benefits among exercising and nonexercising adults with arthritis: results from a qualitative study. Arthritis Rheum 55: 616–627.

44. Boonen A, Braun J, van der Horst Bruinsma IE, Huang F, Maksymowych W, et al. (2010) ASAS/WHO ICF Core Sets for ankylosing spondylitis (AS): how to classify the impact of AS on functioning and health. Ann Rheum Dis 69: 102–107.

45. Boonen A, van Berkel M, Cieza A, Stucki G, van der Heijde D (2009) Which aspects of functioning are relevant for patients with ankylosing spondylitis: results of focus group interviews. J Rheumatol 36. 2501–2511.

46. Boonen A, van Berkel M, Kirchberger I, Cieza A, Stucki G, et al. (2009) Aspects relevant for functioning in patients with ankylosing spondylitis according to the health professionals: a Delphi study with the ICF as reference. Rheumatology (Oxford) 48: 997–1002.

47. Cieza A, Hilfiker R, Boonen A, van der Heijde D, Braun J, et al. (2009) Towards an ICF-based clinical measure of functioning in people with ankylosing spondylitis: a methodological exploration. Disabil Rehabil 31: 528–537.

48. Anonymous (2001) International Classification of Functioning, Disability and Health. Geneva: World Health Organization.

49. Brionez TF, Assassi S, Reveille JD, Learch TJ, Diekman L, et al. (2009) Psychological correlates of self-reported functional limitation in patients with ankylosing spondylitis. Arthritis Res Ther 11: R182.

50. Matthews CE, Ainsworth BE, Thompson RW, Bassett DR Jr (2002) Sources of variance in daily physical activity levels as measured by an accelerometer. Med Sci Sports Exerc 34: 1376–1381.

# 16

# Higher Bone Turnover Is Related to Spinal Radiographic Damage and Low Bone Mineral Density in Ankylosing Spondylitis Patients with Active Disease: A Cross-Sectional Analysis

Suzanne Arends[1,2*⊙], Anneke Spoorenberg[1⊙], Monique Efde[2], Reinhard Bos[2], Martha K. Leijsma[1], Hendrika Bootsma[1], Nic J. G. M. Veeger[3], Elisabeth Brouwer[1], Eveline van der Veer[4]

1 Rheumatology and Clinical Immunology, University of Groningen, University Medical Center Groningen, Groningen, The Netherlands, 2 Rheumatology, Medical Center Leeuwarden, Leeuwarden, The Netherlands, 3 Epidemiology, University of Groningen, University Medical Center Groningen, Groningen, The Netherlands, 4 Laboratory Medicine, University of Groningen, University Medical Center Groningen, Groningen, The Netherlands

## Abstract

*Introduction:* Ankylosing spondylitis (AS) is characterized by excessive bone formation and bone loss. Our aim was to investigate the association of bone turnover markers (BTM) with spinal radiographic damage and bone mineral density (BMD) in AS patients with active disease.

*Methods:* 201 consecutive AS outpatients of the Groningen Leeuwarden AS (GLAS) cohort were included. Serum markers of bone resorption (C-telopeptides of type-I collagen, sCTX) and bone formation (procollagen type-I N-terminal peptide, PINP; bone-specific alkaline phosphatase, BALP) were measured. Z-scores were used to correct for the normal influence that age and gender have on bone turnover. Radiographs were scored by two independent readers according to modified Stoke AS Spinal Score (mSASSS). The presence of complete bridging (ankylosis of at least two vertebrae) was considered as measure of more advanced radiographic damage. Low BMD was defined as lumbar spine and/or hip BMD Z-score ≤ −1.

*Results:* Of the 151 patients with complete data, 52 (34%) had ≥1 complete bridge, 49 (33%) had ≥1 syndesmophyte (non-bridging), and 50 (33%) had no syndesmophytes. 66 (44%) had low BMD. Patients with bridging had significantly higher sCTX and PINP Z-scores than patients without bridging (0.43 vs. −0.55 and 0.55 vs. 0.04, respectively). Patients with low BMD had significantly higher sCTX Z-score than patients with normal BMD (−0.08 vs. −0.61). After correcting for gender, symptom duration, and CRP, sCTX Z-score remained significantly related to the presence of low BMD alone (OR: 1.60), bridging alone (OR: 1.82), and bridging in combination with low BMD (OR: 2.26).

*Conclusions:* This cross-sectional study in AS patients with active and relatively long-standing disease demonstrated that higher serum levels of sCTX, and to a lesser extent PINP, are associated with the presence of complete bridging. sCTX was also associated with low BMD. Longitudinal studies are needed to confirm that serum levels of sCTX can serve as objective marker for bone-related outcome in AS.

**Editor:** Pierre J. Marie, Inserm U606 and University Paris Diderot, France

**Funding:** The GLAS cohort was supported by an unrestricted grant from Pfizer. Pfizer had no role in study design, data collection and analysis, decision to publish, or preparation of the manuscript.

**Competing Interests:** The authors have declared that no competing interests exist.

\* E-mail: s.arends@umcg.nl

⊙ These authors contributed equally to this work.

## Introduction

Ankylosing spondylitis (AS) is an autoinflammatory rheumatic disease that predominantly affects the axial skeleton. The disease is characterized by the combination of inflammation, new bone formation, and bone loss. Spinal radiographic outcome related to excessive bone formation, so called osteoproliferation, comprises the formation of syndesmophytes with as final outcome complete bridging (ankylosis of two vertebrae). Eventually, complete fusion of the entire vertebral column can result in a so-called 'bamboo spine'. [1,2] The natural course of the disease can vary from mild to severe axial involvement and from slow to rapid radiographic progression. [1,3] The presence of syndesmophytes at study entry is the most important predictor for the development of more extensive radiographic damage. [1,3,4] Furthermore, male gender, longer disease duration, smoking, human leukocyte antigen (HLA)-B27 positivity, and increased inflammatory markers were found to be related to spinal osteoproliferation.[5–7].

On the other hand, excessive bone loss can lead to osteopenia and osteoporosis, assessed by bone mineral density (BMD), which can already be observed at early stages of the disease. Severe vertebral bone loss may lead to vertebral fractures with increased spinal deformity. [8,9] The presence of inflammation, low serum vitamin D levels, medication use, and decreased mobility related to pain, stiffness, and radiographic damage may contribute to bone loss in AS patients.[10–13].

There is a clear need for biomarkers reflecting bone-related outcome, which can help physicians in the process of decision-making on the management of AS. Previous studies in AS reported that higher serum levels of matrix metalloproteinase-3 (MMP-3), a marker of tissue remodeling, as well as lower serum levels of sclerostin and dickkopf-1, both regulators of bone turnover, were significantly associated with 2-year radiographic progression of the spine.[14–16] Furthermore, a relation was found between a biochemical marker of type II collagen degradation (urinary CTX-II, reflecting cartilage turnover) and increased radiographic damage or 2-year progression. [17,18] These studies also showed a relation between a biochemical marker of type I collagen degradation (urinary CTX-I, reflecting bone resorption) and lower BMD at the hip. [17,18] In one of our previous studies, we demonstrated that higher serum levels of CTX-I are associated with bone loss in AS patients with active disease. [11].

Bone turnover markers (BTM) may serve as objective markers for bone-related outcome in AS. A challenge of working with BTM is that serum levels change with age and there are differences for gender. Our healthy reference cohort on BTM enables us to correct BTM levels of individual AS patients for the normal influence that age and gender have on bone turnover. The aim of the present cross-sectional study was to investigate the association of BTM with spinal radiographic damage and BMD in AS patients with active disease.

## Methods

### Patients

Data collected before start of tumor necrosis factor-alpha (TNF-α) blocking therapy were used from 201 consecutive AS patients included in the Groningen Leeuwarden Ankylosing Spondylitis (GLAS) cohort [19] between November 2004 and December 2010. Patients with recent fractures or use of bisphosphonates were excluded because of their major influence on the bone metabolism. All patients were over 18 years of age, fulfilled the modified New York criteria for AS, [20] and had active disease defined by Bath AS Disease Activity Index (BASDAI) ≥4 (range 0–10) or based on expert opinion. [21].

### Ethics Statement

The study was approved by the local ethics committees of the Medical Center Leeuwarden (MCL) and University Medical Center Groningen (UMCG). All patients provided written informed consent according to the Declaration of Helsinki to participate in this study.

### BTM Assessments

Bone turnover was studied by assessment of bone resorption marker serum cross-linked telopeptide of type-I collagen (sCTX) and bone formation markers procollagen type-I N-terminal peptide (PINP) and bone-specific alkaline phosphatase (BALP). sCTX was measured by electrochemiluminescence immunoassay (ECLIA; Elecsys 2010 Roche Mannheim, Germany; inter-assay coefficient of variation (IE-CV) 10.8%), PINP by radioimmuno-assay (RIA; Orion Diagnostica, Espoo, Finland; IE-CV 9.0%), and BALP by enzyme-linked immunosorbent assay (ELISA; Metra

Biosystems, Mountain View, CA, USA; IE-CV 5.5%). Serum samples were stored at −20°C until analysis.

BTM Z-scores, the number of standard deviations (SD) from the normal mean corrected for age and gender, were calculated using a Dutch reference group (200 men and 350 women) checked for serum 25-hydroxyvitamin D levels >50 nmol/liter as well as for the absence of osteoporosis (BMD T-score >−2.5) after 50 years of age. Z-scores were calculated as follows: (BTM value of individual patient − mean BTM value of matched 10-year-cohort of reference group)/SD of matched reference cohort.

### Radiological Assessments

The lateral view of radiographs of the cervical and lumbar spine were blinded for patient characteristics and were scored according to the modified Stoke AS Spinal Score (mSASSS) by two trained readers (SA and AS) independent from each other. The anterior corners of lower C2 until upper T1and lower T12 until upper S1 were scored for the presence of erosions, sclerosis, and/or squaring (1 point per site), syndesmophytes (without ankylosis of vertebrae; 2 points per site), and complete bridging (ankylosis of two vertebrae; 3 points per site). The mSASSS was calculated as the sum of the scores at all individual sites (range 0–72). In case ≤3 vertebral sites were missing, these values were substituted by the mean score of the vertebrae of the same spinal segment. If >3 vertebral sites were missing, the patient was excluded from analysis (n = 6). If the mSASSS total score of both readers differed by >5 units, the X-ray was reread by the same readers. When the discrepancy of >5 units persisted following rereading, consensus was reached. [22,23] The average mSASSS total score of both readers was used for analysis.

Inter-observer reliability for mSASSS was very good. The intraclass correlation coefficient (two-way random effects model, single measures, absolute agreement) before consensus was 0.985 (95% confidence interval (CI): 0.979–0.990). Bland-Altman analyses showed that the mean difference in mSASSS between both readers was small (0.7). The 95% limits of agreement were between −5.6 and 7.1, out of a total of 72.

The presence or absence of syndesmophytes and complete bridging was analyzed as measure of definite radiographic damage. Agreement between readers was very good, with Cohen's kappa of 0.88 (0.80–0.96) for the presence of syndesmophytes and 0.91 (0.84–0.98) for the presence of bridging. In case of discrepancy between both readers, the consensus score was used for analysis.

### BMD Measurement

BMD at the lumbar spine (anterior-posterior projection at L1-L4) and hip (total proximal femur) were measured using DXA (Hologic QDR Discovery (UMCG) or Hologic QDR Delphi (MCL), Waltman, MA, USA). Z-scores were calculated using the NHANES reference database. Low BMD was defined as lumbar spine and/or hip BMD Z-score ≤ −1. The International Society for Clinical Densitometry recommends using BMD Z-scores instead of BMD T-scores in premenopausal women and men under the age of 50. [24].

### Clinical Assessments

Demographic data including smoking status, symptom duration, year of diagnosis, HLA-B27 status, history of extra-articular manifestations, presence of peripheral arthritis (defined as ≥1 swollen joint), and use of nonsteroidal anti-inflammatory drugs (NSAIDs) and disease-modifying antirheumatic drugs (DMARDs) were collected. Disease activity was assessed using BASDAI, [25] erythrocyte sedimentation rate (ESR), C-reactive protein (CRP),

**Table 1.** Characteristics of the AS study population (n = 151).

| | | | |
|---|---|---|---|
| Gender (male) (n, %) | 108 (72) | | |
| Age (yrs) | 42.1 ± 11.4 | | |
| Duration of symptoms (yrs) | 15 (1–53) | | |
| Time since diagnosis (yrs) | 7 (0–44) | | |
| HLA-B27+ (n, %) | 120 (82) | | |
| History of IBD (n, %) | 14 (9) | | |
| History of uveitis (n, %) | 44 (29) | | |
| History of psoriasis (n, %) | 9 (6) | | |
| Peripheral arthritis (n, %) | 29 (19) | | |
| Current smoking (n, %)[†] | 45 (41) | | |
| Current NSAID use (n, %) | 108 (72) | | |
| Current DMARD use (n, %) | 36 (24) | | |
| Current steroid use (n, %)‡ | 11 (7) | | |
| BASDAI (range 0–10) | 6.1 ± 1.7 | BASDAI ≥4 (n, %)* | 135 (89) |
| $ASDAS_{CRP}$ | 3.8 ± 0.8 | $ASDAS_{CRP}$ ≥2.1 (n, %)* | 146 (99) |
| ESR (mm/h) | 21 (2–90) | | |
| CRP (mg/l) | 13 (2–99) | | |
| BASFI (range 0–10) | 5.7 (0.4–9.7) | | |
| sCTX Z-score | −0.34 (−2.58–5.38) | | |
| PINP Z-score | 0.23 (−1.75–8.77) | | |
| BALP Z-score | 0.32 (−2.59–10.38) | | |
| mSASSS (range 0–72) | 12 (1–72) | ≥1 syndesmophyte (n, %) | 101 (67) |
| | | ≥1 complete bridge (n, %) | 52 (34) |
| LS BMD Z-score | −0.33 ± 1.49 | LS BMD Z-score ≤−1 (n, %) | 52 (36) |
| | | LS BMD Z-score ≤−2 (n, %) | 16 (11) |
| Hip BMD Z-score | −0.23 ± 1.06 | Hip BMD Z-score ≤−1 (n, %) | 38 (25) |
| | | Hip BMD Z-score ≤−2 (n, %) | 6 (4) |

Values are mean ± SD or median (range) unless otherwise indicated.
[†]Data were available in 72% of the patients.
‡Of these patients, 3 used systemic corticosteroids (prednison 5 mg/d n = 2, budenofalk 6 mg/d n = 1) and 8 used local corticosteroids (nose drops n = 3, eye drops n = 2, inhaled n = 2, skin cream n = 1, injection knee n = 1).
*Active disease based on BASDAI (21) or ASDAS [37].
AS, ankylosing spondylitis; HLA-B27+, human leukocyte antigen B27 positive; IBD, inflammatory bowel disease; NSAID, non-steroidal anti-inflammatory drug; DMARD, disease-modifying antirheumatic drug; BASDAI, Bath AS disease activity index; ASDAS, AS disease activity score; ESR, erythrocyte sedimentation rate; CRP, C-reactive protein; BASFI, Bath AS functional index; PINP, procollagen type I N-terminal peptide; BALP, bone-specific-alkaline phosphatase; sCTX, serum C-telopeptide of type I collagen; mSASSS, modified stoke AS spinal score; LS, lumbar spine; BMD, bone mineral density.

and AS disease activity score (ASDAS) calculated from BASDAI questions 2, 3, and 6, patient's global assessment of disease activity, and CRP. [26,27] Physical function was assessed using Bath AS Functional Index (BASFI; on a scale of 0–10). [28].

Clinical visits including biobanking and radiological and BMD measurements were performed within one year (median difference 1.6 and 0.3 months, respectively).

## Statistical Analysis

Patients with complete data available on BTM, radiology, and BMD were used in all analyses. Results were expressed as mean ± SD or median (range) for normally distributed and non-normally distributed data, respectively. Independent samples t test, Mann-Whitney U test, and Chi-Square test were used to compare differences in patient characteristics between groups.

For BTM comparisons, Kruskal-Wallis test and Mann-Whitney U test were used. Univariable logistic regression was performed to analyze the relation between BTM Z-scores and the presence or absence of complete bridging and low or normal BMD.

Multivariable logistic regression was performed to correct these relations for other variables that were significantly different between these patient groups. Finally, multinomial regression was used for the combined analysis of the presence of bridging and low BMD. Patients without bridging plus normal BMD were used as reference category.

Receiver operating characteristic (ROC) analysis was performed to determine the accuracy of BTM Z-scores to discriminate between patients with or without bridging and low or normal BMD. Area under the curve (AUC) <0.70 was interpreted as poor accuracy, 0.70< AUC <0.90 as moderate accuracy, and AUC > 0.90 as high accuracy. [29].

Spearman's correlation coefficient (ρ) was used to analyze the relation between BTM Z-scores and mSASSS. P values < 0.05 were considered statistically significant. Statistical analysis was performed with IBM SPSS Statistics 20 (SPSS, Chicago, IL, USA).

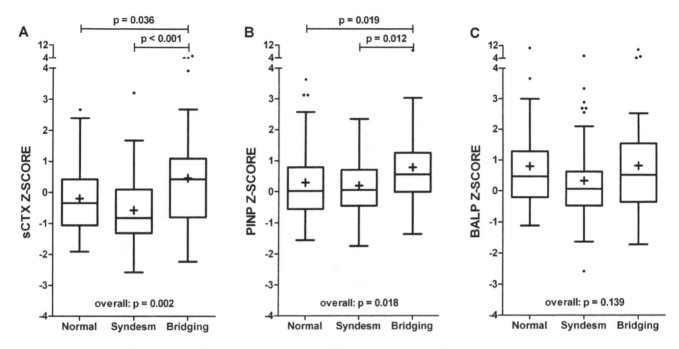

**Figure 1. Bone turnover in AS patients with ≥1 complete bridge (n = 52), ≥1 non-bridging syndesmophyte (n = 49), and without syndesmophytes (n = 50).** A) bone resorption marker sCTX, B) bone formation marker PINP, C) bone formation marker BALP. Box-and-whisker plots (Tukey): boxes indicate medians with interquartile ranges;+indicate means; whiskers indicate 1.5 times the interquartile distances; · indicate outliers.

## Results

In total, 151 of 201 AS patients (75%) had complete data available on BTM, radiology, and BMD. Of these patients, mean age was 42.1 years (SD ±11.4), median symptom duration was 15 years (range 1–53), and 72% were male (Table 1). Patient characteristics were comparable between patients with and without complete data, except for BASFI score (5.7 vs. 6.4, p = 0.048).

### Radiological Damage and BTM

Of the 151 patients, 52 (34%) had at least one complete bridge, 49 (33%) had at least one syndesmophyte (non-bridging), and 50 (33%) had no syndesmophytes. Patients with bridging had significantly higher sCTX and PINP Z-scores than patients with non-bridging syndesmophytes or without syndesmophytes, whereas no significant difference was found in BALP Z-score (Figure 1).

No significant differences in BTM Z-scores were found between patients with and without non-bridging syndesmophytes (Figure 1) and these two categories were combined in further analyses. The presence of complete bridging was considered as measure of more advanced radiographic damage. In these patients, the median number of bridges was 4 (range 1–12). The median difference in Z-score between patients with (n = 52) and without (n = 99) bridging was larger for sCTX than for PINP (0.98 vs. 0.51). In addition, patients with bridging were significantly more often male and had more long-standing disease (Table 2).

In univariable logistic regression, sCTX Z-score (odds ratio (OR): 1.62, 95% CI: 1.22–2.14) and PINP Z-score (OR: 1.43, 1.06–1.93) were significantly associated with the presence of complete bridging. The amount of variance explained by sCTX and PINP was 11.6% and 5.5%, respectively. ROC analysis showed that the AUC discriminating between patients with and without bridging was 0.66 (0.57–0.75) for sCTX Z-score and 0.64 (0.55–0.73) for PINP Z-score. After correcting for gender and

symptom duration, sCTX Z-score (OR: 1.50, 1.09–2.07) remained significantly related to the presence of bridging, while PINP Z-score almost reached significance (OR 1.48, 0.99–2.22). Correcting for time since diagnosis instead of symptom duration yielded similar results (sCTX: OR 1.57, 1.16–2.13; PINP: OR 1.62, 1.12–2.35).

The mSASSS correlated significantly with sCTX Z-score (ρ = 0.200, p = 0.016) and PINP Z-score (ρ = 0.180, p = 0.030); no relation was found with BALP Z-score (ρ = 0.010, p = 0.910).

### Bone Mineral Density and BTM

Of the 151 patients, 66 (44%) had lumbar spine and/or hip BMD Z-score ≤ −1 and 18 (12%) had BMD Z-score ≤ −2. Patients with low BMD (n = 66) had significantly higher sCTX Z-scores than patients with normal BMD (median difference 0.53). No significant difference was found in PINP and BALP Z-scores (Figure 2). In addition, patients with low BMD had significantly higher CRP levels and shorter disease duration (Table 2).

In univariable logistic regression, sCTX Z-score (OR: 1.35, 1.05–1.74) was significantly associated with the presence of low BMD. The amount of variance explained by sCTX Z-score was 5.1%. The AUC of sCTX Z-score was 0.61 (0.52–0.70) to discriminate between patients with low and normal BMD. This relation remained significant (OR: 1.38, 1.04–1.83) after correcting for CRP and symptom duration.

### Combined Analysis

Both complete bridging and low BMD were present in 20 of 151 (13%) patients. 32 (21%) had only bridging, 46 (31%) had only low BMD, and 53 (35%) did not have bridging or low BMD. sCTX Z-score was significantly higher in patients with low BMD, bridging, or both compared to patients without bridging and normal BMD. Furthermore, patients with both bridging and low BMD had significantly higher sCTX Z-scores than patients with only low BMD (Figure 3).

**Table 2.** Characteristics of AS patients with or without complete bridging and with low or normal BMD.

| | Bridging[a] | No bridging | Low BMD[b] | Normal BMD |
|---|---|---|---|---|
| Number of patients | 52 | 99 | 66 | 85 |
| Gender (male) (n, %) | 47 (90) | 61 (62)* | 51 (77) | 57 (67) |
| Duration of symptoms (yrs) | 24 (2–53) | 11 (1–35)* | 13 (2–47) | 18 (1–53)[†] |
| Time since diagnosis (yrs) | 14 (0–44) | 3 (0–26)* | 7 (0–44) | 6 (0–41) |
| HLA-B27+ (n, %) | 43 (88) | 77 (79) | 50 (78) | 70 (84) |
| Current smoking (n, %) | 16 (47) | 29 (39) | 18 (36) | 27 (46) |
| Current NSAID use (n, %) | 40 (77) | 68 (69) | 50 (76) | 58 (68) |
| BASDAI (range 0–10) | 5.9±1.7 | 6.1±1.6 | 5.9±1.8 | 6.2±1.6 |
| ASDAS$_{CRP}$ | 3.8±0.8 | 3.7±0.8 | 3.8±0.9 | 3.7±0.7 |
| ESR (mm/h) | 20 (3–76) | 21 (2–90) | 23 (2–90) | 17 (2–76) |
| CRP (mg/l) | 14 (2–99) | 13 (2–70) | 16 (2–99) | 10 (2–64)[†] |
| BASFI (range 0–10) | 6.2 (1.1–9.7) | 5.6 (0.4–9.3) | 5.5 (0.4–9.7) | 5.7 (0.5–9.3) |
| sCTX Z-score | 0.43 (−2.23–5.38) | −0.55 (−2.58–3.20)* | −0.08 (−1.89–4.01) | −0.61 (−2.58–5.38)[†] |
| sCTX (pg/ml) | 239.4 (31.0–618.7) | 175.8 (13.4–657.1)* | 227.6 (35.6–657.1) | 160.3 (13.4–618.7)[†] |
| PINP Z-score | 0.55 (−1.37–8.77) | 0.04 (−1.75–3.63)* | 0.12 (−1.56–3.63) | 0.28 (−1.75–8.77) |
| PINP (μg/l) | 47.6 (17.9–132.5) | 41.6 (16.0–101.5) | 50.2 (16.4–101.5) | 41.8 (16.0–132.5) |
| BALP Z-score | 0.52 (−1.73–9.68) | 0.28 (−2.59–10.38) | 0.17 (−1.64–10.38) | 0.43 (−2.59–9.68) |
| BALP (U/L) | 18.2 (6.9–67.2) | 17.6 (1.6–41.2) | 18.3 (8.9–41.2) | 17.5 (1.6–67.2) |
| mSASSS (range 0–72) | 40 (11–72) | 7 (1–29)* | 10 (1–72) | 15 (2–72)[†] |
| LS BMD Z-score | 0.09±1.59 | −0.52±1.40* | −1.47±0.93 | 0.60±1.18[†] |
| Hip BMD Z-score | −0.25±0.92 | −0.21±1.13 | −0.97±0.76 | 0.35±0.89[†] |

Values are mean ± SD or median (range) unless otherwise indicated.
[a]Defined as ankylosis of at least two vertebrae.
[b]Defined as lumbar spine and/or hip BMD Z-score ≤ −1.
*p<0.05 compared to patients with at least one complete bridge.
[†]p<0.05 compared to patients with low BMD.
See Table 1 for abbreviations.
No significant differences in extra-articular manifestations or peripheral arthritis were found between patients with or without complete bridging and low or normal BMD (data not shown).

In univariable multinomial logistic regression, sCTX Z-score was significantly associated with the presence of low BMD alone (OR: 1.59), bridging alone (OR: 1.88), and bridging in combination with low BMD (OR: 2.51). The amount of variance explained by sCTX Z-score was 14.4%. The AUC of sCTX Z-score was 0.78 (0.67–0.89) to discriminate between patients with bridging plus low BMD and patients without bridging plus normal BMD.

After correcting for gender, symptom duration, and CRP, sCTX Z-score remained significantly related to the presence of low BMD alone (OR: 1.60), bridging alone (OR: 1.82), and bridging in combination with low BMD (OR: 2.26) (Table 3). The total amount of variance explained by the full model was 45.9%. Correcting for BASDAI, ASDAS, or ESR instead of CRP yielded similar results (data not shown).

## Discussion

The present cross-sectional study within the GLAS cohort showed that higher serum levels of bone resorption marker sCTX and bone formation marker PINP were significantly associated with the presence of complete bridging in AS patients with active disease. The relation of sCTX with bridging remained statistically significant after correcting for gender and disease duration. Our finding that patients with bridging were more often male and had

longer disease duration is in accordance with earlier findings in AS. [4,30,31].

In clinical studies concerning the monitoring of osteoporosis treatment and fracture risk prediction, the use of sCTX and PINP, both products of type I collagen, has been recommended. [32] Neither sCTX nor PINP are specific to bone, but the highest contributions are probably bone derived. BALP, an enzyme that has a central role in the mineralization process after osteoid forming, is specific for bone, but has some cross-reactivity with liver isoform (up to 20%). Although PINP and BALP show smaller circadian rhythm, sCTX was closer related to osteoproliferation than PINP; the median difference in Z-score between AS patients with and without bridging was 0.98 and 0.51, respectively. Surprisingly, no significant association was found for BALP.

Previous studies searching for biomarkers that reflect structural damage in AS have shown that higher serum levels of MMP-3 significantly predicted 2-year radiographic progression in multivariable analysis. [14] Furthermore, lower serum levels of Wnt signalling pathway inhibitors sclerostin and dickkopf-1 were significantly associated with 2-year radiographic progression in univariable analysis. [15,16] Another candidate, cartilage turnover marker urinary cross-linked telopeptide of type-II collagen (uCTX-II) was found to be independently related to radiological damage at baseline and 2-year radiological progression. However, the amount of variance explained by uCTX-II was small (full

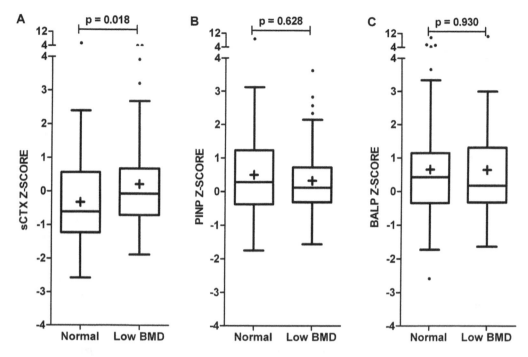

**Figure 2. Bone turnover in AS patients with low (n = 66) and normal (n = 85) BMD.** A) bone resorption marker sCTX, B) bone formation marker PINP, C) bone formation marker BALP. Box-and-whisker plots (Tukey): boxes indicate medians with interquartile ranges;+indicate means; whiskers indicate 1.5 times the interquartile distances; · indicate outliers.

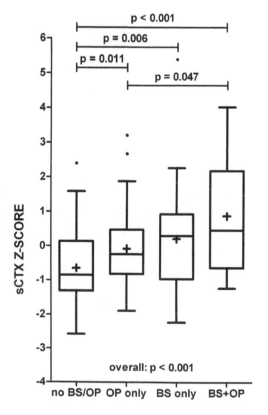

**Figure 3. Bone resorption marker sCTX in AS patients with complete bridging, low BMD or both.** Box-and-whisker plots (Tukey): boxes indicate medians with interquartile ranges;+indicate means; whiskers indicate 1.5 times the interquartile distances; · indicate outliers. BS: complete bridging, OP: low BMD.

model $R^2$ was 6%). [18] In contrast to our findings, Vosse et al. could not demonstrate a relation between uCTX-I and structural damage. [18] The most likely explanation for this difference is that measuring CTX in urine has more variation compared to serum as well as that sCTX levels were not corrected for age and gender in the former study.

Besides osteoproliferation, AS is characterized by bone loss, which can lead to a reduction in BMD and/or vertebral fractures. In the present study, a significant association between sCTX and low BMD was found. Analyzing lumbar spine and hip BMD separately, we found only a significant difference in sCTX for low hip BMD (data not shown). The relation between CTX-I and low hip BMD has been reported before. [17,18] Serum levels of PINP and BALP were comparable between patients with normal and low BMD. These findings are in accordance with two previous studies, which also found no significant correlation between PINP or BALP and BMD in small groups of AS patients. [33,34].

Finally, we analyzed the combination of excessive bone formation (vertebral ankylosis) and bone loss (low BMD). sCTX Z-score was significantly higher in AS patients with low BMD, complete bridging, or both compared to patients without bridging and normal BMD. Interestingly, these differences remained significant after correcting for gender, disease duration, and CRP, suggesting that serum levels of sCTX reflect bone-related outcome in AS. The accuracy of sCTX Z-score to discriminate between patients with bridging plus low BMD and patients without bridging plus normal BMD was moderate (AUC of 0.78).

A striking finding was that AS patients without bridging and normal BMD had a median sCTX Z-score of −0.85. Further exploration of the reduction in this bone resorption marker in this group of AS patients is needed.

With pre-analytical standardization of blood sampling as well as standardization of assays, [32] sCTX and PINP meet most of the requirements of the Outcome Measures in Rheumatology

**Table 3.** Multinomial regression analysis for the relation between bone resorption marker sCTX and the presence of complete bridging and/or low BMD.

| | Low BMD | | Bridging | | Low BMD and bridging | |
|---|---|---|---|---|---|---|
| | OR (95% CI) | p-value | OR (95% CI) | p-value | OR (95% CI) | p-value |
| sCTX Z-score | 1.59 (1.90–2.31) | 0.016 | 1.88 (1.26–2.81) | 0.002 | 2.51 (1.61–3.90) | <0.001 |
| sCTX Z-score (corrected model)‡ | 1.60 (1.04–2.45) | 0.032 | 1.82 (1.12–2.94) | 0.015 | 2.26 (1.37–3.73) | 0.002 |

Patients without bridging and normal BMD were used as reference category.
‡Corrected for gender, symptom duration, and CRP.
See Tables 1 and 2 for abbreviations and definitions, respectively.

(OMERACT) validation criteria for soluble biomarkers reflecting structural damage. [35] Regardless the variation in BTM levels between individual patients, the present cross-sectional study shows that serum levels of sCTX and PINP are higher in AS patients with bridging. Furthermore, both BTM correlate significantly with mSASSS, the structural damage endpoint for AS. These rather weak correlations can probably be explained by the fact that the presence of erosions, sclerosis, and/or squaring can already result in mSASSS scores up to 24, without evidence of bony proliferation on radiographs. To exclude the influence of these relatively minor radiographic changes, we used the presence of complete bridging as measure of more advanced radiographic damage in AS. Interestingly, BTM were found to be associated with the presence of complete bridging, but not with the presence of syndesmophytes. A possible explanation may be that syndesmophytes can vary in size and severity. Complete bridging is considered as the final outcome (ankylosing of two vertebrae).

Although very interesting, our results should be interpreted with some caution due to the cross-sectional design and only AS patients with active and relatively long-standing disease were analyzed. To confirm our results, further studies should include also patients without active disease as well as patients in early stages of the disease. TNF-α blocking agents have shown to be very effective in controlling systemic inflammation and improving clinical outcome in AS. [2] In addition, we found a significant decrease in sCTX after starting TNF-α blocking therapy. [19] In the present analysis, disease activity did not influence the association between sCTX Z-score and the presence of complete bridging or low BMD. However, BTM and inflammatory markers in serum are systemic measurements and the relation with local inflammatory processes was not investigated.

In 50 patients (25%), part of the data on BTM (n = 10), radiology (n = 38), and BMD (n = 15) was missing due to logistic reasons and they were excluded from all analyses. Patient characteristics were comparable between patients with and without complete data, except for somewhat higher BASFI score in patients without complete data. When including all available data per analysis, similar results were found as in the complete case analysis. Similar results were also observed after excluding patients who used corticosteroids (data not shown).

Patients with complete bridging were identified to have significantly longer disease duration and higher lumbar spine BMD compared to patients without bridging. Hip BMD was similar between both groups. On the other hand, patients with low lumbar spine BMD had significantly shorter disease duration than patients with normal BMD. These findings suggest that bridging causes an overestimation in lumbar spine BMD measured by

DXA in patients with advanced AS. This is in line with our previous finding that the difference between lumbar spine and hip BMD correlated positively with disease duration. [11] Furthermore, Karberg et al. showed that in AS patients with short disease duration (<5 years), low BMD was found more frequently in the spine, whereas in patients with longer disease duration (>10 years), osteoporosis was more frequent found in the hip. [36] For this reason, we used both lumbar spine and hip to define low BMD in our study. However, since we analyzed a group of AS patients with relatively long-standing disease (median symptom duration of 15 years), the percentage of patients with low BMD may be underestimated. BMD Z-scores were used because of the young age (mean 42 years) of the AS population [24].

The prevalence of low BMD found in our cohort was high compared to the general population. Of the AS patients, 44% had lumbar spine and/or hip BMD Z-score ≤ −1 and 12% had BMD Z-score ≤ −2. Due to the small number of patients with BMD Z-score ≤ −2, separate analyses using this threshold could not be performed, which may limit the clinical interpretation of our results. Patients who used bisphosphonates (because of severe osteoporosis) were excluded because of the large reduction in BTM.

## Conclusion

This cross-sectional analysis in AS patients with active disease demonstrated that higher serum levels of sCTX, and to a lesser extent PINP, are associated with the presence of complete bridging. Higher serum levels of sCTX were also associated with low BMD. Longitudinal studies are needed to confirm that BTM, especially sCTX, can serve as objective markers for bone-related outcome as well as to investigate whether BTM can predict spinal radiographic progression and decrease in BMD in AS.

## Acknowledgments

The authors wish to acknowledge Mrs. W. Gerlofs, Mrs. S. Katerbarg, Mrs. A. Krol, and Mrs. R. Rumph for their contribution to clinical data collection; and Mrs. J. Hoving-Ensing, Mrs. M. Inia, Mrs. H. Kamminga-Rasker, Mrs. K. Koerts, and Mrs. L. Wagenmakers for their contribution to BTM assessments.

## Author Contributions

Conceived and designed the experiments: SA AS HB EB EV. Performed the experiments: SA AS ME RB MKL EB EV. Analyzed the data: SA AS NJGMV EV. Wrote the paper: SA AS EB EV.

# References

1. Baraliakos X, Listing J, Rudwaleit M, Haibel H, Brandt J, et al. (2007) Progression of radiographic damage in patients with ankylosing spondylitis: defining the central role of syndesmophytes. Ann Rheum Dis 66: 910–915.
2. Braun J, Sieper J (2007) Ankylosing spondylitis. Lancet 369: 1379–1390.
3. Baraliakos X, Listing J, von der Recke A, Braun J (2009) The natural course of radiographic progression in ankylosing spondylitis–evidence for major individual variations in a large proportion of patients. J Rheumatol 36: 997–1002.
4. van Tubergen A, Ramiro S, van der Heijde D, Dougados M, Mielants H, et al. (2012) Development of new syndesmophytes and bridges in ankylosing spondylitis and their predictors: a longitudinal study. Ann Rheum Dis 71: 518–523.
5. Ramiro S, Stolwijk C, van Tubergen A, van der Heijde D, Dougados M, et al. (2013) Evolution of radiographic damage in ankylosing spondylitis: a 12 year prospective follow-up of the OASIS study. Ann Rheum Dis doi: 10.1136/annrheumdis-2013-204055. [Epub ahead of print].
6. Poddubnyy D, Haibel H, Listing J, Marker-Hermann E, Zeidler H, et al. (2012) Baseline radiographic damage, elevated acute-phase reactant levels, and cigarette smoking status predict spinal radiographic progression in early axial spondylarthritis. Arthritis Rheum 64: 1388–1398.
7. Haroon N, Inman RD, Learch TJ, Weisman MH, Lee M, et al. (2013) The impact of tumor necrosis factor alpha inhibitors on radiographic progression in ankylosing spondylitis. Arthritis Rheum 65: 2645–2654.
8. Geusens P, Vosse D, van der Linden S (2007) Osteoporosis and vertebral fractures in ankylosing spondylitis. Curr Opin Rheumatol 19: 335–339.
9. Vosse D, Landewe R, van der Heijde D, van der Linden S, van Staa TP, et al. (2009) Ankylosing spondylitis and the risk of fracture: results from a large primary care-based nested case-control study. Ann Rheum Dis 68: 1839–1842.
10. Ghozlani I, Ghazi M, Nouijai A, Mounach A, Rezqi A, et al. (2009) Prevalence and risk factors of osteoporosis and vertebral fractures in patients with ankylosing spondylitis. Bone 44: 772–776.
11. Arends S, Spoorenberg A, Bruyn GA, Houtman PM, Leijsma MK, et al. (2011) The relation between bone mineral density, bone turnover markers, and vitamin D status in ankylosing spondylitis patients with active disease: a cross-sectional analysis. Osteoporos Int 22: 1431–1439.
12. Lange U, Teichmann J, Strunk J, Muller-Ladner U, Schmidt KL (2005) Association of 1.25 vitamin D3 deficiency, disease activity and low bone mass in ankylosing spondylitis. Osteoporos Int 16: 1999–2004.
13. El Maghraoui A (2004) Osteoporosis and ankylosing spondylitis. Joint Bone Spine 71: 291–295.
14. Maksymowych WP, Landewe R, Conner-Spady B, Dougados M, Mielants H, et al. (2007) Serum matrix metalloproteinase 3 is an independent predictor of structural damage progression in patients with ankylosing spondylitis. Arthritis Rheum 56: 1846–1853.
15. Appel H, Ruiz-Heiland G, Listing J, Zwerina J, Herrmann M, et al. (2009) Altered skeletal expression of sclerostin and its link to radiographic progression in ankylosing spondylitis. Arthritis Rheum 60: 3257–3262.
16. Heiland GR, Appel H, Poddubnyy D, Zwerina J, Hueber A, et al. (2012) High level of functional dickkopf-1 predicts protection from syndesmophyte formation in patients with ankylosing spondylitis. Ann Rheum Dis 71: 572–574.
17. Park MC, Chung SJ, Park YB, Lee SK (2008) Bone and cartilage turnover markers, bone mineral density, and radiographic damage in men with ankylosing spondylitis. Yonsei Med J 49: 288–294.
18. Vosse D, Landewe R, Garnero P, van der Heijde D, van der Linden S, et al. (2008) Association of markers of bone- and cartilage-degradation with radiological changes at baseline and after 2 years follow-up in patients with ankylosing spondylitis. Rheumatology (Oxford) 47: 1219–1222.
19. Arends S, Spoorenberg A, Houtman PM, Leijsma MK, Bos R, et al. (2012) The effect of three years of TNFalpha blocking therapy on markers of bone turnover and their predictive value for treatment discontinuation in patients with ankylosing spondylitis: a prospective longitudinal observational cohort study. Arthritis Res Ther 14: R98.

20. van der Linden S, Valkenburg HA, Cats A (1984) Evaluation of diagnostic criteria for ankylosing spondylitis. A proposal for modification of the New York criteria. Arthritis Rheum 27: 361–368.
21. Braun J, Davis J, Dougados M, Sieper J, van der Linden S, et al. (2006) First update of the international ASAS consensus statement for the use of anti-TNF agents in patients with ankylosing spondylitis. Ann Rheum Dis 65: 316–320.
22. Spoorenberg A, de Vlam K, van der Linden S, Dougados M, Mielants H, et al. (2004) Radiological scoring methods in ankylosing spondylitis. Reliability and change over 1 and 2 years. J Rheumatol 31: 125–132.
23. Wanders AJ, Landewe RB, Spoorenberg A, Dougados M, van der Linden S, et al. (2004) What is the most appropriate radiologic scoring method for ankylosing spondylitis? A comparison of the available methods based on the Outcome Measures in Rheumatology Clinical Trials filter. Arthritis Rheum 50: 2622–2632.
24. The International Society for Clinical Densitometry. Available at: http://www.iscd.org/official-positions/2013-iscd-official-positions-adult/. Accessed 2014 January 15.
25. Garrett S, Jenkinson T, Kennedy LG, Whitelock H, Gaisford P, et al. (1994) A new approach to defining disease status in ankylosing spondylitis: the Bath Ankylosing Spondylitis Disease Activity Index. J Rheumatol 21: 2286–2291.
26. Lukas C, Landewe R, Sieper J, Dougados M, Davis J, et al. (2009) Development of an ASAS-endorsed disease activity score (ASDAS) in patients with ankylosing spondylitis. Ann Rheum Dis 68: 18–24.
27. van der Heijde D, Lie E, Kvien TK, Sieper J, Van den Bosch F, et al. (2009) ASDAS, a highly discriminatory ASAS-endorsed disease activity score in patients with ankylosing spondylitis. Ann Rheum Dis 68: 1811–1818.
28. Calin A, Garrett S, Whitelock H, Kennedy LG, O'Hea J, et al. (1994) A new approach to defining functional ability in ankylosing spondylitis: the development of the Bath Ankylosing Spondylitis Functional Index. J Rheumatol 21: 2281–2285.
29. Swets JA (1988) Measuring the accuracy of diagnostic systems. Science 240: 1285–1293.
30. Lee W, Reveille JD, Davis JC Jr, Learch TJ, Ward MM, et al. (2007) Are there gender differences in severity of ankylosing spondylitis? Results from the PSOAS cohort. Ann Rheum Dis 66: 633–638.
31. Boonen A, vander Cruyssen B, de Vlam K, Steinfeld S, Ribbens C, et al. (2009) Spinal radiographic changes in ankylosing spondylitis: association with clinical characteristics and functional outcome. J Rheumatol 36: 1249–1255.
32. Vasikaran S, Eastell R, Bruyere O, Foldes AJ, Garnero P, et al. (2011) Markers of bone turnover for the prediction of fracture risk and monitoring of osteoporosis treatment: a need for international reference standards. Osteoporos Int 22: 391–420.
33. Acebes C, de la Piedra C, Traba ML, Seibel MJ, Garcia Martin C, et al. (1999) Biochemical markers of bone remodeling and bone sialoprotein in ankylosing spondylitis. Clin Chim Acta 289: 99–110.
34. Mitra D, Elvins DM, Collins AJ (1999) Biochemical markers of bone metabolism in mild ankylosing spondylitis and their relationship with bone mineral density and vertebral fractures. J Rheumatol 26: 2201–2204.
35. Maksymowych WP, Landewe R, Tak PP, Ritchlin CJ, Ostergaard M, et al. (2009) Reappraisal of OMERACT 8 draft validation criteria for a soluble biomarker reflecting structural damage endpoints in rheumatoid arthritis, psoriatic arthritis, and spondyloarthritis: the OMERACT 9 v2 criteria. J Rheumatol 36: 1785–1791.
36. Karberg K, Zochling J, Sieper J, Felsenberg D, Braun J (2005) Bone loss is detected more frequently in patients with ankylosing spondylitis with syndesmophytes. J Rheumatol 32: 1290–1298.
37. Machado P, Landewe R, Lie E, Kvien TK, Braun J, et al. (2011) Ankylosing Spondylitis Disease Activity Score (ASDAS): defining cut-off values for disease activity states and improvement scores. Ann Rheum Dis 70: 47–53.

# 17

# Increased Risk of Ischemic Stroke in Young Patients with Ankylosing Spondylitis: A Population-Based Longitudinal Follow-Up Study

**Chia-Wei Lin[1], Ya-Ping Huang[2], Yueh-Hsia Chiu[3], Yu-Tsun Ho[1], Shin-Liang Pan[1,4]\***

1 Department of Physical Medicine and Rehabilitation, National Taiwan University Hospital, Taipei, Taiwan, 2 Department of Physical Medicine and Rehabilitation, National Taiwan University Hospital Yu-Lin Branch, Yunlin, Taiwan, 3 Department and Graduate Institute of Health Care Management, Chang Gung University, Tao-Yuan, Taiwan, 4 Department of Physical Medicine and Rehabilitation, National Taiwan University College of Medicine, Taipei, Taiwan

## Abstract

*Background:* Prospective data on the association between ischemic stroke and ankylosing spondylitis (AS) in the young are sparse. The purpose of this population-based, age- and sex-matched longitudinal follow-up study was to investigate the risk of developing ischemic stroke in young patients with AS.

*Methods:* A total of 4562 patients aged 18- to 45-year-old with at least two ambulatory visits in 2001 with a principal diagnosis of AS were enrolled in the AS group. The non-AS group consisted of 22810 age- and sex-matched, randomly sampled subjects without AS. The two-year ischemic stroke-free survival rate for each group were calculated using the Kaplan-Meier method. Cox proportional hazards regression analysis was used to estimate the hazard ratio of ischemic stroke after adjusting for demographic and clinical covariates.

*Results:* During follow-up, 21 patients in the AS group and 53 in the non-AS group developed ischemic stroke. The ischemic stroke-free survival rate over the 2 year follow-up was lower in the AS group than the non-AS group (p = 0.0021). The crude hazard ratio of ischemic stroke for the AS group was 1.98 (95% CI, 1.20–3.29; p = 0.0079) and the adjusted hazard ratio after controlling for demographic and comorbid medical disorders was 1.93 (95% CI, 1.16–3.20; p = 0.0110).

*Conclusion:* Our study showed an increased risk of developing ischemic stroke in young patients with AS.

**Editor:** James T. Rosenbaum, Oregon Health & Science University, United States of America

**Funding:** This work was supported by grants DOH93-TD-M-113-030, DOH94-TD-M-113-004, and DOH95-TD-M-113-002 from the Department of Health (DOH), Executive Yuan, Republic of China and grant NSC101-2314-B-002-088 from the National Science Council, Executive Yuan, Republic of China. This study used the complete National Health Insurance Research Database provided by the Bureau of National Health Insurance, Department of Health. The conclusions in our study are not necessarily those of the Department of Health, Executive Yuan, Republic of China. The funders had no role in study design, data collection and analysis, decision to publish, or preparation of the manuscript.

**Competing Interests:** The authors have declared that no competing interests exist.

\* E-mail: panslcb@gmail.com

## Introduction

Ankylosing spondylitis (AS), an autoimmune disease with systemic inflammation, predominantly involves the axial skeleton [1]. AS has been associated with an increased risk of ischemic heart disease [2–8], but whether AS patients are at a higher risk of ischemic stroke remains controversial. Two observational studies have reported an increased risk of cerebrovascular disease in AS patients [9,10], whereas another study found that AS patients had no increased prevalence of stroke compared to non-AS patients [11]. In addition, two of these studies were based on a cross-sectional survey [9,11] and prospective data on the relationship between AS and cerebrovascular diseases are sparse. Moreover, these studies were carried out mainly on middle-aged or older AS patients, and little is known about cerebrovascular risk in young AS patients. Thus, the aim of this population-based, age- and sex-matched longitudinal follow-up study was to evaluate the risk of developing ischemic stroke in young patients with AS.

## Materials and Methods

### Data source

The data used in this study were obtained from the complete National Health Insurance (NHI) claim database in Taiwan for the period 2000 to 2003. The NHI program, a single-payer compulsory social insurance program, has been implemented in Taiwan since 1995, and the coverage rate was 96% of the whole population in 2000 and 97% at the end of 2003, at which time more than 21.9 million inhabitants were enrolled. It should be noted that the rationale for using the NHI database after 2000 is that, from Jan 1st, 2000, according to the rules of the Bureau of NHI, NHI claim data have been encoded using the standardized International Classification of Disease, 9th Revision, Clinical Modification (ICD-9-CM).

## Ethics Statement

To keep individual information confidential so as to satisfy regulations on personal privacy in Taiwan, all personal identification numbers in the data were encrypted by converting them into scrambled numbers before data processing. This study was exempt from full review by the National Taiwan University Hospital Research Ethics Committee, and the need for informed consent was waived because the data used consisted of de-identified secondary data released for research purposes and were analyzed anonymously, thus complying with the regulations of the Department of Health, Executive Yuan, Republic of China.

## Study Design and Subjects

We used an age- and sex-matched cohort study design to investigate the risk of ischemic stroke in young patients with AS. The study population included an AS group and a non-AS group. The AS group consisted of subjects aged between 18 to 45 years who had received a principal diagnosis of AS (ICD-9-CM code 720.0) in ambulatory medical care visits between January 1, 2001 and December 31, 2001. The index visit was defined as the first ambulatory visit during which the principal diagnosis of AS was made. In order to maximize case ascertainment, only patients with at least two ambulatory visits (including the index visit) with a principal diagnosis of AS in this period were considered for inclusion in the AS group (n = 11428). The exclusion criteria for the recruitment of subjects into the AS group were: (1) a previous diagnosis of AS during year 2000 (n = 6473) to increase the likelihood of identifying AS cases newly diagnosed in 2001; (2) a previous diagnosis of any type of stroke (ICD-9-CM codes 430-438) (n = 91) before the index visit; and (3) a diagnosis of diffuse diseases of connective tissue (ICD-9-CM code 710, n = 252) or rheumatoid arthritis (ICD-9-CM code 714, n = 765) before the index visit; 6866 subjects were excluded because of one or more of these criteria, leaving 4562 subjects in the final AS group.

The non-AS group was constructed by sampling the subjects without a diagnosis of AS in the same 2001 NHI claim database. We assigned the first ambulatory visit during 2001 as the index visit. The exclusion criteria for recruiting subjects into the non-AS group were: (1) a previous diagnosis of AS before the index visit; (2) a previous diagnosis of stroke before the index visit; and (3) a diagnosis of diffuse diseases of connective tissue or rheumatoid arthritis before the index visit. We randomly sampled 5 age- and sex-matched subjects for each subject in the AS group. A total of 22810 subjects was included in the non-AS group.

## Outcome

All ambulatory medical care and inpatient records for each subject in the two groups for the 2 year follow-up period were retrieved and the mortality data for those subjects who died during follow-up were obtained from the mortality registry. These medical records and mortality data were linked through a unique encrypted identification number for each subject. We identified the date of the first principal diagnosis of ischemic stroke (ICD-9-CM codes 433–437) during follow-up as the primary endpoint. All subjects were followed from the index visit to the first occurrence of ischemic stroke, death, or end of follow-up (whichever occurred first). We evaluated the effect of AS on the ischemic stroke-free survival, adjusting for the demographic features of age and sex and for the cardiovascular comorbidities of hypertension (ICD-9-CM code 401–405), diabetes (ICD-9-CM code 250), dyslipidemia (ICD-9-CM code 272), coronary heart disease (ICD-9-CM codes 410–414, and 429.2), and other types of heart disease (ICD-9-CM code 393-398, 420–429). Information on these preexisting comorbid medical disorders was obtained by retrieving all the ambulatory medical care and inpatients records in the NHI database for the year before the index visit.

## Statistical analysis

The Chi-square test and Student's $t$ test were used to compare differences in demographic characteristics and comorbid medical disorders between the AS and non-AS groups. The ischemic stroke-free survival probabilities for the two groups were estimated using the Kaplan-Meier method and differences in ischemic stroke-free survival between the two groups were tested using the log rank test. Cox proportional hazards regression analysis was used to estimate the effect of AS on the subsequent occurrence of ischemic stroke after adjusting for medical comorbidities. Univariate analysis was initially performed for each variable, then the best subset selection method was used to obtain the final multiple regression model. An alpha level of 0.05 was considered statistically significant. The analyses were performed using SAS 9.2 software (SAS Institute, Cary, NC).

## Results

Table 1 shows the distribution of demographic characteristics and medical comorbidities in the AS and non-AS groups. Men made up 73.8% of the AS group, which had a mean age of 31.3 years (SD = 7.6). The AS group had a higher prevalence of dyslipidemia (p = 0.0157), coronary heart disease (p<0.0001), and other types of heart disease (p<0.0001). There was no significant difference between the two groups in the prevalence of diabetes mellitus (p = 0.3755) or hypertension (p = 0.7527).

Of the 4562 subjects with AS, 21 (0.46%) developed ischemic stroke during the 2-year follow-up compared to 53 (0.23%) of the 22810 subjects in the non-AS group. Comparison of the ischemic stroke-free survival curves showed that the stroke-free survival rate for the AS group was significantly lower than that for the non-AS group (p = 0.0021, Figure 1).

The results of the Cox proportional hazards regression analysis are shown in Table 2. The left column shows the crude hazard ratio (HR) for each variable based on the univariate analysis. The covariates with a p value less than 0.05 were age, AS, hypertension, coronary heart disease, and other heart diseases. Compared to the non-AS group, the crude HR of ischemic stroke for the AS group was 1.98 (95% CI, 1.20 to 3.29; p = 0.0079). The middle column shows the results using the full multivariate model; age and sex were not included in the multiple regression analysis, since the AS and non-AS groups were matched for these variables. The right column shows the result of the final best subset selected model; the variables included in the final model were AS, hypertension, and coronary heart disease. The adjusted HR of developing ischemic stroke during the 2-year follow-up was 1.93 (95% CI, 1.16 to 3.20; p = 0.0110) for the AS group compared to the non-AS group. It should also be noted that hypertension and coronary heart disease were also associated with a higher risk of ischemic stroke.

Of the 21 AS patients who developed stroke, 15 (71.4%) were male. The mean age of these 21 AS patients was 38.0 years (SD = 6.9), elder than that (31.3 years, SD = 7.6) of the remaining 4541 AS patients who did not develop stroke (p<0.0001). The prevalence of diabetes mellitus, hypertension, dyslipidemia, coronary heart disease, and other heart disease of these 21 AS patients at baseline were 0%, 4.8%, 9.5%, 4.8%, and 4.8%, respectively. There was lack of significant difference in the prevalence of the above medical co-morbidities between the AS patients who developed stroke or not.

**Table 1.** Demographic and clinical characteristics of the AS and non-AS groups.

| Variable | AS group | Non-AS group | p value |
|---|---|---|---|
| | N = 4562 | N = 22810 | |
| Men | 3365 (73.8) | 16825 (73.8) | 1.0000 |
| Age (years) | 31.3±7.6 | 31.2±7.6 | 0.2866 |
| Diabetes | 72 (1.6) | 321 (1.4) | 0.3755 |
| Hypertension | 102 (2.2) | 493 (2.2) | 0.7527 |
| Dyslipidemia | 122 (2.7) | 479 (2.1) | 0.0157 |
| Coronary heart disease | 61 (1.3) | 171 (0.8) | <0.0001 |
| Other heart diseases | 122 (2.7) | 285 (1.2) | <0.0001 |

Values are expressed as the mean ± SD or n (%).

## Sensitivity analysis

In order to assess the robustness of our results, we carried out the following sensitivity analyses. First, in the present study, the diagnosis of AS was entirely determined by ICD codes from the insurance database, and may be less accurate than those obtained through a standardized procedure. Moreover, the radiographic data are not available in the NHI database. Therefore, we performed additional analysis, using a more rigorous definition that included only AS patients who received two principal diagnosis of AS with at least one being made by a rheumatologist, orthopedist, or physiatrist. The results showed that 3719 (82%) out of the original 4562 patients in the AS group fit this more rigorous case definition. The estimated adjusted HR obtained from this analysis was 1.79 (95% CI, 1.01 to 3.18), consistent with the estimates from the original analysis (Table 2, right column, adjusted HR 1.93, 95% CI, 1.16 to 3.20). Second, while AS patients who had at least 2 ambulatory visits in 2001 were considered for inclusion, the non-AS group consisted of age and gender matched patients who had at least one ambulatory visit in 2001. It may raise a concern that the non-AS group would consist of a potentially healthier population requiring fewer ambulatory visits, which may have had an influence on the risk of stroke. Therefore, we performed additional analysis restricting the non-AS group inclusion criteria to only subjects with at least 2 ambulatory visits in 2001. The majority of the subjects in the non-AS group (21649 out of 22810, 94.9%) had two or more ambulatory visits in 2001. The adjusted HR of ischemic stroke for AS was 1.89 (95% CI, 1.14 to 3.14), which is almost unchanged compared to the original estimates (adjusted HR 1.93, 95% CI, 1.16 to 3.20). Third, as shown in Table 1, the AS group had a higher prevalence of dyslipidemia, coronary heart disease, and other types of heart disease compared to the non-AS group. As these co-morbidities may also contribute to the risk of ischemic stroke, we conducted an analysis excluding all patients (in both the AS and non-AS groups) with any one of the co-morbidities listed in Table 1 (i.e. diabetes mellitus, hypertension, dyslipidemia,

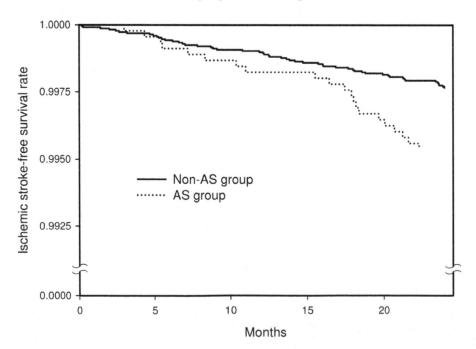

**Figure 1. Two-year ischemic stroke-free survival rates for the ankylosing spondylitis (AS) group (dotted line) and non-AS group (solid line).**

**Table 2.** Crude and adjusted hazard ratio (HR) for the occurrence of ischemic stroke during the two-year follow-up period in the AS and non-AS groups.

| | Occurrence of ischemic stroke | | | | | |
| | Univariate analysis | | Full multivariate model | | Best subset selected model | |
| Variable | Crude HR (95% CI) | p value | Adjusted HR (95% CI) | p value | Adjusted HR (95% CI) | p value |
|---|---|---|---|---|---|---|
| Age (years) | 1.12 (1.08 to 1.16) | <0.0001 | NA | NA | NA | NA |
| Sex (female vs. male) | 0.97 (0.58 to 1.63) | 0.9060 | NA | NA | NA | NA |
| AS (AS vs. non-AS) | 1.98 (1.20 to 3.29) | 0.0079 | 1.92 (1.16 to 3.19) | 0.0116 | 1.93 (1.16 to 3.20) | 0.0110 |
| Hypertension (yes vs. no) | 6.32 (3.18 to 12.69) | <0.0001 | 4.55 (2.02 to 10.23) | 0.0002 | 4.66 (2.15 to 10.09) | <0.0001 |
| Diabetes mellitus (yes vs. no) | 0.96 (0.13 to 6.86) | 0.9633 | 0.42 (0.06 to 3.19) | 0.4031 | NA | NA |
| Dyslipidemia (yes vs. no) | 2.56 (0.93 to 7.01) | 0.0677 | 1.39 (0.47 to 4.13) | 0.5490 | NA | NA |
| Coronary heart disease (yes vs. no) | 8.55 (3.45 to 21.19) | <0.0001 | 3.78 (1.27 to 11.24) | 0.0170 | 4.18 (1.53 to 11.46) | 0.0053 |
| Other heart diseases (yes vs. no) | 3.80 (1.39 to 10.40) | 0.0095 | 1.42 (0.45 to 4.48) | 0.5467 | NA | NA |

Abbreviations: AS, ankylosing spondylitis; CI, confidence interval; NA, not applicable.

coronary heart disease, and other heart disease). The adjusted HR of ischemic stroke for AS was 2.20 (95% CI, 1.25 to 3.90, p = 0.0065), still supporting that AS is associated with a higher risk of developing ischemic stroke. Fourth, we performed a competing risk analysis accounting for death due to causes other than stroke as a competing risk. The adjusted HR of ischemic stroke for AS is 1.84 (95% CI, 1.10 to 3.08), which is very close to the original estimates (adjusted HR 1.93, 95% CI, 1.16 to 3.20).

## Discussion

The major finding in our study was that, in young patients with AS, AS was associated with a 1.9-fold increased risk of ischemic stroke. This association was still seen after controlling for common vascular risk factors. The 2-year ischemic stroke-free survival rate for the AS subjects was lower than that for the non-AS group. Our findings are consistent with two previous observational studies carried out in the US (prevalence ratio: 1.7, 95% CI, 1.3 to 2.3) [9] and in Quebec (prevalence ratio: 1.25, 95% CI, 1.15 to 1.35) [10]. The mechanism responsible for the association between AS and ischemic stroke is unclear; however, we propose the following explanations.

Inflammation plays an important role in the pathogenesis and progression of atherosclerosis [3,12–15]. Previous studies have shown that, compared to patients without AS, AS patients have higher levels of inflammatory markers, such as interleukin 6, tumor necrosis factor alpha, and C-reactive protein [3,16,17]. In addition, AS patients have been reported to show early features of atherosclerosis, such as an increase in intima media thickness in the carotid arteries [18–22] and impaired flow-mediated dilatation in the brachial arteries [19,23]. Thus, the increased risk of ischemic stroke in the AS group may result from accelerated atherosclerosis caused by systemic inflammation.

Heart disorders, such as aortic insufficiency, mitral valve disease, and cardiomyopathy, are part of the extraskeletal manifestations of AS [24,25]. These heart disorders may also contribute to a higher risk of ischemic stroke [26,27]. However, in our study, although the AS group had a higher prevalence of coronary heart disease and other heart diseases, AS remained an independent risk factor of ischemic stroke after controlling for vascular risk factors and heart diseases in the multivariate analysis. The adjusted hazard ratio of ischemic stroke for the AS group (adjusted HR: 1.93, 95% CI: 1.16 to 3.20) in the multivariate

analysis is very close to the crude HR (1.98, 95% CI: 1.20 to 3.29) in the univariate analysis (Table 2). These findings suggest that the increased risk of ischemic stroke in the AS group is independent of the heart involvement in AS.

Non-steroidal anti-inflammatory drugs (NSAIDs) are widely used for treating AS [28,29]. However, the use of NSAID was not evaluated in our study because observational studies on the effects of NSAID exposure on vascular risks are potentially confounded by indication, as patients with more severe rheumatic diseases are likely to receive higher NSAID doses and also to be at higher disease-related vascular risk. In addition, since NSAIDs are widely available as over the counter medications, their use is not readily assessable in the insurance database. It is therefore difficult to separate the effects of NSAIDs from the biological impacts resulting from AS. Moreover, it remains controversial whether NSAIDs is associated with an increased risk of stroke. A recent large-scale meta-analysis of 280 trials of NSAIDs versus placebo and 474 trials of one NSAID versus another NSAID showed there was no evidence that any NSAID, including selective COX-2 inhibitors and traditional NSAIDs, significantly increased the risk of stroke [30]. Therefore, the use of NSAID was not included in our analysis.

In the present population-based study, the estimated prevalence of AS was 0.12% using case definition that requires at least two ambulatory visits with a principal diagnosis of AS in 2001. This prevalence estimate is relatively lower than that obtained from a community-based survey on the prevalence of rheumatic diseases in Taiwan [31] which used a 2-stage screening process in 1992. In that study, the estimated prevalence of AS in the adult Taiwanese population ranged from 0.19 to 0.54% [31]. Since some AS patients with mild symptoms who did not seek medical service would not be recorded in the NHI database, our study may tend to recruit patients with more severe or active AS, and it can be expected that the estimated prevalence of AS in our study would be lower than that reported from the previous community-based survey.

The strength of the present study was the use of a longitudinal population-based NHI database. The NHI program is a single-payer compulsory social insurance program with considerably high coverage rate in Taiwan. The barrier to medical access is negligible because the NHI system allows patients to visit any clinic or hospital freely without referral by a general practitioner, and patients pay only about $5–$15 USD at each visit.

Considering the neurological deficit and functional disability related to stroke, and the minimal barrier to medical access in Taiwan, it can be expected that most patients who developed stroke would seek medical help and would be captured in the NHI database, which enabled us to identify all incident cases of stroke and establish a temporal relationship between AS and ischemic stroke. Nevertheless, several limitations should be acknowledged. First, the diagnoses of AS, ischemic stroke, and medical comorbidities were determined using the ICD codes from the NHI claim database, and there may be concern about the diagnostic accuracy of the database. However, the Bureau of NHI has formed different audit committees that make it a rule to randomly sample the claims data from every hospital and to review charts on a regular basis to verify the diagnostic validity and quality of care. In addition, one validation study that evaluated the validity of the NHI database for patients with a principal diagnosis of ischemic stroke showed that the NHI database appears to be a valid resource for population-based research in ischemic stroke [32]. Accordingly, the NHI claim database is an established research database and independent studies have demonstrated the validity of the data [33]. Furthermore, we performed sensitivity analyses using various case definitions, and found that AS was consistently linked to an increased risk of developing ischemic stroke, suggesting that our results are robust to different case definitions. Second, although we excluded subjects with a previous diagnosis of AS during year 2000 to increase the likelihood of identifying AS patients newly diagnosed in 2001, it was possible that some prevalent AS cases with more longstanding AS who had not sought medical care in 2000 but coded for the first time in

2001 based on our database, were included in the AS group. Third, due to the inherent limitation of the NHI database, information was lacking regarding lifestyle factors, such as smoking, alcohol consumption, and obesity. Moreover, since traditional vascular risk factors, such as diabetes, hypertension and dyslipidemia, are disorders with an insidious onset, some asymptomatic vascular risk factors may not be captured in the NHI database. Therefore, the prevalence of vascular risk factors may be underestimated in both the AS and non-AS groups. These potential confounders may lead to residual confounding and may affect the interpretation of our findings. Fourth, the follow-up time was only 2 years and the long-term effects of AS on the development of ischemic stroke cannot therefore be evaluated. Finally, since Taiwanese are mainly of Chinese ethnicity, it is uncertain whether our findings can be generalized to other ethnic groups.

In conclusion, the present population-based longitudinal follow-up study demonstrates there is an increased risk of ischemic stroke in young patients with AS and highlights the importance of early risk assessment for ischemic stroke in such patients. Further long-term follow-up study would be required to validate our findings and to investigate the underlying pathophysiological mechanism.

## Author Contributions

Conceived and designed the experiments: CWL YPH YHC YTH SLP. Performed the experiments: CWL YPH YHC YTH SLP. Analyzed the data: CWL YPH YHC SLP. Contributed reagents/materials/analysis tools: CWL YPH YHC SLP. Wrote the paper: CWL YPH YHC YTH SLP.

## References

1. Braun J, Sieper J (2007) Ankylosing spondylitis. Lancet 369: 1379–1390.
2. El Maghraoui A (2011) Extra-articular manifestations of ankylosing spondylitis: prevalence, characteristics and therapeutic implications. Eur J Intern Med 22: 554–560.
3. Divecha H, Sattar N, Rumley A, Cherry L, Lowe GD, et al. (2005) Cardiovascular risk parameters in men with ankylosing spondylitis in comparison with non-inflammatory control subjects: relevance of systemic inflammation. Clin Sci (Lond) 109: 171–176.
4. Peters MJ, van der Horst-Bruinsma IE, Dijkmans BA, Nurmohamed MT (2004) Cardiovascular risk profile of patients with spondylarthropathies, particularly ankylosing spondylitis and psoriatic arthritis. Semin Arthritis Rheum 34: 585–592.
5. Roman MJ, Salmon JE (2007) Cardiovascular manifestations of rheumatologic diseases. Circulation 116: 2346–2355.
6. Mathieu S, Gossec L, Dougados M, Soubrier M (2011) Cardiovascular profile in ankylosing spondylitis: a systematic review and meta-analysis. Arthritis Care Res (Hoboken) 63: 557–563.
7. Bremander A, Petersson IF, Bergman S, Englund M (2011) Population-based estimates of common comorbidities and cardiovascular disease in ankylosing spondylitis. Arthritis Care Res (Hoboken) 63: 550–556.
8. Huang YP, Wang YH, Pan SL (2013) Increased risk of ischemic heart disease in young patients with newly diagnosed ankylosing spondylitis—a population-based longitudinal follow-up study. PLoS One 8: e64155.
9. Han C, Robinson DW Jr, Hackett MV, Paramore LC, Fraeman KH, et al. (2006) Cardiovascular disease and risk factors in patients with rheumatoid arthritis, psoriatic arthritis, and ankylosing spondylitis. J Rheumatol 33: 2167–2172.
10. Szabo SM, Levy AR, Rao SR, Kirbach SE, Lacaille D, et al. (2011) Increased risk of cardiovascular and cerebrovascular diseases in individuals with ankylosing spondylitis: A population-based study. Arthritis Rheum 63: 3294–3304.
11. Kang JH, Chen YH, Lin HC (2010) Comorbidity profiles among patients with ankylosing spondylitis: a nationwide population-based study. Ann Rheum Dis 69: 1165–1168.
12. Ross R (1999) Atherosclerosis—an inflammatory disease. N Engl J Med 340: 115–126.
13. Pearson TA, Mensah GA, Alexander RW, Anderson JL, Cannon RO 3rd, et al. (2003) Markers of inflammation and cardiovascular disease: application to clinical and public health practice: A statement for healthcare professionals from the Centers for Disease Control and Prevention and the American Heart Association. Circulation 107: 499–511.
14. Verma S, Anderson TJ (2002) Fundamentals of endothelial function for the clinical cardiologist. Circulation 105: 546–549.
15. Stoll G, Bendszus M (2006) Inflammation and atherosclerosis: novel insights into plaque formation and destabilization. Stroke 37: 1923–1932.
16. Gratacos J, Collado A, Filella X, Sanmarti R, Canete J, et al. (1994) Serum cytokines (IL-6, TNF-alpha, IL-1 beta and IFN-gamma) in ankylosing spondylitis: a close correlation between serum IL-6 and disease activity and severity. Br J Rheumatol 33: 927–931.
17. Lange U, Teichmann J, Stracke H (2000) Correlation between plasma TNF-alpha, IGF-1, biochemical markers of bone metabolism, markers of inflammation/disease activity, and clinical manifestations in ankylosing spondylitis. Eur J Med Res 5: 507–511.
18. Hamdi W, Chelli Bouaziz M, Zouch I, Ghannouchi MM, Haouel M, et al. (2012) Assessment of preclinical atherosclerosis in patients with ankylosing spondylitis. J Rheumatol 39: 322–326.
19. Bodnar N, Kerekes G, Seres I, Paragh G, Kappelmayer J, et al. (2011) Assessment of subclinical vascular disease associated with ankylosing spondylitis. J Rheumatol 38: 723–729.
20. Cece H, Yazgan P, Karakas E, Karakas O, Demirkol A, et al. (2011) Carotid intima-media thickness and paraoxonase activity in patients with ankylosing spondylitis. Clin Invest Med 34: E225.
21. Peters MJ, van Eijk IC, Smulders YM, Serne E, Dijkmans BA, et al. (2010) Signs of accelerated preclinical atherosclerosis in patients with ankylosing spondylitis. J Rheumatol 37: 161–166.
22. Gonzalez-Juanatey C, Vazquez-Rodriguez TR, Miranda-Filloy JA, Dierssen T, Vaqueiro I, et al. (2009) The High Prevalence of Subclinical Atherosclerosis in Patients With Ankylosing Spondylitis Without Clinically Evident Cardiovascular Disease. Medicine 88: 358–365.
23. Sari I, Okan T, Akar S, Cece H, Altay C, et al. (2006) Impaired endothelial function in patients with ankylosing spondylitis. Rheumatology (Oxford) 45: 283–286.
24. O'Neill TW, Bresnihan B (1992) The heart in ankylosing spondylitis. Ann Rheum Dis 51: 705–706.
25. Ribeiro P, Morley KD, Shapiro LM, Garnett RA, Hughes GR, et al. (1984) Left ventricular function in patients with ankylosing spondylitis and Reiter's disease. Eur Heart J 5: 419–422.
26. Avierinos JF, Brown RD, Foley DA, Nkomo V, Petty GW, et al. (2003) Cerebral ischemic events after diagnosis of mitral valve prolapse: a community-based study of incidence and predictive factors. Stroke 34: 1339–1344.
27. Cohen A, Tzourio C, Chauvel C, Bertrand B, Crassard I, et al. (1997) Mitral valve strands and the risk of ischemic stroke in elderly patients. The French Study of Aortic Plaques in Stroke (FAPS) Investigators. Stroke 28: 1574–1578.

28. Braun J, van den Berg R, Baraliakos X, Boehm H, Burgos-Vargas R, et al. (2011) 2010 update of the ASAS/EULAR recommendations for the management of ankylosing spondylitis. Ann Rheum Dis 70: 896–904.

29. van den Berg R, Baraliakos X, Braun J, van der Heijde D (2012) First update of the current evidence for the management of ankylosing spondylitis with non-pharmacological treatment and non-biologic drugs: a systematic literature review for the ASAS/EULAR management recommendations in ankylosing spondylitis. Rheumatology (Oxford) 51: 1388–1396.

30. Bhala N, Emberson J, Merhi A, Abramson S, Arber N, et al. (2013) Vascular and upper gastrointestinal effects of non-steroidal anti-inflammatory drugs: meta-analyses of individual participant data from randomised trials. Lancet 382: 769–779.

31. Chou CT, Pei L, Chang DM, Lee CF, Schumacher HR, et al. (1994) Prevalence of rheumatic diseases in Taiwan: a population study of urban, suburban, rural differences. J Rheumatol 21: 302–306.

32. Cheng CL, Kao YH, Lin SJ, Lee CH, Lai ML (2011) Validation of the National Health Insurance Research Database with ischemic stroke cases in Taiwan. Pharmacoepidemiol Drug Saf 20: 236–242.

33. Wu CH, Wang YH, Huang YP, Pan SL (2012) Does adhesive capsulitis of the shoulder increase the risk of stroke? A population-based propensity score-matched follow-up study. PLoS One 7: e49343.

# rs10865331 Associated with Susceptibility and Disease Severity of Ankylosing Spondylitis in a Taiwanese Population

**Ya-Feng Wen[1,7◐], James Cheng-Chung Wei[2,3◐], Yu-Wen Hsu[1,7◐], Hung-Yi Chiou[4,7],
Henry Sung-Ching Wong[7], Ruey-Hong Wong[5], Shiro Ikegawa[7,8], Wei-Chiao Chang[1,6,7]\***

**1** Department of Clinical Pharmacy, School of Pharmacy, Taipei Medical University, Taipei, Taiwan, **2** Division of Allergy, Immunology and Rheumatology, Department of Medicine, Chung Shan Medical University Hospital, Taichung, Taiwan, **3** Institute of Medicine, Chung Shan Medical University, Taichung, Taiwan, **4** School of Public Health, Taipei Medical University, Taipei, Taiwan, **5** Department of Public Health, Chung Shan Medical University, Taichung, Taiwan, **6** Department of Pharmacy, Taipei Medical University-Wanfang Hospital, Taipei, Taiwan, **7** Master Program for Clinical Pharmacogenomics and Pharmacoproteomics, School of Pharmacy, Taipei Medical University, Taipei, Taiwan, **8** Laboratory for Bone and Joint Diseases, RIKEN Center for Integrative Medical Science, Yokohama, Japan

## Abstract

Ankylosing spondylitis (AS) is a highly familial rheumatic disorder and is considered as a chronic inflammatory disease. Genetic factors are involved in the pathogenesis of AS. To identify genes which render people susceptible to AS in a Taiwanese population, we selected six single-nucleotide polymorphisms (SNPs) from previous genome-wide association studies (GWASs) which were associated with AS in European descendants and Han Chinese. To assess whether the six SNPs contributed to AS susceptibility and severity in Taiwanese population, 475 AS patients fulfilling the modified New York Criteria and 527 healthy subjects were recruited. We found that rs10865331 was significantly associated with AS susceptibility and with Bath AS Function Index (BASFI). The AA and AG genotypes of rs10865331 were also significantly associated with a higher erythrocyte sedimentation rate. Our findings provided evidence that rs10865331 is associated AS susceptibility and with disease activity (BASFI) in a Taiwanese population.

**Editor:** Yu-Jia Chang, Taipei Medicine University, Taiwan

**Funding:** This work was supported by the funding from an Excellence for Cancer Research Center grant, Department of Health, Executive Yuan, Taiwan, R.O.C. (DOH102-TD-C-111-002) and grants from the National Science Council, Taiwan, ROC (NSC101-2628-B038-001-MY2; NSC101-2320-B038-029-MY3). The funders had no role in study design, data collection and analysis, decision to publish, or preparation of the manuscript.

**Competing Interests:** The authors have declared that no competing interests exist.

\* Email: wcc@tmu.edu.tw

◐ These authors contributed equally to this work.

## Background

Ankylosing spondylitis (AS) is a systemic, autoimmune disease that causes inflammation of the area where ligaments and tendons insert into the bone, and includes sacroiliitis, spondylitis, spondylodiscitis, and spondylarthritis. The prevalence of AS in Taiwan is about 0.2%~0.3% which is similar to those in Europe and USA [1,2]. The male-to-female ratio is about 3:1 in AS. Twin and family studies have indicated that genetic factors contribute over 90% to the overall AS susceptibility [3,4]. *Human leucocyte antigen-B 27* (*HLA-B27*) gene is the best-known genetic susceptibility marker for AS, and frequencies of *HLA-B27* are approximately 5.7% and 95% in the general Taiwanese population and Taiwanese AS patients, respectively [5]. Wei et al., showed that HLA-B60 and HLA-B61 are associated with AS in HLA-B27-negative patients in Taiwan [6]. Despite the strong association between HLA and AS, only 1%~5% of HLA-B27 carriers develop AS [4]. Many non-major histocompatibility complex (non-MHC) regions were found to be significantly associated to AS in genome-wide association studies (GWASs) [7–9]. Additionally, genetic polymorphisms of *ORAI1* (rs12313273 and rs7135617) and *STIM1* (rs3750996) were

reported to be associated with the pathogenesis of HLA-B27-positive (HLA-B27(+)) AS patients [10,11].

Previous GWAS reports in European descent indicated that AS development was strongly associated with the 2p15 (rs10865331), 21q22 (rs2242944), *anthrax toxin receptor 2* (*ANTXR2*) (rs4333130), and *interleukin (IL)-23 receptor* (*IL23R*) (rs2310173) loci [7]. John Reveille et al. confirmed the associations of *IL23R* (rs11209026) and *endoplasmic reticulum aminopeptidase 1* (*ERAP1*) (rs27037 and rs27434) with AS [12]. Other significant loci, including *RUNX3* (rs11249215), *LTBR-TNFRSF1A* (rs11616188), and *IL12B* (rs6556416), were also found in a combined discovery and replication study of Europeans [8]. Furthermore, Evans et al., showed a new susceptibility loci of *PTGER4* (rs10440635), *TBKBP1* (10781500), *ANTXR2* (rs4389526), and *CARD9* (rs10781500) that were also involved in the disease pathogenesis. In addition, the *ERAP1* polymorphisms (rs30187) was found to associate with the risk of HLA-B27(+) AS patients [8].

The GWAS conducted in Han Chinese identified new AS susceptibility loci at 6q21 (rs13210693), *HAPLN1-EDIL3* (rs4552569), and *ANO6* (rs17095830). However, there is no strong evidence to indicate the association between *ANTXR2* and

**Table 1.** Six previously reported single nucleotide polymorphisms associated with ankylosing spondylitis.

| SNP | Population | Chr.[a] position | Candidate gene | No. Sample (Case/Control) | Trend p value | Ref.[b] |
|------|-----------|-----------|----------------|---------------------------|---------------|------|
| rs27434 | Han Chinese | 5p15 | ERAP1 | 1,837/4,231 | 6.68E-4 | 9 |
| rs3734523 | European | 6p22.2 | MHC | 2,053/5,140 | 1.60E-8 | 7 |
| rs4672495 | European | 2p15 | - | 2,053/5,140 | 3.30E-9 | 7 |
| rs10865331 | Han Chinese | 2p15 | - | 1,837/4,231 | 1.98E-8 | 9 |
| rs11209032 | British, Australian | 1p31 | IL23R | 4,810/13,579 | 2.3E-17 | 8 |
| rs13210693 | Han Chinese | 6q21 | - | 1,837/4,231 | 9.31E-7 | 9 |

[a]. Chr., Chromosome.
[b]. Reference number (Ref.) is the same as that in the text.

*IL23R* polymorphisms and AS in Han Chinese population [9,13]. Wang *et al.* confirmed the findings of previous studies [14–16] that *ERAP1* is a risk factor for AS susceptibility in a Taiwanese population [17]. However, susceptibility loci between *EDIL3*, *HAPLN1* at 5q14.3 and within *ANO6* at 12q12 discovered in a Han Chinese GWAS were negatively associated with Taiwanese population [18], suggesting that genetic factors underlying the susceptibility may differ between these two populations. In this study, we selected SNPs from previous GWAS reports to test whether candidate genetic variations contribute to AS susceptibility and severity in a Taiwanese population.

## Methods

### Subjects

The design of the work was conformed to the *Declaration of Helsinki*. The study was approved by the Institute Review Board of Chung Shan Medical University Hospital. Before any data were collected, we received informed consent from all subjects. All subjects provided a written consent form. AS patients who fulfilled the selection criteria were sequentially solicited at Chung Shan Medical University Hospital in Taichung, Taiwan. The criteria included (a) patients being aged 17~82 years; (b) cognitive performance not being influenced by other diseases such as dementia; and (c) an AS diagnosis having been made by modified New York criteria developed in 1984. AS diagnosed by qualified rheumatologist. Patients with sacroiliitis were confirmed by a qualified radiologist. The detailed clinical history included extraspinal manifestations, age on initial symptoms, and laboratory parameters of inflammation, i.e., the erythrocyte sedimentation rate (ESR), and C-reactive protein (CRP). Family history of AS was also recorded. The age of onset of AS symptom was defined as the time when the first symptom (axial symptom, peripheral arthritis, uveitis, or enthesitis) was noted. Peripheral arthritis was

defined as the presence of at least one swollen joint. All AS patients in this study had sacroiliitis. These symptoms were recorded in medical record reviews, and were ascertained by a rheumatologist, ophthalmologist, and gastroenterologist.

Potential controls were randomly selected from sequential patients with no significant medical histories or abnormal laboratory results. To exclude controls with potential risks of getting AS, we used the *HLA-B* (rs13202464) polymorphism as a screening factor. Forty-three control subjects carrying the heterozygous AG genotype were excluded. Meanwhile, our data confirmed that *HLA-B* was significantly associated with AS in a Taiwanese population ($P<0.0001$). The Bath AS Disease Activity Index (BASDAI), Bath AS Functional Index (BASFI), and Bath AS Global (BAS-G) were respectively applied to evaluate disease activity, physical function, and global wellbeing. Modified Chinese versions of the BASDAI, BASFI, and BAS-G had good intra-class correlations and Cronbach's alpha values.

### Candidate SNPs

We included SNPs which showed a significant association with AS in three previous GWAS studies (with trend *P*-values of less than or near $10^{-7}$) [7–9] and excluded those hadpublished on Taiwanese populations. The reason for including *ERAP1* (rs27434) is because the other three SNPs on ERAP1 are reported as predisposing factors for AS in Taiwanese [17]; therefore, we test whether SNP, rs27434, has the same effect or not.

### DNA extraction

Blood cells were subjected to DNA extraction by first treating them with 0.5% sodium dodecylsulfate lysis buffer and then protease K (1 mg/ml) to digest nuclear proteins for 4 h at 60°C. Total DNA was harvested using a Gentra (Qiagen, Valencia, CA) extraction kit followed by 70% alcohol precipitation.

**Table 2.** Characteristics of the Taiwanese population.

| Characteristic | AS patient | Control |
|----------------|-----------|---------|
| Number of subjects | 475 | 527 |
| Gender: male No (%) | 323 (68.0) | 365 (69.3) |
| Age: mean ± SD (years) | 39.0±11.3 | 39.0±11.9 |
| BASDAI | 4.3±2.2 | |
| BASFI | 2.1±2.2 | |
| BAS-G | 4.4±2.8 | |

**Table 3.** Association risk SNPs in previous study and current study.

| SNP | Minor allele | European cohort[7] Allele frequency[a] | British, Australia cohort[8] Allele frequency[a] | Han Chinese cohort[9] Allele frequency[a] | Current study Allele frequency[a] | OR (95% CI)[b] | P-value[b] | HWE[c] |
|---|---|---|---|---|---|---|---|---|
| rs3734523 | A | 0.09/0.12 | | | 0.02/0.04 | 0.58 (0.33–1.00) | 0.052 | 0.265 |
| rs4672495 | G | 0.36/0.32 | | | 0.17/0.19 | 0.89 (0.67–1.17) | 0.400 | 0.632 |
| rs10865331 | A | 0.43/0.36 | 0.45/0.37 | 0.54/0.48 | 0.53/0.47 | 1.65 (1.21–2.23) | **0.001**\*\* | 0.817 |
| rs11209032 | G | | 0.36/0.33 | | 0.49/0.49 | 1.04 (0.26–1.96) | 0.794 | 0.073 |
| rs27434 | G | 0.26/0.21 | | 0.55/0.53 | 0.46/0.50 | 0.86 (0.94–1.96) | 0.347 | 0.336 |
| rs13210693 | G | | | 0.47/0.44 | 0.52/0.48 | 1.38 (1.96–2.06) | 0.039 | 0.867 |

$\chi^2$-test was applied for testing genotype frequencies of SNPs in controls and patients with AS.

\*\*Significant (p<0.0017) value is in bold.

[a]Allele frequency in case/control.

[b]The OR and P-value were showed for dominant model of SNPs.

[c]HWE were performed by chi-square.

[7,8,9]The reference numbers are as the same as that in the text.

## Genotyping

Genotyping for the seven SNPs was carried out using the TaqMan Allelic Discrimination Assay (Applied Biosystems, Foster City, CA). A polymerase chain reaction (PCR) used a 96-well micro-plate with an ABI9700 Thermal Cycler (Applied Biosystems). After the PCR, StepOne software vers. 2.2.2 (Applied Biosystems) was used to detect and analyze the fluorescence. Possession of the *HLA-B27* polymorphism was assessed by flow cytometry as previously described [19].

## Statistical analysis

JMP, Version 8.0 SAS Institute Inc., Cary, NC, 1989–2007 was applied for statistical analyses. Hardy-Weinberg equilibrium (HWE) was used to test the SNPs' allelic frequencies by using $\chi^2$-test. Statistical differences between the patient and control groups in genotype frequencies were evaluated by $\chi^2$-test with one degree of freedom or Fisher's exact test. Kruskal-Wallis test was applied to compare the mean of continuous variables (BASDAI, BASFI, and BAS-G). Differences in the values of the ESR, and CRP among AS patients stratified by different genotypes were computed by Wilcoxon rank sum test. Analysis of covariance (ANCOVA) was used to adjust for age, gender, and disease duration. The correlation coefficient was examined between inflammatory biochemical results (ESR and CRP) and BASDI, BASFI, BAS-G. *P*-value of <0.05 was considered statistical significant.

## Results

### Clinical features

Six selected SNPs are shown in Table 1. 475 patients with AS and 527 control subjects were recruited (Table 2). All AS patients were diagnosed according to the modified New York criteria. Their mean age was 39 years; 69.3% were men and 90.7% were HLA-B27 (+). Their mean BASDAI, BASFI and BAS-G scores were 4.3±2.2, 2.1±2.2, and 4.4±2.8, respectively. No significant different distribution of genotypes was found between HapMap CHB population and our control subjects (Table S1 in File S1).

### rs10865331 is associated with AS susceptibility

All genotype distributions of the polymorphisms fulfilled the criteria of HWE (*P*>0.05). Table 3 showed a comparison between AS cases and controls for each genotype and individual allele for all six SNPs. The rs10865331 A allele carrier (contained AA and AG genotypes) had 1.65 fold risk compared with GG genotype carrier (OR (95% CI) = 1.65 (1.21–2.23), *P*-value = 0.001). G allele of rs13210693 at 6q21, had a significant correlation with AS susceptibility (OR (95% CI) = 1.38 (1.96–2.06), *P*-value = 0.039). Since *P*-value was considered significant when it was less than 0.0083, after applying Bonferroni correction, only rs10865331 polymorphism showed significant association with AS.

### rs10865331 is associated with AS severity

We investigated the relationship between genetic polymorphisms and clinical phenotypes including the BASDAI, BASFI, and BAS-G. We found that rs10865331 was highly associated with the BASFI (*P*-value = 0.033). However, the results showed no statistical significance after applying the Bonferroni correction and adjusting for gender and disease duration (Table 4). We further analyzed the association between inflammatory biochemical results (ESR and CRP) and the rs10865331 genetic polymorphism. rs10865331 AA and AG genotypes were significantly correlated with an increased ESR compared to the GG genotype in AS patients (*P*-value = 0.021) (Figure 1). The means±standard

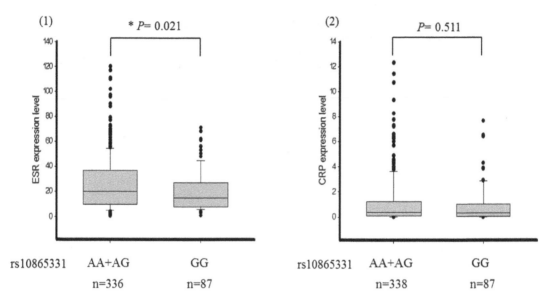

**Figure 1. Comparison of the erythrocyte sedimentation rate (ESR) and C-reactive protein (CRP) levels among different genotypes of rs10865331 in ankylosing spondylitis (AS) patients.**

deviations of the ESR for the combined AA and AG genotypes and GG genotype were $26.00 \pm 21.74$ and $20.07 \pm 16.26$, respectively. However, the risk allele (A allele) of rs10865331 showed no correlation with CRP ($P$-value $= 0.511$). CRP values were $1.17 \pm 1.89$ for the combined AA and AG genotypes and $0.96 \pm 1.49$ for the GG genotype. In addition, the A allele of rs10865331 in HLA-B27(+) AS patients had a significant association with the ESR ($P$-value $= 0.010$) (Figure 2).

### ESR and CRP showed positive correlations with the Bath indices

Table 4 indicated the relationship between rs10865331 and BASFI. We, therefore, further tested the correlation between inflammatory biochemical data (ESR and CRP) and disease activity (BASDI, BASFI, BAS-G). As shown in Figure 3A, ESR associated with BASDI ($R = 0.1671$, $P$-value $= 0.0004$), BASFI ($R = 0.3047$, $P$-value $< 0.0001$), and BAS-G ($R = 0.1932$, $P$-value $< 0.0001$). Regarding to CRP, positive correlations between CRP and BASDI ($R = 0.178$, $P$-value $< 0.0001$), BASFI ($R = 0.3061$, $P$-value $< 0.0001$), BAS-G ($R = 0.2420$, $P$-value $< 0.0001$) were found. (Figure 3B)

### Discussion

In the case-control study, rs10865331 was significantly associated with a genetic predisposition for AS and also affected patients' daily functional activities represented by BASFI. However, the

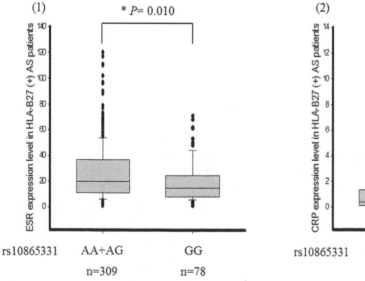
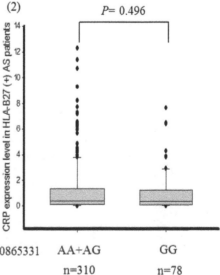

**Figure 2. Comparison of the erythrocyte sedimentation rate (ESR) and C-reactive protein (CRP) levels among different genotypes of rs10865331 in ankylosing spondylitis (AS) patients positive for HLA-B27.**

**Table 4.** Difference in disease activity scores in the AS patients stratified by genotypes.

| SNP | Genotype | BASDAI | BASFI | BAS-G |
|---|---|---|---|---|
| rs3734523 | AA | 3.84 | 4.01 | 5.00 |
| | AG | 3.61±2.48 | 1.35±2.23 | 3.79±3.07 |
| | GG | 4.32±2.19 | 2.03±2.16 | 4.41 ± 2.73 |
| Unadjusted p value | | 0.289 | 0.170 | 0.538 |
| Adjusted p value | | 0.361[†] | 0.194[§] | 0.573[†] |
| rs4672495 | GG | 3.99±2.63 | 0.79±0.82 | 4.13 ± 2.80 |
| | GT | 4.22±2.31 | 2.06±2.25 | 4.31 ± 2.76 |
| | TT | 4.32±2.15 | 2.08±2.24 | 4.42 ± 2.76 |
| Unadjusted p value | | 0.847 | 0.210 | 0.862 |
| Adjusted p value | | 0.737[†] | 0.275[§] | 0.888[†] |
| rs10865331 | AA | 4.66±2.09 | 2.35±2.34 | 4.66 ± 2.73 |
| | AG | 4.16±2.22 | 2.13±2.32 | 4.31 ± 2.75 |
| | GG | 4.22±2.25 | 1.47±1.69 | 4.22 ± 2.68 |
| Unadjusted p value | | 0.132 | **0.033***  | 0.391 |
| Adjusted p value | | 0.104[†] | 0.133[§] | 0.500[†] |
| rs11209032 | AA | 4.61±2.10 | 2.11±2.36 | 4.56 ± 2.55 |
| | AG | 4.09±2.10 | 1.97±2.12 | 4.32 ± 2.77 |
| | GG | 4.34±2.44 | 2.12±2.32 | 4.36 ± 2.90 |
| Unadjusted p value | | 0.096 | 0.941 | 0.604 |
| Adjusted p value | | 0.156[†] | 0.467[§] | 0.737[†] |
| rs27434 | GG | 4.56±2.12 | 2.05±2.08 | 4.53 ± 2.50 |
| | AG | 4.17±2.28 | 2.03±2.14 | 4.50 ± 2.85 |
| | AA | 4.33±2.11 | 1.61±1.92 | 3.84 ± 2.60 |
| Unadjusted p value | | 0.593 | 0.364 | 0.083 |
| Adjusted p value | | 0.407[†] | 0.331[§] | 0.125[†] |
| rs13210693 | AA | 4.37±2.30 | 1.93±2.20 | 4.10 ± 2.79 |
| | AG | 4.18±2.20 | 1.95±2.21 | 4.26 ± 2.66 |
| | GG | 4.60±2.07 | 2.28±2.09 | 4.83±2.75 |
| Unadjusted p value | | 0.203 | 0.209 | 0.127 |
| Adjusted p value | | 0.271[†] | 0.368[§] | 0.100[†] |

BAS, Bath Ankylosing Spondylitis; DAI, Disease Activity Index; FI, Function Index; G, Global. Data are presented as the mean ± standard deviation. The Kruskal-Wallis test is applied to exam the difference in disease activity scores in the AS patients stratified by genotypes.
[†]Adjusted for the effects of age and gender.
[§]Adjusted for the effects of age, gender, and disease duration. Significant ($p<0.05$) values are in bold.

association between AS and the BASFI became insignificance after adjusting for age, gender, and the duration of the disease, this is possibly caused by the variation of scores among patients. We, therefore, used clinically important measures, including the ESR and CRP, to support the correlation between candidate SNPs and disease severity. We found an association between inflammatory biochemical lab data, i.e., the ESR, and disease severity in AS patients. After excluding HLA-B27(−) AS patients, the same trend was also found. This is the first study to confirm that the intergenic SNP, rs10865331, on chromosome 2p15 is highly associated with AS disease in a Taiwanese population.

The intergenic region, 2p15, of the associated rs10865331 SNP was replicated in several studies of Spanish, Korean and Han Chinese populations [14,15,20]. The rs10865331 polymorphism located 99 kb upstream of *B3GNT2* and 182 kb downstream of *TMEM17*. Although the mechanism and functions leading to progression of AS still need to be elucidated, an SNP on *B3GNT2* was found to be a susceptibility marker for rheumatoid arthritis in

a Japanese GWAS meta-analysis [21]. In addition, a polymorphism (rs6545946) at 2p15 could be a plausible candidate SNP for Crohn's disease, which is a common comorbid condition of AS in Ashkenazi Jewish patients [22]. The evidence implies that intergenic regions of chromosomes 2p15 are somehow associated with certain immune diseases.

*ERAP1* involves peptide trimming as presented by HLA class I molecules within the endoplasmic reticulum and only affects AS risk in HLA-B(+) individuals [23]. *ERAP1* may play an important role in the shedding of proinflammatory cytokine receptors and downregulation of inflammatory responses [24]. Nonetheless, the association between *ERAP1* polymorphisms and AS is divergent in different ethnic groups in genetic studies. In a meta-analysis study, rs27434 showed no significant correlation with AS, which corresponded with our results [16]. Wang et al. identified another *ERAP1* SNP, rs27037, which can predict AS susceptibility and syndesmophyte formation [17]. rs27434 is a synonymous SNP, and rs27037 is located in the intron possibly affecting the

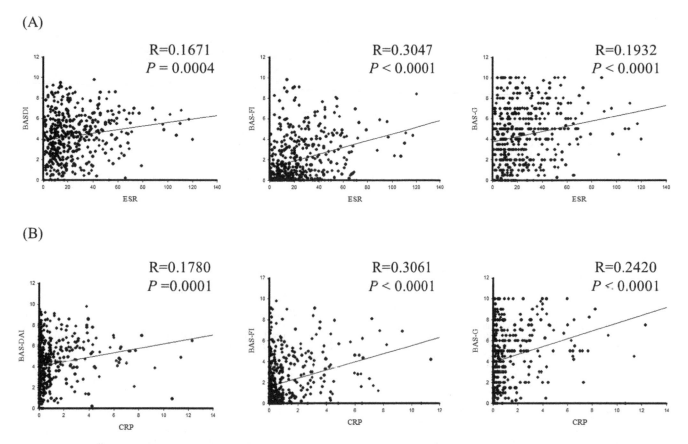

**Figure 3. Correlation analysis between erythrocyte sedimentation rate (ESR), C-reactive protein (CRP) and Bath Indices (BASDI, BASFI and BAS-G).**

regulation of MHC I heavy chain homodimers leading to unfolded protein responses [25]. This may explain the different effects of the two SNPs.

In 2013, evidence from high-density genotyping of immune-related loci indicated that major histocompatibility complex (MHC) class I presentation and IL-23 pathway are key elements in the development of ankylosing spondylitis [26]. Indeed, previous studies also confirmed an important role of *IL23R* gene in AS [27]. IL23R belongs to the hemopoietin receptor family for IL-23, a proinflammatory cytokine, and is involved in the production and differentiation of memory T-cells [27]. rs11209032 showed a significant correlation with AS in a UK case-control study and meta-analysis [28]. Another meta-analysis showed that rs11209032 was significantly associated with AS in European but not Asian populations [29]. Genetic differences between different ethnic groups may explain why rs11209032 had no statistical association with AS in a Taiwanese population. Interestingly, many studies reported that variations in *IL23R* were not associated with AS [15,30] but were correlated with inflammatory bowel disease (IBD) which is clinically related to AS [31]. Our previous results also indicated that two susceptibility SNPs identified from Han Chinese GWAS study [9], *HAPLN1-EDIL3* (rs4552569) and *ANO6* (rs17095830), were not associated with AS severity but IBD in a Taiwanese population [18]. Further studies are needed to clarify the mechanism by which MHC and IL-23 involve the pathogenesis of AS and IBD.

By a systemic overview of genetic variations of the risk in three previous GWASs, we were better able to understand the high-risk polymorphisms in the Taiwanese population. A new susceptibility polymorphism at 2p15 (rs10865331) was associated with AS and disease severity. However, even with large-scale screening of candidate susceptibility loci, the exact pathological mechanism and interactions between AS genes, e.g., *ERAP1* and *HLA-B*, are still unknown. Furthermore, examination of epigenetic factors and copy number variations are required, and functional studies that show how susceptible genes actually affect AS should be conducted. Combining all the functional causal alleles in Taiwanese populations may improve our understanding of the genetic basis of the disease and lead to novel treatment approaches.

## Supporting Information

**File S1  Supporting tables.** Table S1, Comparison between HapMap CHB population and Taiwanese population. Table S2, Genotype and allele frequencies in controls and patients among HLA-B27 (+) with AS.

## Author Contributions

Conceived and designed the experiments: WCC HYC HSCW RHW. Performed the experiments: YFW YWH. Analyzed the data: YWH HSCW. Contributed reagents/materials/analysis tools: JCCW. Wrote the paper: YFW SI WCC.

## References

1.  Reveille JD (2011) Epidemiology of spondyloarthritis in North America. Am J Med Sci 341: 284–286.
2.  Zochling J, Smith EU (2010) Seronegative spondyloarthritis. Best Pract Res Clin Rheumatol 24: 747–756.
3.  Brown M, Laval S, Brophy S, Calin A (2000) Recurrence risk modelling of the genetic susceptibility to ankylosing spondylitis. Annals of the rheumatic diseases 59: 883–886.
4.  Brown MA, Kennedy LG, Macgregor AJ, Darke C, Duncan E, et al. (1997) Susceptibility to ankylosing spondylitis in twins the role of genes, HLA, and the environment. Arthritis & Rheumatism 40: 1823–1828.
5.  Yang KL, Chen IH, Hsiao CK, Cherng JM, Yang KZ, et al. (2004) Polymorphism of HLA-B27 in Taiwanese Chinese. Tissue Antigens 63: 476–479.
6.  Wei JC, Tsai WC, Lin HS, Tsai CY, Chou CT (2004) HLA-B60 and B61 are strongly associated with ankylosing spondylitis in HLA-B27-negative Taiwan Chinese patients. Rheumatology (Oxford) 43: 839–842.
7.  Australo-Anglo-American Spondyloarthritis Consortium (TASC), Reveille JD, Sims AM, Danoy P, Evans DM, et al. (2010) Genome-wide association study of ankylosing spondylitis identifies non-MHC susceptibility loci. Nat Genet 42: 123–127.
8.  Evans DM, Spencer CC, Pointon JJ, Su Z, Harvey D, et al. (2011) Interaction between ERAP1 and HLA-B27 in ankylosing spondylitis implicates peptide handling in the mechanism for HLA-B27 in disease susceptibility. Nat Genet 43: 761–767.
9.  Lin Z, Bei JX, Shen M, Li Q, Liao Z, et al. (2012) A genome-wide association study in Han Chinese identifies new susceptibility loci for ankylosing spondylitis. Nat Genet 44: 73–77.
10. Wei JC, Yen JH, Juo SH, Chen WC, Wang YS, et al. (2011) Association of ORAI1 haplotypes with the risk of HLA-B27 positive ankylosing spondylitis. PLoS One 6: e20426.
11. Wei JC, Hung KS, Hsu YW, Wong RH, Huang CH, et al. (2012) Genetic Polymorphisms of Stromal Interaction Molecule 1 Associated with the Erythrocyte Sedimentation Rate and C-Reactive Protein in HLA-B27 Positive Ankylosing Spondylitis Patients. PLoS One 7: e49698.
12. Wellcome Trust Case Control Consortium, Australo-Anglo-American Spondylitis Consortium (TASC), Burton PR, Clayton DG, Cardon LR, et al. (2007) Association scan of 14,500 nonsynonymous SNPs in four diseases identifies autoimmunity variants. Nat Genet 39: 1329–1337.
13. Chen C, Zhang X, Wang Y (2012) ANTXR2 and IL-1R2 polymorphisms are not associated with ankylosing spondylitis in Chinese Han population. Rheumatol Int 32: 15–19.
14. Bang SY, Kim TH, Lee B, Kwon E, Choi SH, et al. (2011) Genetic studies of ankylosing spondylitis in Koreans confirm associations with ERAP1 and 2p15 reported in white patients. J Rheumatol 38: 322–324.
15. Davidson SI, Liu Y, Danoy PA, Wu X, Thomas GP, et al. (2011) Association of STAT3 and TNFRSF1A with ankylosing spondylitis in Han Chinese. Ann Rheum Dis 70: 289–292.
16. Chen R, Yao L, Meng T, Xu W (2012) The association between seven ERAP1 polymorphisms and ankylosing spondylitis susceptibility: a meta-analysis involving 8,530 cases and 12,449 controls. Rheumatol Int 32: 909–914.
17. Wang CM, Ho HH, Chang SW, Wu YJ, Lin JC, et al. (2012) ERAP1 genetic variations associated with HLA-B27 interaction and disease severity of syndesmophytes formation in Taiwanese ankylosing spondylitis. Arthritis Res Ther 14: R125.
18. Wei JC, Hsu YW, Hung KS, Wong RH, Huang CH, et al. (2013) Association study of polymorphisms rs4552569 and rs17095830 and the risk of ankylosing spondylitis in a Taiwanese population. PLoS One 8: e52801.
19. Chou CT, Tsai YF, Liu J, Wei JC, Liao TS, et al. (2001) The detection of the HLA-B27 antigen by immunomagnetic separation and enzyme-linked immunosorbent assay-comparison with a flow cytometric procedure. J Immunol Methods 255: 15–22.
20. Sanchez A, Szczypiorska M, Juanola X, Bartolome N, Gratacos J, et al. (2010) Association of the intergenic single-nucleotide polymorphism rs10865331 (2p15) with ankylosing spondylitis in a Spanish population. J Rheumatol 37: 2345–2347.
21. Suzuki T, Ikari K, Yano K, Inoue E, Toyama Y, et al. (2013) *PADI4* and HLA-DRB1 Are Genetic Risks for Radiographic Progression in RA Patients, Independent of ACPA Status: Results from the IORRA Cohort Study. PLoS One 8: e61045.
22. Kenny EE, Pe'er I, Karban A, Ozelius L, Mitchell AA, et al. (2012) A Genome-Wide Scan of Ashkenazi Jewish Crohn's Disease Suggests Novel Susceptibility Loci. PLoS Genet 8: e1002559.
23. Evans DM, Spencer CC, Pointon JJ, Su Z, Harvey D, et al. (2011) Interaction between ERAP1 and HLA-B27 in ankylosing spondylitis implicates peptide handling in the mechanism for HLA-B27 in disease susceptibility. Nat Genet 43: 761–767.
24. Cui X, Rouhani FN, Hawari F, Levine SJ (2003) Shedding of the type II IL-1 decoy receptor requires a multifunctional aminopeptidase, aminopeptidase regulator of TNF receptor type 1 shedding. J Immunol 171: 6814–6819.
25. Colbert RA, DeLay ML, Klenk EI, Layh-Schmitt G (2010) From HLA-B27 to spondyloarthritis: a journey through the ER. Immunol Rev 233: 181–202.
26. Cortes A, Hadler J, Pointon JP, Robinson PC, Karaderi T, et al. (2013) Identification of multiple risk variants for ankylosing spondylitis through high-density genotyping of immune-related loci. Nat Genet 45: 730–738.
27. Trinchieri G, Pflanz S, Kastelein RA (2003) The IL-12 family of heterodimeric cytokines: new players in the regulation of T cell responses. Immunity 19: 641–644.
28. Karaderi T, Harvey D, Farrar C, Appleton LH, Stone MA, et al. (2009) Association between the interleukin 23 receptor and ankylosing spondylitis is confirmed by a new UK case-control study and meta-analysis of published series. Rheumatology (Oxford) 48: 386–389.
29. Lee YH, Choi SJ, Ji JD, Song GG (2012) Associations between interleukin-23R polymorphisms and ankylosing spondylitis susceptibility: a meta-analysis. Inflamm Res 61: 143–149.
30. Davidson SI, Wu X, Liu Y, Wei M, Danoy PA, et al. (2009) Association of ERAP1, but not IL23R, with ankylosing spondylitis in a Han Chinese population. Arthritis Rheum 60: 3263–3268.
31. Tremelling M, Cummings F, Fisher SA, Mansfield J, Gwilliam R, et al. (2007) IL23R variation determines susceptibility but not disease phenotype in inflammatory bowel disease. Gastroenterology 132: 1657–1664.

# 19

# Bone Morphogenetic Protein 6 Polymorphisms Are Associated with Radiographic Progression in Ankylosing Spondylitis

Young Bin Joo[1]⑨, So-Young Bang[1]⑨, Tae-Hwan Kim[1]*, Seung-Cheol Shim[2], Seunghun Lee[3], Kyung Bin Joo[3], Jong Heon Kim[4], Hye Joon Min[5], Proton Rahman[6], Robert D. Inman[7]

1 Department of Rheumatology, Hanyang University Hospital for Rheumatic Diseases, Seoul, Republic of Korea, 2 Division of Rheumatology, Daejeon Rheumatoid & Degenerative Arthritis Center, Chungnam National University Hospital, Daejeon, Republic of Korea, 3 Department of Radiology, Hanyang University Hospital for Rheumatic Diseases, Seoul, Republic of Korea, 4 Department of Orthopedics, Hanyang University Hospital for Rheumatic Diseases, Seoul, Republic of Korea, 5 Department of anthropology, Cornell University, Ithaca, New York, United States of America, 6 Department of Rheumatology, Memorial University, St. Clare's Mercy Hospital, St. John's, Newfoundland, Canada, 7 Division of Rheumatology, University of Toronto, Toronto Western Hospital, Toronto, Ontario, Canada

## Abstract

*Background and Object:* Nearly 25 genetic loci associated with susceptibility to ankylosing spondylitis (AS) have been identified by several large studies. However, there have been limited studies to identify the genes associated with radiographic severity of the disease. Thus we investigated which genes involved in bone formation pathways might be associated with radiographic severity in AS.

*Methods:* A total of 417 Korean AS patients were classified into two groups based on the radiographic severity as defined by the modified Stoke' Ankylosing Spondylitis Spinal Score (mSASSS) system. Severe AS was defined by the presence of syndesmophytes and/or fusion in the lumbar or cervical spine (n = 195). Mild AS was defined by the absence of any syndesmophyte or fusion (n = 170). A total of 251 single nucleotide polymorphisms (SNPs) within 52 genes related to bone formation were selected and genotyped. Odds ratios (OR) and 95% confidence interval (95% CI) were analysed by multivariate logistic regression controlling for age at onset of symptoms, sex, disease duration, and smoking status as covariates.

*Results:* We identified new loci of bone morphogenetic protein 6 (*BMP6*) associated with radiographic severity in patients with AS that passed false discovery rate threshold. Two SNPs in *BMP6* were significantly associated with radiologic severity [*rs270378* (OR 1.97, p = $6.74 \times 10^{-4}$) and *rs1235192* [OR 1.92, p = $1.17 \times 10^{-3}$]) adjusted by covariates.

*Conclusion:* This is the first study to demonstrate that *BMP6* is associated with radiographic severity in AS, supporting the role wingless-type like/BMP pathway on radiographic progression in AS.

**Editor:** Shervin Assassi, University of Texas Health Science Center at Houston, United States of America

**Funding:** The authors have no support or funding to report.

**Competing Interests:** The authors have declared that no competing interests exist.

* Email: thkim@hanyang.ac.kr

⑨ These authors contributed equally to this work.

## Introduction

Ankylosing spondylitis (AS) is a chronic inflammatory disease that preferentially affects the axial structures causing spinal ankylosis [1]. The process of ankylosis is closely associated with permanent work disability as well as decreased quality of life [2]

AS is a highly heritable (>90%), and human leukocyte antigen B27 (HLA-B27) is the strongest genetic association with AS, with >80% of patients being positive for HLA-B27 [3,4]. However, HLA-B27 contributes only 16–50% of genetic risk [5], reflecting the fact that other non-HLA-B27 variants likely influence disease susceptibility. Recently, the International Genetics of Ankylosing

Spondylitis Consortium confirmed the association of 25 loci at genome-wide significance in addition to HLA-B27. This included 12 of the 13 previously reported loci associated with AS in Europeans and 13 additional loci [1].

Although radiologic severity is also largely heritable (>60%) [6], there has been limited studies addressing the genetic influence on severity in contrast to studies of susceptibility to AS. A few studies confirmed the positive association with severity of AS, which have reported that that large multifunctional peptidase (LMP) 2, major histocompatibility complex and in endoplasmic reticulum amino-peptidases (ERAP) 1 have been reported to affect radiographic severity in AS [7–11]. These studies generally used candidate

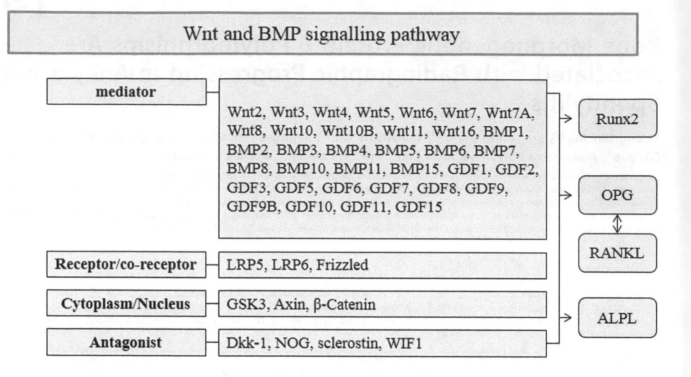

**Figure 1. 52 Gene lists analyzed in our study.** Genes were selected from public databases including the SNP database of the National Centre for Biotechnology Information (NCBI; http://www.ncbi.nlm.nih.gov/SNP/) and the International HapMap Project (http://www.hapmap.org/).

susceptibility gene of AS for analysis of possible associated genetic markers with severity. Two studies did not identify any significant genetic markers showing significant association with radiographic severity in AS [12,13].

Underlying mechanism of new bone formation in AS remain incompletely understood. Current concepts propose a complex interaction between chronic inflammation and wingless-type like (WNT) pathway [14]. A recent study demonstrated that uncoupled interaction of WNT pathway with inflammation may play a key role in the development of new bone formation in AS. The effect of anti-tumor necrosis factor alpha agents on radiographic progression in AS has led to differing conclusions [15,16]. The effect of increased C-reactive protein (CRP) or erythrocyte sedimentation rate (ESR) on structural change in AS is also inconclusive; some report its positive relationship [17,18], but others are not, especially in longstanding AS [19,20]. Some studies showed Dickkopf-1 and sclerostin is associated with radiographic severity independently inflammation, implicating complex molecular mechanisms, which can directly inhibit or enhance the WNT pathway, and which could be significantly impacting new bone formation in AS [21–23].

Based on these data, we hypothesized that genetic factors related to bone formation could be responsible for differential radiographic severity amongst AS. To test this hypothesis, we investigated the potential association of radiographic severity with the polymorphisms of genes involved in bone formation in Korean patients with AS.

## Materials and Methods

### Study Population and Clinical Data

We included a total of 417 patients with AS who are all of Korean ethnicity, recruited from the Hanyang University Hospital for Rheumatic Disease. All patients with AS satisfied the 1984 modified New York criteria for AS [24]. Clinical data collected included age, gender, age at disease onset, which means the onset age of axial symptoms, disease duration, smoking status, nonsteroidal anti-inflammatory drugs (NSAIDs) dose and duration used, HLA-B27 positivity, baseline ESR, and CRP. NSAIDs used was scored by the method which Dougados et al. suggested [25].

### Radiographic Scoring

The modified Stoke Ankylosing Spondylitis Spinal Score (mSASSS), which is considered the standard for quantification of chronic spinal changes in AS, was used for assessing radiographic severity. [26,27] In mSASSS, scoring evaluates the anterior radiographic changes of the lumbar spine and cervical spine in lateral radiographic view: 0 - normal, 1 - erosion, squaring, or sclerosis, 2 -syndesmophyte or 3– bridging syndesmophyte (maximum 72) [28] In the cases with less than 3 vertebral site missing, the missing scores were substituted by the mean score of the vertebra of the same spinal segment of the patients. Two expert radiologists (SL, KBJ) scored independently. Then, discordant scores were reevaluated by both readers. Their interclass and intraclass correlation coefficients were 0.95 and 0.97, respectively.

**Table 1.** Clinical characteristics of study cohort.

| | All patients (n = 365) | Severe AS (n = 195) | Mild AS (n = 170) | p |
|---|---|---|---|---|
| Age at onset, year | 37.0±8.6 | 41.6±8.1 | 33.0±6.8 | <0.001 |
| Male | 340 (93.2) | 174 (89.2) | 166 (97.6) | 0.001 |
| Disease duration, year | 14.1±6.8 | 16.7±7.3 | 11.9±5.4 | <0.001 |
| Smoker (n = 322) | 201 (62.4) | 114 (74.0) | 87 (51.8) | <0.001 |
| HLA-B27 (n = 344) | 334 (97.1) | 151 (98.7) | 183 (95.8) | 0.195 |
| ESR, mm/hr (n = 197) | 20.5±23.9 | 23.2±26.4 | 18.1±21.4 | 0.135 |
| CRP, mg/dL (n = 194) | 1.2±2.2 | 1.4±2.7 | 1.1±1.6 | 0.381 |
| mSASSS, range 0–72 | | | | |
|   Cervical spine | 12.2±11.0 | 19.4±12.5 | 6.0±2.7 | <0.001 |
|   Lumbar spine | 10.8±13.1 | 21.9±11.5 | 1.2±2.1 | <0.001 |
|   Total | 23.1±21.9 | 41.5±19.7 | 7.2±3.6 | <0.001 |
| *Continuous NSAID intake (n = 161) | 44 (27.3) | 24 (33.3) | 20 (22.5) | 0.124 |

Data were shown to mean ± SD or n (%).
*Continuous NSAID intake was defined as 70 or more the score. AS; ankylosing spondylitis, HLA-B27: human leukocyte antigen-B27; ESR: erythrocyte sedimentation rate; CRP: C-reactive protein; Msasss: modified stokes AS spine score; NSAID: non-steroidal anti-inflammatory drugs.

## Severity Classification

The patients with AS are classified into two groups-mild or severe-based on the radiographic severity as follows. Within the measurement error of mSASSS, that scores of 1 is intermediate, and perhaps of indeterminate significance. Also, since a syndesmophyte at only 1 level can be seen in other state than AS, severe AS was defined by three or more syndesmophytes and/or fusion at the lumbar spine or cervical spine. Mild AS was defined by the absence of any syndesmophyte. Patients who had only 1 or 2 syndesmophytes or fusion were excluded from the analysis to allow a clear differentiation of severity between mild and severe.

## Genotyping

In this study, 52 candidate genes (see **Figure 1** and **Table S1**) associated with involved in bone formation pathways were selected from public databases including the SNP database of the National Centre for Biotechnology Information (NCBI; http://www.ncbi.nlm.nih.gov/SNP/) and the International HapMap Project (http://www.hapmap.org/). SNP genotyping using the Sequenom MassARRAY® system (iPLEX GOLD) was performed according to the manufacturer's instructions (Sequenom, San Diego, CA, USA). Briefly, PCR and single-base extension (SBE) primers were designed using MassARRAY assay design software (Sequenom, San Diego, CA, USA). Manufacturer's instructions for the multiplex reaction were followed for the PCR amplification, the shrimp alkaline phosphatase (SAP) enzyme treatment, the SBE reactions using an iPLEX GOLD assay, and the clean-up with a resin kit (Sequenom, San Diego, CA, USA). The multiplex assays were designed using Sequenom's Assay Design Suite 1.0. Only 251 SNPs of 52 genes were genotyped due to problems inherent with designing multiplex reactions. PCR and SBE primers sequences and all protocols are available upon request. Reaction products were dispensed onto a SpectroCHIP bioarray (Sequenom, San Diego, CA, USA) using a MassARRAY nanodispenser (Sequenom, San Diego, CA, USA) and assayed on the MassARRAY platform (Sequenom, San Diego, CA, USA). Differences in mass were detected with matrix-assisted laser desorption/ionization time-of-flight mass spectrometry (MALDI-TOF MS). MassAR-RAY Workstation software was used to process and analyse the

iPLEX SpectroCHIP bioarray. Typer Analyzer software was used to analyse all genotypes obtained from the assays.

## Statistical Analysis

We eliminated SNPs that had insufficient call rates (<90% and minor allele frequency <1%) in cases and controls, Hardy-Weinberg disequilibrium in controls ($p < 1 \times 10^{-5}$), and samples that were less than 90% sequenced. To determine the association of respective SNPs with radiologic severity, odds ratio (OR) and 95% confidence interval were calculated using logistic analysis (allelic model), controlling for age of disease onset, sex, disease duration, and smoking status. Given the large number of tests, there was high potential for false discovery. Thus, we used a false discovery rate (FDR) method to control the error inherent in multiple comparisons [29]. The association of genotype of significant genes with total mSASSS was analyzed using Kruskal-Wallis test with Mann Whitney P. Statistical analyses were conducted in PLINK v1.07 and SPSS17 software (Chicago, IL, USA).

## Ethics Statement

The Institutional Review Board of Hanyang University approved the protocol. All patients gave written informed consent.

## Results

### Clinical Characteristics of Patients with AS

In this study, we included the AS patient with longstanding disease; the mean disease duration from symptoms onset to the time when radiograph was taken was 14.1±6.8 years, and the mean score of mSASSS was 23.1±21.9 (**Table 1**). After excluding the patients who had only 1 or 2 syndesmophyte or fusion, a total of 365 patients were classified into 2 groups such as severe (n = 195) or mild AS (n = 170). Patients with severe AS were older at onset of symptoms (41.6±8.1 vs 33.0±6.8), had higher percentage of males (97.6 vs 89.2) and smokers (74.0 vs 51.8), and had longer disease duration (16.7±7.3 vs 11.9±5.4) compared with those with mild AS. The percentage of HLA-B27, NSAID used, ESR, and CRP were not significantly different between the two groups. Total mSASSS (range 0–72) was 41.5±19.7 in

**Table 2.** Significant association between polymorphism associated with bone formation in AS patients.

| SNP | Gene | Chr | Position | Risk Allele | Allele Freq. (Cases) | Allele Freq. (Controls) | OR | 95% CI | p | FDR thresholds |
|---|---|---|---|---|---|---|---|---|---|---|
| rs270378 | BMP6 | 6 | 7762715 | C | 0.585 | 0.497 | 1.97 | 1.33 - 2.90 | $6.74 \times 10^{-4}$ | $1.56 \times 10^{-3}$ |
| rs1235192 | BMP6 | 6 | 7867046 | G | 0.716 | 0.606 | 1.92 | 1.30-2.86 | $1.17 \times 10^{-3}$ | $1.61 \times 10^{-3}$ |

AS: ankylosing spondylitis; SNP: single nucleotide polymorphism; Chr: chromosome; Freq: frequency; OR: odds ratio; CI: confidence interval; FDR: false discovery rate; BMP6: bone morphogenetic protein 6.

patients with severe AS, and $7.2 \pm 3.6$ in that with mild AS ($p < 0.001$).

## Associations of SNPs Related to Bone Formation Mechanism with Radiologic Severity

To control the clinical differences between two groups, logistic regression analysis was adjusted for age at onset of symptoms, sex, disease duration, and smoking status. Among 52 genes analyzed, only BMP6-related SNPs were associated with radiographic severity (**Table 2 and Table S2**). SNP *rs270378* of BMP6 showed the strongest association with severe AS (OR 1.97, p = $6.74 \times 10^{-4}$, Table 2). *rs1235192* of BMP6 was also associated with severe AS (OR 1.92, p = $1.17 \times 10^{-3}$), although these SNPs did not reach significance after Bonferroni correction. These two SNPs were not in linkage disequilibrium (LD) (R2 = 0.004, D' = 0.106, Distance: 104 kb).

## Association of Allele Frequency (Genotype) of BMP6 with Total mSASSS

We looked at the trend of the allele with the actual mSASSS. In this study, it appears that the presence of risk allele in *rs1235192* was associated with markedly increased total mSASSS. As shown in **figure 2**, mSASSS in the group with G (TG or GG) was much higher than that in the group without it (p = 0.046). But the allele difference of SNP rs270378 for mSASSS was not statistically significant (P>0.05).

## Discussion

Our results highlight the role of certain biological pathways in the pathogenesis of AS. Recently, new hypothesis have been proposed that WNTs and BMPs are likely to play an important role in new bone formation in AS [14]. However, genetic studies that were examined this hypothesis are few, although genetic factors are likely playing a key role in defining new bone formation [14]. In this study, we specifically examined SNPs of genes related to bone formation, and most of which were related to WNTs and BMPs pathways. Among them, risk alleles at *rs270378* and *rs1235192* in *BMP6* were found to increase the risk of syndesmophyte formation. These relationships remained significant even after adjusted *P* value by FDR was applied to the multiple comparisons. We demonstrated for the first time that SNPs in *BMP6* likely play a contributory role in syndesmophyte formation or ankylosis in AS.

Recently, several genetic association studies were done to identify the risk variant for radiographic severity in AS. Haroon et al reported that *LMP2* variants in Caucasian AS affected baseline mSASSS, but not radiographic progression [7]. ERAP1 variants was reported to be associated with syndesmophyte formation in Taiwanese patients with AS, as reported by Wang et al [8]. This study compared the polymorphisms of genes between patients with at least one syndesmophyte vs those with no syndesmophytes. Two studies have suggested that prediction of radiographic severity was improved by genetic variants by showing prediction model of radiographic severity using the bath ankylosing spondylitis radiology index (BASRI) [10,30].

Our results add to the knowledge about the genetic factors of AS radiographic severity in above results. The present study used the mSASSS to define severe AS, since the mSASSS had been accepted as the optimal method for quantification of chronic spinal changes [26] Other method such as BASRI is difficult to differentiate less or more severe spinal disease as its ceiling effect, But the mSASSS method could. The study addressed specifically severe cases, thereby eliminating cases of intermediate severity

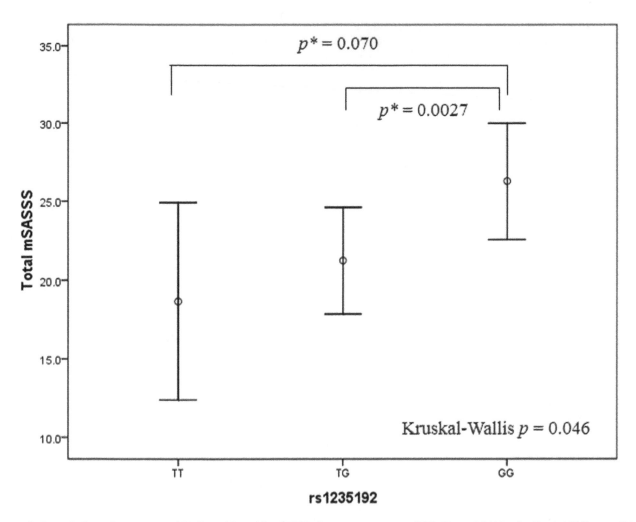

**Figure 2. Association of genotype of BMP6 with total mSASSS.** Data represent mean (95% CI). p = 0.046 by the Kruskal-Wallis test. *Mann Whitney P.

which may confound clear stratification for severity. There are reports of successfully identifying the risk variant using extremely high or low levels of interest [31,32]. We also adjusted for smoking status, which is known to important environmental risk factor for radiographic progression, as well as age, sex, and disease duration. These points considered in our study may lead to accurate prediction of genetic markers of radiographic severity.

We found that the two (rs270378 and rs1235192) SNPs in BMP6 are associated with increased risk of syndesmophyte formation. These SNPs were not in LD (R2 = 0.004, D′ = 0.106, Distance: 104 kb). Interestingly, stronger effect on syndesmophytes was found in the group carrying double risk SNPs, rs270378 C and rs1235192 G (P = 3.48×10−4). There were two separate signals at this locus. The association at each SNP in the locus was with a common variant. All these findings suggest that these two SNPs confer the risk for syndesmophytes through independent contribution.

In this study, it appears that the presence of risk allele in rs1235192 was associated with markedly increased total mSASSS. As shown in figure 2, the mSASSS score in the group with G was much higher than that in the group without it (P = 0.046). But the allele difference of SNP rs270378 for mSASSS score was not statistically significant (P>0.05).

BMPs play an important role in bone morphogenesis and remodeling in health and disease. BMPs, including BMP6, are important in bone metabolism and can induce ectopic osteogenesis [33]. It has been known that BMP6 messenger RNA is localized in hypertrophic cartilage [34], and BMP6 has an important role in the maintenance and repair of human articular cartilage [35]. Polymorphisms in BMP6 were independently associated with risk for sickle cell osteonecrosis [36,37], pulmonary hypertension in sickle cell disease, [38] breast cancer growth and progression [39]. However, there was no report about variants in BMP genes and their association with new bone formation in AS.

In AS, two process of endochondral and direct bone formation contribute to ankylosis process. WNTs and BMP signaling play a role in endochondral bone formation and WNTs also play in direct bone formation [14]. In WNT pathway, WNT bind to low-density lipoprotein receptor-related protein 5 and 6 (LRP5 and 6) on mesenchymal cells followed by activation of intracellular β-catenin involve in bone formation proceeds. During this process, other key molecules such as BMP, axin, glycogen synthase kinase 3 beta (GSK3β), pronounced like the toy Frisbee (FRZB) interact each other to enhance or inhibit to bone formation [14]. WNT signaling elements such as Wnt3a and Wnt10b are associated with direct membranous bone formation, whereas, over-expression of β-catenin in late stage of chondrogenesis is associated with endochondral bone formation through stimulation of the chondrocytes maturation [40]. We investigated the polymorphisms in genes associated with WNT pathway but we did not identify the risk variant affecting the differential radiographic severity in AS.

BMPs are also important for signaling in bone formation process in AS. In the presence of BMPs, progenitor cells first differentiate into chondrocytes building a cartilaginous template that is subsequently replaced by bone [41–43]. Three specific BMPs have been studied in human AS. The levels of BMP2, BMP4, and BMP7 increased in AS patients with spinal fusion compared with patients without fusion [44]. However, these changes in BMP2 and BMP7 are not specific to AS, since BMP2 and BMP7 also increased in RA patients [45]. Until now, there is no report regarding to the level of BMP6 and its association with radiographic severity in human AS.

An Interesting observation on ankylosis in experimental models was seen in the study of Lories et al. [46]. They demonstrated that different BMPs are expressed during the process of ankylosis in male DBA/1 mice. BMP2 was induced in the early stage, BMP7 affects prehypertrophic chondrocytes, and BMP6 affects to hypertrophic chondrocytes in later stage. By immunohistochemistry staining, BMP6 was positive in hypertrophic chondrocyte-like cell showing later stage of endochondral bone formation in ankylosing enthesitis. This is interpreted as indicating that BMP6 is necessary to complete bone formation. This finding supports to our results that polymorphisms of BMP6 could affect to the bone formation, especially syndesmophyte formation in AS. However, further study investigating human histologic finding is needed to demonstrate the biologic role of BMP6 in syndesmophyte or ankylosis formation in human AS.

There is some limitation in this study. We used the cross-sectional data not longitudinal data. To determine the radiographic severity, it would be optimal to compare the radiographs between baseline and later follow-up. To address this in part, we selected primarily longstanding AS patients. The mean disease duration is 14.1±6.8 years, and more than 75% had disease duration of 10 years or more. Considering that significant radiographic progression commonly occurs in the first 10 years of disease [47] and that the strongest predictor of radiologic spinal progression is the presence of syndesmophytes at baseline [19,48–50], mild AS patients who have no syndesmophyte over a course

of 11.9±5.4 years of disease are likely to how minimal progression over time. In contrast, patients with severe AS who have already three more syndesmophytes at entry to the clinic are likely to show increased radiographic progression during further follow-up. We had not included functional data in the study. However, our result was supported by the experimental study of Lories et al discussed above [46]. As mentioned above, BMP6, which was associated with increased risk of development of syndesmophyte in our study, has been found in the early course of bone formation in animal immunohistochemistry study. However, future functional study in patients with AS is needed for better understanding of the role of BMP6 in bone formation. Finally, type 1 error of our result was controlled with the FDR method, not Bonferroni correction as our sample size was small. Despite the perception of small sample size, this is the largest racially and ethnically homogeneous AS population with mSASSS reported to date. Thus our results are meaningful and acceptable as type 1 error of result was controlled with the FDR method.

In summary, we show that certain BMP6 polymorphisms, especially *rs270378* and *rs1235192*, are possible risk factors for the development of syndesmophyte and ankylosis in AS. These variants could be excellent candidates for further investigation although replication in larger sample and in different ethnic groups is needed.

## Supporting Information

**Table S1** This table contains the 366 single nucleotide polymorphisms (SNPs) analyzed in our study.

**Table S2** SNPs Association between polymorphism associated with bone formation in AS patients (p<0.05, adjusted by age at onset of symptom, sex, disease duration, and smoking).

## Author Contributions

Conceived and designed the experiments: YBJ SYB THK SCS JHK. Performed the experiments: HJM PR RDI KBJ SHL. Analyzed the data: SYB YBJ THK. Contributed reagents/materials/analysis tools: THK PR RDI. Contributed to the writing of the manuscript: YBJ SYB SCS THK.

## References

1. Cortes A, Hadler J, Pointon JP, Robinson PC, Karaderi T, et al. (2013) Identification of multiple risk variants for ankylosing spondylitis through high-density genotyping of immune-related loci. Nat Genet 45: 730–738.
2. Chen HA, Chen CH, Liao HT, Lin YJ, Chen PC, et al. (2011) Factors associated with radiographic spinal involvement and hip involvement in ankylosing spondylitis. Semin Arthritis Rheum 40: 552–558.
3. Brown MA, Kennedy LG, MacGregor AJ, Darke C, Duncan E, et al. (1997) Susceptibility to ankylosing spondylitis in twins: the role of genes, HLA, and the environment. Arthritis Rheum 40: 1823–1828.
4. Brown MA (2008) Breakthroughs in genetic studies of ankylosing spondylitis. Rheumatology (Oxford) 47: 132–137.
5. Khan MA, Ball EJ (2002) Genetic aspects of ankylosing spondylitis. Best Pract Res Clin Rheumatol 16: 675–690.
6. Brophy S, Hickey S, Menon A, Taylor G, Bradbury L, et al. (2004) Concordance of disease severity among family members with ankylosing spondylitis? J Rheumatol 31: 1775–1778.
7. Haroon N, Maksymowych WP, Rahman P, Tsui FW, O'Shea FD, et al. (2012) Radiographic severity of ankylosing spondylitis is associated with polymorphism of the large multifunctional peptidase 2 gene in the Spondyloarthritis Research Consortium of Canada cohort. Arthritis Rheum 64: 1119–1126.
8. Wang CM, Ho HH, Chang SW, Wu YJ, Lin JC, et al. (2012) ERAP1 genetic variations associated with HLA-B27 interaction and disease severity of syndesmophytes formation in Taiwanese ankylosing spondylitis. Arthritis Res Ther 14: R125.
9. Lian Z, Chai W, Shi LL, Chen C, Liu J, et al. (2013) Analysis of PPARGC1B, RUNX3 and TBKBP1 Polymorphisms in Chinese Han Patients with Ankylosing Spondylitis: A Case-Control Study. PLoS One 8: e61527.
10. Bartolome N, Szczypiorska M, Sanchez A, Sanz J, Juanola-Roura X, et al. (2012) Genetic polymorphisms inside and outside the MHC improve prediction of AS radiographic severity in addition to clinical variables. Rheumatology (Oxford) 51: 1471–1478.
11. Szczypiorska M, Sanchez A, Bartolome N, Arteta D, Sanz J, et al. (2011) ERAP1 polymorphisms and haplotypes are associated with ankylosing spondylitis susceptibility and functional severity in a Spanish population. Rheumatology (Oxford) 50: 1969–1975.
12. Pimentel-Santos FM, Ligeiro D, Matos M, Mourao AF, Vieira de Sousa E, et al. (2012) ANKH and susceptibility to and severity of ankylosing spondylitis. J Rheumatol 39: 131–134.
13. Seo JS, Lee SS, Kim SI, Ryu WH, Sa KH, et al. (2005) Influence of VEGF gene polymorphisms on the severity of ankylosing spondylitis. Rheumatology (Oxford) 44: 1299–1302.
14. Lories RJ, Luyten FP, de Vlam K (2009) Progress in spondylarthritis. Mechanisms of new bone formation in spondyloarthritis. Arthritis Res Ther 11: 221.
15. van der Heijde D, Salonen D, Weissman BN, Landewe R, Maksymowych WP, et al. (2009) Assessment of radiographic progression in the spines of patients with ankylosing spondylitis treated with adalimumab for up to 2 years. Arthritis Res Ther 11: R127.
16. van der Heijde D, Landewe R, Einstein S, Ory P, Vosse D, et al. (2008) Radiographic progression of ankylosing spondylitis after up to two years of treatment with etanercept. Arthritis Rheum 58: 1324–1331.
17. Ramiro S, van der Heijde D, van Tubergen A, Stolwijk C, Dougados M, et al. (2014) Higher disease activity leads to more structural damage in the spine in

ankylosing spondylitis: 12-year longitudinal data from the OASIS cohort. Ann Rheum Dis.

18. Poddubnyy D, Haibel H, Listing J, Marker-Hermann E, Zeidler H, et al. (2012) Baseline radiographic damage, elevated acute-phase reactant levels, and cigarette smoking status predict spinal radiographic progression in early axial spondylarthritis. Arthritis Rheum 64: 1388–1398.

19. van Tubergen A, Ramiro S, van der Heijde D, Dougados M, Mielants H, et al. (2012) Development of new syndesmophytes and bridges in ankylosing spondylitis and their predictors: a longitudinal study. Ann Rheum Dis 71: 518–523.

20. Kroon F, Landewe R, Dougados M, van der Heijde D (2012) Continuous NSAID use reverts the effects of inflammation on radiographic progression in patients with ankylosing spondylitis. Ann Rheum Dis 71: 1623–1629.

21. Heiland GR, Appel H, Poddubnyy D, Zwerina J, Hueber A, et al. (2012) High level of functional dickkopf-1 predicts protection from syndesmophyte formation in patients with ankylosing spondylitis. Ann Rheum Dis 71: 572–574.

22. Appel H, Ruiz-Heiland G, Listing J, Zwerina J, Herrmann M, et al. (2009) Altered skeletal expression of sclerostin and its link to radiographic progression in ankylosing spondylitis. Arthritis Rheum 60: 3257–3262.

23. Schett G, Rudwaleit M (2010) Can we stop progression of ankylosing spondylitis? Best Pract Res Clin Rheumatol 24: 363–371.

24. van der Linden S, Valkenburg HA, Cats A (1984) Evaluation of diagnostic criteria for ankylosing spondylitis. A proposal for modification of the New York criteria. Arthritis Rheum 27: 361–368.

25. Dougados M, Braun J, Szanto S, Combe B, Geher P, et al. (2012) Nonsteroidal antiinflammatory drug intake according to the Assessment of SpondyloArthritis International Society Score in clinical trials evaluating tumor necrosis factor blockers: example of etanercept in advanced ankylosing spondylitis. Arthritis Care Res (Hoboken) 64: 290–294.

26. Wanders AJ, Landewe RB, Spoorenberg A, Dougados M, van der Linden S, et al. (2004) What is the most appropriate radiologic scoring method for ankylosing spondylitis? A comparison of the available methods based on the Outcome Measures in Rheumatology Clinical Trials filter. Arthritis Rheum 50: 2622–2632.

27. van der Heijde D, Landewe R (2005) Selection of a method for scoring radiographs for ankylosing spondylitis clinical trials, by the Assessment in Ankylosing Spondylitis Working Group and OMERACT. J Rheumatol 32: 2048–2049.

28. Creemers MC, Franssen MJ, van't Hof MA, Gribnau FW, van de Putte LB, et al. (2005) Assessment of outcome in ankylosing spondylitis: an extended radiographic scoring system. Ann Rheum Dis 64: 127–129.

29. Benjamini Y, Drai D, Elmer G, Kafkafi N, Golani I (2001) Controlling the false discovery rate in behavior genetics research. Behav Brain Res 125: 279–284.

30. Ward MM, Hendrey MR, Malley JD, Learch TJ, Davis JC Jr, et al. (2009) Clinical and immunogenetic prognostic factors for radiographic severity in ankylosing spondylitis. Arthritis Rheum 61: 859–866.

31. Edmondson AC, Braund PS, Stylianou IM, Khera AV, Nelson CP, et al. (2011) Dense genotyping of candidate gene loci identifies variants associated with high-density lipoprotein cholesterol. Circ Cardiovasc Genet 4: 145–155.

32. Bandarian F, Hedayati M, Daneshpour MS, Naseri M, Azizi F (2013) Genetic Polymorphisms in the APOA1 Gene and their Relationship with Serum HDL Cholesterol Levels. Lipids 48: 1207–1216.

33. Jane JA, Jr., Dunford BA, Kron A, Pittman DD, Sasaki T, et al. (2002) Ectopic osteogenesis using adenoviral bone morphogenetic protein (BMP)-4 and BMP-6 gene transfer. Mol Ther 6: 464–470.

34. Gitelman SE, Kobrin MS, Ye JQ, Lopez AR, Lee A, et al. (1994) Recombinant Vgr-1/BMP-6-expressing tumors induce fibrosis and endochondral bone formation in vivo. J Cell Biol 126: 1595–1609.

35. Bobacz K, Gruber R, Soleiman A, Erlacher L, Smolen JS, et al. (2003) Expression of bone morphogenetic protein 6 in healthy and osteoarthritic human articular chondrocytes and stimulation of matrix synthesis in vitro. Arthritis Rheum 48: 2501–2508.

36. Baldwin C, Nolan VG, Wyszynski DF, Ma QL, Sebastiani P, et al. (2005) Association of klotho, bone morphogenic protein 6, and annexin A2 polymorphisms with sickle cell osteonecrosis. Blood 106: 372–375.

37. Ulug P, Vasavda N, Awogbade M, Cunningham J, Menzel S, et al. (2009) Association of sickle avascular necrosis with bone morphogenic protein 6. Ann Hematol 88: 803–805.

38. Ashley-Koch AE, Elliott L, Kail ME, De Castro LM, Jonassaint J, et al. (2008) Identification of genetic polymorphisms associated with risk for pulmonary hypertension in sickle cell disease. Blood 111: 5721–5726.

39. Slattery ML, John EM, Torres-Mejia G, Herrick JS, Giuliano AR, et al. (2013) Genetic variation in bone morphogenetic proteins and breast cancer risk in hispanic and non-hispanic white women: The breast cancer health disparities study. Int J Cancer 132: 2928–2939.

40. Macsai CE, Foster BK, Xian CJ (2008) Roles of Wnt signalling in bone growth, remodelling, skeletal disorders and fracture repair. J Cell Physiol 215: 578–587.

41. Carter S, Braem K, Lories RJ (2012) The role of bone morphogenetic proteins in ankylosing spondylitis. Ther Adv Musculoskelet Dis 4: 293–299.

42. Urist MR (1965) Bone: formation by autoinduction. Science 150: 893–899.

43. Hall BK, Miyake T (2000) All for one and one for all: condensations and the initiation of skeletal development. Bioessays 22: 138–147.

44. Chen HA, Chen CH, Lin YJ, Chen PC, Chen WS, et al. (2010) Association of bone morphogenetic proteins with spinal fusion in ankylosing spondylitis. J Rheumatol 37: 2126–2132.

45. Park MC, Park YB, Lee SK (2008) Relationship of bone morphogenetic proteins to disease activity and radiographic damage in patients with ankylosing spondylitis. Scand J Rheumatol 37: 200–204.

46. Lories RJ, Derese I, Luyten FP (2005) Modulation of bone morphogenetic protein signaling inhibits the onset and progression of ankylosing enthesitis. J Clin Invest 115: 1571–1579.

47. Carette S, Graham D, Little H, Rubenstein J, Rosen P (1983) The natural disease course of ankylosing spondylitis. Arthritis Rheum 26: 186–190.

48. Baraliakos X, Listing J, Rudwaleit M, Haibel H, Brandt J, et al. (2007) Progression of radiographic damage in patients with ankylosing spondylitis: defining the central role of syndesmophytes. Ann Rheum Dis 66: 910–915.

49. Maksymowych WP, Landewe R, Conner-Spady B, Dougados M, Mielants H, et al. (2007) Serum matrix metalloproteinase 3 is an independent predictor of structural damage progression in patients with ankylosing spondylitis. Arthritis Rheum 56: 1846–1853.

50. Baraliakos X, Listing J, von der Recke A, Braun J (2009) The natural course of radiographic progression in ankylosing spondylitis–evidence for major individual variations in a large proportion of patients. J Rheumatol 36: 997–1002.

# 20

# A Functional Variant of PTPN22 Confers Risk for Vogt-Koyanagi-Harada Syndrome but Not for Ankylosing Spondylitis

Qi Zhang[1][9], Jian Qi[1][9], Shengping Hou[1], Liping Du[1], Hongsong Yu[1], Qingfeng Cao[1], Yan Zhou[1], Dan Liao[1], Aize Kijlstra[2], Peizeng Yang[1]*

1 The First Affiliated Hospital of Chongqing Medical University, Chongqing Key Laboratory of Ophthalmology and Chongqing Eye Institute, Chongqing, P. R. China, 2 University Eye Clinic Maastricht, Maastricht, The Netherlands

## Abstract

*Background:* Protein tyrosine phosphatase non-receptor 22 (*PTPN22*) is a key negative regulator of T lymphocytes and has emerged as an important candidate susceptibility factor for a number of immune-related diseases. This study aimed to examine the predisposition of PTPN22 SNPs to Vogt-Koyanagi-Harada (VKH) syndrome and acute anterior uveitis (AAU) associated with ankylosing spondylitis (AS).

*Methods:* A total of 1005 VKH syndrome, 302 AAU⁺AS⁺ patients and 2010 normal controls among the Chinese Han population were enrolled in the study. Genotyping, PTPN22 expression, cell proliferation, cytokine production and cell activation were examined by PCR-RFLP, Real-time PCR, CCK8, ELISA and Flow cytometry.

*Results:* The results showed significantly increased frequencies of the rs2488457 CC genotype and C allele but a decreased frequency of the GG genotype in VKH syndrome patients ($P_{Bonferroni\ correction}$ ($P_c$) $= 3.47 \times 10^{-7}$, OR $= 1.54$; $P_c = 3.83 \times 10^{-8}$, OR $= 1.40$; $P_c = 6.35 \times 10^{-4}$, OR $= 0.62$; respectively). No significant association of the tested SNPs with AAU⁺AS⁺ patients was observed. Functional studies showed a decreased PTPN22 expression, impaired cell proliferation and lower production of IL-10 in rs2488457 CC cases compared to GG cases ($P_c = 0.009$, $P_c = 0.015$ and $P_c = 0.048$ respectively). No significant association was observed concerning T cell activation and rs2488457 genotype.

*Conclusions:* The study showed that a functional variant of PTPN22 confers risk for VKH syndrome but not for AAU⁺AS⁺ in a Chinese Han population, which may be due to a modulation of the PTPN22 expression, PBMC proliferation and IL-10 production.

**Editor:** Graham R. Wallace, University of Birmingham, United Kingdom

**Funding:** This work was supported by Key Project of Natural Science Foundation (81130019), National Basic Research Program of China (973 Program) (2011CB510200), National Natural Science Foundation Project (81300754, 81270990, 81070722), Clinic Key Project of Ministry of Health, Basic Research program of Chongqing (cstc2013jcyjC10001), Chongqing Key Laboratory of Ophthalmology (CSTC, 2008CA5003), Key Project of Health Bureau of Chongqing (2012-1-003) and Fund for PAR-EU Scholars Program. The funders had no role in study design, data collection and analysis, decision to publish, or preparation of the manuscript.

**Competing Interests:** The authors have declared that no competing interests exist.

* E-mail: peizengycmu@126.com

[9] These authors contributed equally to this work.

## Introduction

Uveitis occurring in the context of systemic inflammatory diseases accounts for approximately half of the uveitis entities seen at a specialty clinic [1]. In Asia, the most three common systemic inflammatory diseases associated with uveitis are ankylosing spondylitis (AS), Vogt-Koyanagi-Harada (VKH) syndrome and Behcet's disease [2,3,4]. AS is known as a common inflammatory rheumatic disorder associated with characteristic inflammatory back pain, enthesitis, asymmetrical peripheral oligoarthritis, and specific organ attacks related to acute anterior uveitis (AAU), psoriasis and chronic inflammatory bowel disease [5]. VKH syndrome, a systemic granulomatous inflammatory illness, usually manifests as bilateral panuveitis associated with extraocular findings involved in tegumentary, hairy, auditory, and central nervous system signs [6]. Behcet's disease, a multisystem inflammatory disease, is usually characterized by recurrent uveitis, oral ulceration, arthritis, genital ulceration, skin lesions, and vascular inflammation [7]. The three are usually considered to be immune-related diseases. The pathogenesis of these disorders are yet indistinct, but genetic predisposition, environmental factors and the innate immune system are presumed to be interactively involved in their complex pathogenesis [8,9,10,11,12]. Human leukocyte antigen (*HLA*) genes, such as *HLA-B27*, *HLA-DR4* and *HLA-B51*, have been shown to be genetic predisposing factors for certain uveitis entities. However their contribution to the genetic risk is still limited and does not fully explain the genetic association. This has been the reason for a further analysis of non-*HLA* genes, with an emphasis on genes involved in the immunological and inflammatory response.

The protein tyrosine phosphatase non-receptor 22 (*PTPN22*) gene encodes the lymphoid-specific phosphatase known as Lyp, which contains a non-catalytic C-terminus composed of four proline-rich domains and a catalytic N-terminal domain. By interacting with Csk (C-terminal Src kinase), ZAP70 (zeta-associated protein-70) and Vav (a guanine-nucleotide exchange factor for the GTPases) involved in the TCR (T-cell receptor) signaling pathway, Lyp plays an important suppressive role of T cell responses [13,14,15,16,17]. *PTPN22* has been shown to be one of the strongest non-HLA susceptibility genes for various autoimmune diseases, such as rheumatoid arthritis (RA), type 1diabetes (T1D), systemic lupus erythematosus (SLE), and Graves' disease (GD) [18,19,20,21,22]. In several earlier studies, the main point of these association studies is the *PTPN22* SNP +1858C/T (rs2476601). The *PTPN22* 1858C/T polymorphism shows a large variation among ethnic groups and appears to be low in Asian and African populations and is virtually absent in Chinese Han [23,24,25,26]. In these latter populations it is possible that SNPs that are in linkage disequilibrium with the 1858C/T SNP (rs2476601) or even functional variants of *PTPN22* might be involved in the pathogenesis of autoimmune disease [27,28]. In Asian populations, SNPs named rs2488457, rs3789604 and rs1310182, have been associated with several immune diseases, such as T1D, GD, RA and primary immune thrombocytopenia (ITP) [21,29,30,31].

We recently evaluated the contribution of *PTPN22* gene polymorphisms (rs2488457, rs1310182 and rs3789604) to ocular Behcet's disease in Chinese and were not able to detect a significant association [32]. We now extend these studies on *PTPN22* gene polymorphisms in two other frequently observed uveitis entities in China, namely VKH syndrome and anterior uveitis associated with ankylosing spondylitis. For this study we chose three SNPs (rs2488457, rs1310182 and rs3789604) based on earlier literature and allele frequency in the Chinese Han population and showed that rs2488457 (-1123G/C) confers a significant risk for VKH syndrome. Functional analysis of this allele suggested that the polymorphism of SNP rs2488457 may involved in the development of VKH disease.

## Materials and Methods

### Study subjects

A total of 302 AAU+AS+ patients and 1005 VKH syndrome patients of Chinese Han ethnicity, were gathered from the Uveitis Study Center of the Sun Yat-sen University (Guangzhou, China) and the First Affiliated Hospital of Chongqing Medical University (Chongqing, China) between January 2005 and February 2013. The diagnoses of AS and VKH syndrome were strictly according to the Modified New York Criteria 1984 for AS and the Revised diagnostic criteria 2001 for VKH syndrome [33,34]. We included 2010 healthy individuals, matched with the patients in gender, age, race and geographical origin. Genotype frequencies of the tested SNPs in the controls are complied with the Hardy-Weinberg equilibrium (HWE).

### Ethics statement

The study protocol was approved by the Ethics Committee of the First Affiliated Hospital of Chongqing Medical University, Chongqing, China (Permit Number: 2009-201008), and all processes were in agreement with the Declaration of Helsinki. Blood samples could not be collected until informed consent was signed by each participant.

### Genomic DNA extraction and genotyping

All peripheral blood samples were gathered in EDTA tubes and stored at $-70°C$. The methods for DNA extraction and genotyping were described in our previous study [32]. Direct sequencing was performed for approximately randomly selected 5% of samples to confirm the validity of the genotyping method used.

### Cells isolation and culture

Peripheral blood mononuclear cells (PBMCs) were separated by Ficoll-Hypaque density gradient centrifugation. The PBMCs were resuspended at a concentration of $1 \times 10^6$ cells/ml and treated with LPS (100 ng/ml, Sigma, Missouri, USA) for 24 h to stimulate TNF-$\alpha$, IL-1$\beta$, IL-6, IL-8 and MCP-1 production. For stimulation of IFN-$\gamma$, IL-10 and IL-17 production, the PBMCs were treated with anti-CD3 (OKT3, 0.5 µg/ml) and anti-CD28 antibodies (15E8, 0.1 µg/ml) (Miltenyi Biotec, Palo Alto, CA) for 72 h.

### RNA preparation and real-time quantitative PCR

Total RNA was extracted from PBMCs with TRIzol (Invitrogen, Carlsbad, CA) according to the manufacturer's instructions. Real-time PCR was performed on the ABI7500 Fast System (Applied Biosystems). The primers used for PTPN22 and β-actin detection have been described elsewhere [32,35]. The relative expression of PTPN22 was normalized to the expression of the internal control β-actin using the $2^{-\Delta\Delta CT}$ method.

### Cell proliferation assay

PBMCs stimulated with anti-CD3/CD28 antibodies (5:1) (Miltenyi Biotec, Palo Alto, CA) were incubated for 72 h. Cell proliferation was examined with Cell Counting Kit-8 (CCK8) (Sigma-Aldrich, St Louis, MO) according to the manufacturer's instructions. The absorbance was determined at 450 nm using a Microplate Reader (SpectraMax M2e, Molecular Devices, USA).

### Measurement of cytokines

Supernatants of the stimulated PBMCs were collected for cytokine detection. The production of TNF-$\alpha$, IL-1$\beta$, IL-6, IL-8, MCP-1, IFN-$\gamma$, IL-10 and IL-17 was measured with Duoset ELISA development kits (R&D Systems, Minneapolis, MN) according to the manufacturer instructions.

### Flow cytometry analysis

In order to determine the activation of CD4+ T cells, PBMCs were incubated with FITC-conjugated anti-human CD4, APC-conjugated anti-human CD44, PE-conjugated anti-human CD25, PE-cy7-conjugated anti-human CD69 or appropriate isotypes (eBioscience, San Diego, CA) for 30 minutes at 4°C. FACScan flow cytometer (BD Biosciences, San Diego, CA) and FlowJo software (Tree Star, Inc. Ashland, USA) were used for flow cytometry analysis.

### Statistical analysis

Genotype frequencies were calculated by direct counting. HWE was examined with the chi-square test. Allele and genotype frequencies in patients and controls were compared by the chi-square test with SPSS (v. 17.0; SPSS Inc., Chicago, IL). The P values were corrected (Pc) with the Bonferroni correction by multiplying with the number of comparisons performed. The results of gene expression, cytokine expression, cell proliferation and the activation of CD4+T cells were analyzed by Student's t test or Nonparametric Mann-Whitney U-test. Values were considered to be significantly different when P<0.05. Data are expressed as mean ± SD or mean ± SEM.

## Results

### Clinical feature of AAU+AS+ and VKH syndrome patients

The demographic characteristics and clinical features of the enrolled VKH syndrome and AAU+AS+ patients are shown in Table S1-S3 (Supporting Tables).

### Genotype and allele frequencies of PTPN22 polymorphisms in patients and controls

Three SNPs of PTPN22 (rs2488457, rs1310182 and rs3789604) were genotyped in 302 AAU+AS+ patients, 1005 VKH syndrome patients, and 2010 healthy controls. A significantly increased frequency of the CC genotype and C allele of rs2488457, and a decreased frequency of the GG genotype in VKH syndrome patients    ($P_c = 3.47 \times 10^{-7}$,     OR = 1.54;     $P_c = 3.83 \times 10^{-8}$, OR = 1.40;  $P_c = 6.35 \times 10^{-4}$,  OR = 0.62; respectively) (Table 1) were identified. No significant association was found for the other two SNPs and VKH syndrome patients (Table 1). Similarly, we failed to find a significant association of the three PTPN22 SNPs with AAU+AS+ (Table S4).

### Linkage disequilibrium (LD) data of the SNPs used

The LD data for the three SNPs (rs2488457, rs1310182 and rs3789604) investigated in this study showed no linkage disequilibrium. Values of the pair-wise D' and $r^2$ are shown in blocks (Figure S1).

### The influence of rs2488457 on the expression of PTPN22

To investigate whether the expression of PTPN22 was affected by the different genotypes of rs2488457 we performed the following experiments. PBMCs were isolated for PTPN22 detection from 58 unrelated genotyped healthy individuals (CC = 18, CG = 31, GG = 9). Our results showed a significantly decreased expression of PTPN22 in CC cases compared to CG and GG cases (Figure 1. $P_c = 0.015$; $P_c = 0.009$, respectively).

### The influence of rs2488457 on the proliferation of PBMCs

Since the role of PTPN22 on immune cell proliferation is still controversial, we examined the influence of rs2488457 on the proliferation of PBMCs. PBMCs used for proliferation experiments were obtained from 58 unrelated genotyped healthy individuals (CC = 18, CG = 31, GG = 9). The results showed a significantly decreased proliferation in CC cases compared to GG cases following in vitro stimulation with anti-CD3/CD28 antibodies (Figure 2. $P_c = 0.015$).

### The influence of rs2488457 on the cytokine production

Cytokines play a critical role in the pathogenesis of uveitis and we therefore investigated whether the different genotypes of rs2488457 affected production cytokines such as TNF-α, IL-1β, IL-6, IL-8, MCP-1, IFN-γ, IL-10 and IL-17. PBMCs were obtained from 58 unrelated genotyped healthy individuals (CC = 18, CG = 31, GG = 9) and stimulated with LPS or anti-CD3/CD28 antibodies, then supernatants were collected for cytokine analysis. A significantly decreased production of IL-10 by stimulated PBMCs was observed in CC cases compared to CG or GG cases (Figure 3. A  $P_c = 0.048$;  $P_c = 0.048$,  respectively). Although a decreased IL-8 and an increased IL-6 production by stimulated PBMCs were observed in CC cases compared to GG cases (Figure 3. B–C), significance was lost after correction for multiple comparisons. No significant association was observed concerning IFN-γ, IL-17, TNF-α, IL-1β and MCP-1 production by stimulated PBMCs with the different genotypes of rs2488457 (Figure 3. D–H).

### The influence of rs2488457 on the activation of CD4+ T cells

Previous studies showed that PTPN22 knockout mice accumulate activated T cells. To investigate the role of rs2488457 on T cell activation, we examined the early and late activation markers of CD4+ T cells in carriers of the different genotypes of rs2488457. PBMCs used for the detection of T cell activation were obtained from 31 unrelated genotyped healthy individuals (CC = 9, CG = 18,  GG = 4). No significant association was observed concerning the frequencies of CD4+CD44+CD69+ and CD4+CD44+CD25+ T cells in the different genotypes of rs2488457 (Figure 4).

## Discussion

In the present study, we show that a functional variant rs2488457 of PTPN22 is associated with a higher risk for the development of VKH syndrome. A functional rationale is provided since the risk genotype modulates PTPN22 expression, PBMC proliferation and IL-10 production. Our study confirms earlier findings whereby PTPN22 has emerged as a critical candidate susceptibility gene for amount of immune-related diseases [36,37,38]. Most studies on the association between immune disorders and PTPN22 showed an association with the 1858C/T rs2476601 polymorphism [37,39]. This polymorphism is absent in Chinese Han, but the rs2488457 (-1123G/C) has been shown to be in linkage disequilibrium (LD) with rs2476601 and this area of the gene may have functional consequences [25,28]. Further studies are needed to clarify the exact molecular mechanisms involved.

We showed that rs2488457 had an effect on the PTPN22 expression, PBMCs proliferation and cytokine production. We only investigated the effect of rs2488457 in healthy controls since the patients do not represent a homogenous sample due to a variable disease course and the fact that they are often treated with immunosuppressive agents. We observed a decreased expression of PTPN22 in individuals carrying the rs2488457 CC genotype. Although the exact mechanism whereby rs2488457 modulates disease susceptibility remains unknown, our results indicate that this SNP may change the transcriptional activity of the PTPN22 gene. Of interest is the fact that the DNA sequence around rs2488457 exactly matches with the binding site for the transcription factor activator protein 4 (AP-4) [27]. Further studies are needed to examine whether AP-4 affects the transcription activities of PTPN22. PTPN22 is critically involved in the TCR signaling pathway [13,16] and proliferation is one of consequences of TCR signaling. We therefore studied whether rs2488457 could affect the proliferation of PBMCs. The results showed that a decreased proliferation of PBMCs in rs2488457 CC cases as compared to GG cases when the cells were stimulated in vitro with a combination of anti-CD3/CD28 antibodies. Others have shown a decreased proliferation of CD4+T cell in 1858C/T which would be in agreement with our findings when considering that this locus is in linkage disequilibrium with rs2488457 [40]. Our results also revealed that the production of IL-10 from individuals carrying the rs2488457 CC genotype was significantly decreased compared to CG and GG carriers. A similar association of the 1858C/T polymorphism with a decreased IL-10 production has been demonstrated in a previous study [41]. The report showed that

**Table 1.** Effects of PTPN22 SNPs on VKH syndrome risk.

| Genotype | VKH (N=1005) | | Controls (N=2010) | | P value | Pc value | OR (95%CI) |
|---|---|---|---|---|---|---|---|
| | N | % | N | % | | | |
| rs2488457 | | | | | | | |
| GG | 102 | 10.1 | 310 | 15.4 | $7.06 \times 10^{-5}$ | $6.35 \times 10^{-4}$ | 0.62(0.49–0.79) |
| CG | 454 | 45.2 | 1009 | 51.2 | 0.009 | NS | 0.82(0.70–0.95) |
| CC | 449 | 44.7 | 691 | 34.4 | $3.86 \times 10^{-8}$ | $3.47 \times 10^{-7}$ | 1.54(1.32–1.80) |
| G Allele | 658 | 32.7 | 1629 | 40.5 | $4.25 \times 10^{-9}$ | $3.83 \times 10^{-8}$ | 0.71(0.64–0.80) |
| C Allele | 1352 | 67.3 | 2391 | 59.5 | $4.25 \times 10^{-9}$ | $3.83 \times 10^{-8}$ | 1.40(1.25–1.57) |
| rs1310182 | | | | | | | |
| CC | 48 | 4.8 | 84 | 4.2 | 0.450 | NS | 1.15(0.80–1.65) |
| CT | 292 | 29 | 589 | 29.3 | 0.887 | NS | 0.99(0.84–1.17) |
| TT | 665 | 66.2 | 1337 | 66.5 | 0.849 | NS | 0.99(0.84–1.16) |
| C Allele | 388 | 19.3 | 757 | 18.8 | 0.659 | NS | 1.03(0.90–1.18) |
| T Allele | 1622 | 80.7 | 3263 | 81.2 | 0.659 | NS | 0.97(0.85–1.11) |
| rs3789604 | | | | | | | |
| TT | 648 | 64.5 | 1254 | 62.4 | 0.262 | NS | 1.09(0.94–1.28) |
| GT | 303 | 30.1 | 651 | 32.4 | 0.231 | NS | 0.90(0.77–1.06) |
| GG | 54 | 5.4 | 105 | 5.2 | 0.863 | NS | 1.03(0.74–1.44) |
| T Allele | 1599 | 79.6 | 3159 | 78.6 | 0.384 | NS | 1.06(0.96–1.21) |
| G Allele | 411 | 20.4 | 861 | 21.4 | 0.384 | NS | 0.94(0.83–1.08) |

$P_c$ = Bonferroni corrected P value. NS = Not significant. OR = odds ratio. 95% CI = 95% confidence interval.

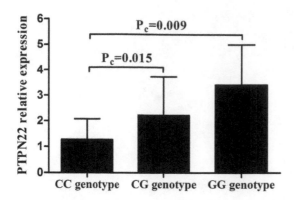

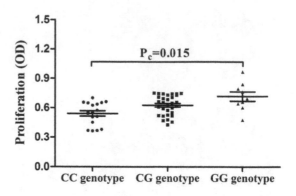

**Figure 1. The influence of rs2488457 on the mRNA expression of PTPN22.** The mRNA expression of PTPN22 in PBMCs from normal controls carrying different genotypes of rs2488457 (CC = 18, CG = 31, GG = 9). Data are represented as the mean ± SD.

**Figure 2. The influence of rs2488457 on the proliferation of PBMCs.** The proliferation of anti-CD3/CD28 stimulated PBMCs from normal controls carrying different genotypes of rs2488457 (CC = 18, CG = 31, GG = 9). Data are represented as the mean ± SEM.

IL-10 gene knockout mice develop autoimmune disease which indicated that IL-10 played a critical role in autoimmunity [42]. The decreased production of IL-10 from individuals carrying the rs2488457 CC genotype fits in with the predisposing role of this genotype for VKH syndrome. Although the important role of *PTPN22* in the activation of T cells has been reported in a transgenic animal model [43], our results failed to find an association of rs2488457 with the activation of T cells. One possible reason for this discrepancy could be due to species differences (human versus mouse).

AS, VKH syndrome and Behcet's disease are three common systemic inflammatory diseases associated with uveitis seen in Asia [2,3,4]. Very recently, our group revealed that *PTPN22* gene polymorphism did not confer risk for ocular Behcet's disease [32], but the role of *PTPN22* gene polymorphisms in other uveitis entities such as AAU⁺AS⁺ and VKH syndrome in Chinese Han was not yet clear.

For several autoimmune diseases characterized by specific autoantibodies like rheumatoid arthritis, type 1 diabetes and

systemic lupus erythematosus, a significant association with PTPN22 gene polymorphisms has been demonstrated by several groups [18,19,20]. However, a number of other immune diseases without specific autoantibodies did not show an association with *PTPN22* gene polymorphisms, such as multiple sclerosis, ulcerative colitis, Crohn's disease and systemic sclerosis [44,45,46,47]. *PTPN22* +1858C/T SNP was also not associated with AS in a Spanish population nor with AAU⁺AS⁺ in American patients [48,49]. On the other hand a Taiwanese study recently showed that the PTPN22 CC and GC genotypes of rs2488457 had a higher risk of AS than individuals with the GG genotype [relative risk = 1.39, 95% confidence interval (95% CI) 1.03–1.88) [50]. We were not able to find an association with PTPN22 gene polymorphisms (including rs2488457) and AAU+AS+. The reason for the discrepancy with the Taiwanese study is not clear but may be caused by the fact that we only included AS patients with uveitis. Furthermore the Taiwanese patients originated China's South-East coastal areas, while our cases mainly came from China's Midwest areas. Six other SNPs (rs3811021, rs1217413, rs1237682, rs3761935, rs3789608, and rs2243471) were reported

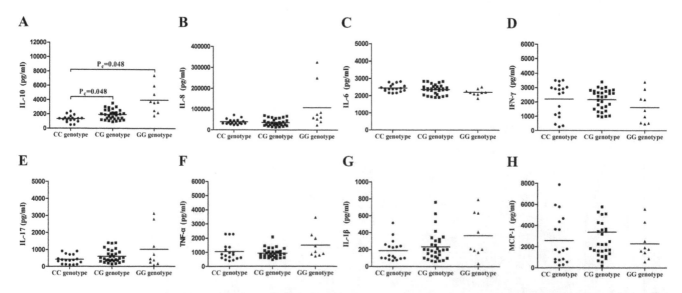

**Figure 3. The influence of rs2488457 on the cytokine production.** The production of IL-10(A), IL-8(B), IL-6(C), IFN-γ(D), IL-17(E), TNF-α(F), IL-1β(G) and MCP-1(H) by PBMCs from normal controls carrying different genotypes of rs2488457 (CC = 18, CG = 31, GG = 9). Data are represented as the mean.

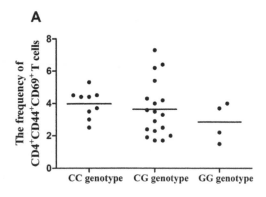
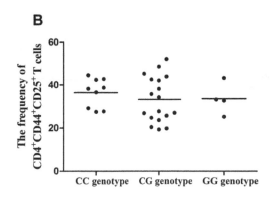

**Figure 4. The influence of rs2488457 on the activation of CD4+ T cells.** (A) The frequency of $CD4^+CD44^+CD69^+$ T cells from normal controls carrying different genotypes of rs2488457 (CC = 9, CG = 18, GG = 4). (B) The frequency of $CD4^+CD44^+CD25^+$ T cells from normal controls carrying different genotypes of rs2488457 (CC = 9, CG = 18, GG = 4). Data are represented as the mean.

not associated with VKH disease in Japan [51]. These results did not include the associated SNP rs2488457 found in our study. The different conclusions between the Japanese study and ours might be due to differences in ethnicity or due to differences in sample size.

As mentioned above, our study showed a strong association of *PTPN22*/rs2488457 with VKH syndrome but not with $AAU^+AS^+$. Why certain uveitis entities are associated with PTPN22 gene polymorphisms and others are not remains unclear. AS is currently classified as an autoinflammatory disease, whereas VKH syndrome is considered as an autoimmune disease directed against melanocytes [11,52]. In an earlier study, we failed to find an association between *PTPN22* polymorphisms and ocular Behcet' disease[32]. Behcet' disease is also thought to be an autoinflammatory disease. The lack of an association between *PTPN22* polymorphisms with both $AAU^+AS^+$ and ocular Behcet's disease suggests that the PTPN22 association with uveitis may be confined to those entities that involve an autoimmune pathogenesis.

There are also several limitations to consider in this study. First of all, the enrolled patients and controls all belong to a Chinese Han population. Further multi-ethnic and multicenter studies should be performed in the future to confirm our data. Secondly, the enrolled patients in this study were all recruited from our uveitis clinic. In view of the multiple organ involvement in VHK syndrome and AS, further studies are needed to examine the association of *PTPN22*/rs2488457 with VKH syndrome and AS patients recruited from other medical departments. It would be interesting to study the functional effect of the other SNPs used in our study. Since we only found an association of SNP rs2488457 with VKH disease and since there was no linkage disequilibrium among the three SNPs used in our study (rs2488457, rs1310182 and rs3789604), we confined the functional analysis to rs2488457.

In conclusion, our results show that a functional variant rs2488457 of the *PTPN22* gene is associated with an increased risk for the development of VKH syndrome by modulating the gene expression, PBMC proliferation and IL-10 production.

## Supporting Information

**Figure S1 Pair-wise linkage disequilibrium values of PTPN22 SNPs in a Chinese Han population.** (A) Values of the pair-wise D' ($\times$100) are shown in blocks. (B) Values of the pair-wise $r^2$ ($\times$100) are shown in blocks.

**Table S1 Characteristics of the investigated healthy controls.**

**Table S2 Clinical features of the VKH syndrome patients.**

**Table S3 Clinical features of the AS patients.**

**Table S4 Effects of PTPN22 SNPs on $AAU^+AS^+$ risk.**

## Acknowledgments

We would like to thank all donors enrolled in the present study.

## Author Contributions

Conceived and designed the experiments: QZ PY. Performed the experiments: QZ JQ SH DL. Analyzed the data: QZ JQ SH LD. Contributed reagents/materials/analysis tools: QZ JQ HY QC YZ. Wrote the paper: QZ JQ PY AK.

## References

1. Smith JR, Rosenbaum JT (2002) Management of uveitis: a rheumatologic perspective. Arthritis and rheumatism 46: 309–318.
2. Yang P, Zhang Z, Zhou H, Li B, Huang X, et al. (2005) Clinical patterns and characteristics of uveitis in a tertiary center for uveitis in China. Current eye research 30: 943–948.
3. Ohguro N, Sonoda KH, Takeuchi M, Matsumura M, Mochizuki M (2012) The 2009 prospective multi-center epidemiologic survey of uveitis in Japan. Japanese journal of ophthalmology 56: 432–435.
4. Goto H, Mochizuki M, Yamaki K, Kotake S, Usui M, et al. (2007) Epidemiological survey of intraocular inflammation in Japan. Japanese journal of ophthalmology 51: 41–44.
5. Braun J, Sieper J (2007) Ankylosing spondylitis. Lancet 369: 1379–1390.

6. Yang P, Ren Y, Li B, Fang W, Meng Q, et al. (2007) Clinical characteristics of Vogt-Koyanagi-Harada syndrome in Chinese patients. Ophthalmology 114: 606–614.
7. Yang P, Fang W, Meng Q, Ren Y, Xing L, et al. (2008) Clinical features of chinese patients with Behcet's disease. Ophthalmology 115: 312–318 e314.
8. Lin Z, Bei JX, Shen M, Li Q, Liao Z, et al. (2012) A genome-wide association study in Han Chinese identifies new susceptibility loci for ankylosing spondylitis. Nature genetics 44: 73–77.
9. Reveille JD, Sims AM, Danoy P, Evans DM, Leo P, et al. (2010) Genome-wide association study of ankylosing spondylitis identifies non-MHC susceptibility loci. Nature genetics 42: 123–127.
10. Shu Q, Yang P, Hou S, Li F, Chen Y, et al. (2010) Interleukin-17 gene polymorphism is associated with Vogt-Koyanagi-Harada syndrome but not with

Behcet's disease in a Chinese Han population. Human immunology 71: 988–991.

11. Yamaki K, Gocho K, Hayakawa K, Kondo I, Sakuragi S (2000) Tyrosinase family proteins are antigens specific to Vogt-Koyanagi-Harada disease. Journal of immunology 165: 7323–7329.

12. Mizuki N, Meguro A, Ota M, Ohno S, Shiota T, et al. (2010) Genome-wide association studies identify IL23R-IL12RB2 and IL10 as Behcet's disease susceptibility loci. Nature genetics 42: 703–706.

13. Behrens TW (2011) Lyp breakdown and autoimmunity. Nature genetics 43: 821–822.

14. Siminovitch KA (2004) PTPN22 and autoimmune disease. Nature genetics 36: 1248–1249.

15. Gregersen PK (2005) Gaining insight into PTPN22 and autoimmunity. Nature genetics 37: 1300–1302.

16. Rhee I, Veillette A (2012) Protein tyrosine phosphatases in lymphocyte activation and autoimmunity. Nature immunology 13: 439–447.

17. Fousteri G, Liossis SN, Battaglia M (2013) Roles of the protein tyrosine phosphatase PTPN22 in immunity and autoimmunity. Clin Immunol 149: 556–565.

18. Begovich AB, Carlton VE, Honigberg LA, Schrodi SJ, Chokkalingam AP, et al. (2004) A missense single-nucleotide polymorphism in a gene encoding a protein tyrosine phosphatase (PTPN22) is associated with rheumatoid arthritis. American journal of human genetics 75: 330–337.

19. Bottini N, Musumeci L, Alonso A, Rahmouni S, Nika K, et al. (2004) A functional variant of lymphoid tyrosine phosphatase is associated with type I diabetes. Nature genetics 36: 337–338.

20. Kyogoku C, Langefeld CD, Ortmann WA, Lee A, Selby S, et al. (2004) Genetic association of the R620W polymorphism of protein tyrosine phosphatase PTPN22 with human SLE. American journal of human genetics 75: 504–507.

21. Ichimura M, Kaku H, Fukutani T, Koga H, Mukai T, et al. (2008) Associations of protein tyrosine phosphatase nonreceptor 22 (PTPN22) gene polymorphisms with susceptibility to Graves' disease in a Japanese population. Thyroid: official journal of the American Thyroid Association 18: 625–630.

22. Orru V, Tsai SJ, Rueda B, Fiorillo E, Stanford SM, et al. (2009) A loss-of-function variant of PTPN22 is associated with reduced risk of systemic lupus erythematosus. Hum Mol Genet 18: 569–579.

23. Mori M, Yamada R, Kobayashi K, Kawaida R, Yamamoto K (2005) Ethnic differences in allele frequency of autoimmune-disease-associated SNPs. Journal of human genetics 50: 264–266.

24. Lee YH, Rho YH, Choi SJ, Ji JD, Song GG, et al. (2007) The PTPN22 C1858T functional polymorphism and autoimmune diseases—a meta-analysis. Rheumatology 46: 49–56.

25. Zhang ZH, Chen F, Zhang XL, Jin Y, Bai J, et al. (2008) PTPN22 allele polymorphisms in 15 Chinese populations. International journal of immunogenetics 35: 433–437.

26. Lee HS, Korman BD, Le JM, Kastner DL, Remmers EF, et al. (2009) Genetic risk factors for rheumatoid arthritis differ in Caucasian and Korean populations. Arthritis and rheumatism 60: 364–371.

27. Kawasaki E, Awata T, Ikegami H, Kobayashi T, Maruyama T, et al. (2006) Systematic search for single nucleotide polymorphisms in a lymphoid tyrosine phosphatase gene (PTPN22): association between a promoter polymorphism and type 1 diabetes in Asian populations. American journal of medical genetics Part A 140: 586–593.

28. Viken MK, Olsson M, Flam ST, Forre O, Kvien TK, et al. (2007) The PTPN22 promoter polymorphism -1123G>C association cannot be distinguished from the 1858C>T association in a Norwegian rheumatoid arthritis material. Tissue antigens 70: 190–197.

29. Taniyama M, Maruyama T, Tozaki T, Nakano Y, Ban Y (2010) Association of PTPN22 haplotypes with type 1 diabetes in the Japanese population. Human immunology 71: 795–798.

30. Huang JJ, Qiu YR, Li HX, Sun DH, Yang J, et al. (2012) A PTPN22 promoter polymorphism -1123G>C is associated with RA pathogenesis in Chinese. Rheumatology international 32: 767–771.

31. Ge J, Li H, Gu D, Du W, Xue F, et al. (2012) PTPN22 -1123G > C polymorphism is associated with susceptibility to primary immune thrombocytopenia in Chinese population. Platelets.

32. Zhang Q, Hou S, Jiang Z, Du L, Li F, et al. (2012) No association of PTPN22 polymorphisms with susceptibility to ocular Behcet's disease in two Chinese Han populations. PloS one 7: e31230.

33. van der Linden S, Valkenburg HA, Cats A (1984) Evaluation of diagnostic criteria for ankylosing spondylitis. A proposal for modification of the New York criteria. Arthritis and rheumatism 27: 361–368.

34. Read RW, Holland GN, Rao NA, Tabbara KF, Ohno S, et al. (2001) Revised diagnostic criteria for Vogt-Koyanagi-Harada disease: report of an international committee on nomenclature. American journal of ophthalmology 131: 647–652.

35. Hou S, Xiao X, Li F, Jiang Z, Kijlstra A, et al. (2012) Two-stage association study in Chinese Han identifies two independent associations in CCR1/CCR3 locus as candidate for Behcet's disease susceptibility. Human genetics 131: 1841–1850.

36. Burn GL, Svensson L, Sanchez-Blanco C, Saini M, Cope AP (2011) Why is PTPN22 a good candidate susceptibility gene for autoimmune disease? FEBS letters 585: 3689–3698.

37. Zheng J, Ibrahim S, Petersen F, Yu X (2012) Meta-analysis reveals an association of PTPN22 C1858T with autoimmune diseases, which depends on the localization of the affected tissue. Genes and immunity 13: 641–652.

38. Chew GY, Sinha U, Gatenby PA, Demalmanche T, Adelstein S, et al. (2013) Autoimmunity in primary antibody deficiency is associated with protein tyrosine phosphatase nonreceptor type 22 (PTPN22). The Journal of allergy and clinical immunology 131: 1130–1135 e1131.

39. Tang S, Peng W, Wang C, Tang H, Zhang Q (2012) Association of the PTPN22 gene (+1858C/T, -1123G/C) polymorphisms with type 1 diabetes mellitus: a systematic review and meta-analysis. Diabetes research and clinical practice 97: 446–452.

40. Aarnisalo J, Treszl A, Svec P, Marttila J, Oling V, et al. (2008) Reduced CD4+T cell activation in children with type 1 diabetes carrying the PTPN22/Lyp 620Trp variant. Journal of autoimmunity 31: 13–21.

41. Rieck M, Arechiga A, Onengut-Gumuscu S, Greenbaum C, Concannon P, et al. (2007) Genetic variation in PTPN22 corresponds to altered function of T and B lymphocytes. Journal of immunology 179: 4704–4710.

42. Anderson AC, Reddy J, Nazareno R, Sobel RA, Nicholson LB, et al. (2004) IL-10 plays an important role in the homeostatic regulation of the autoreactive repertoire in naive mice. Journal of immunology 173: 828–834.

43. Zhang J, Zahir N, Jiang Q, Miliotis H, Heyraud S, et al. (2011) The autoimmune disease-associated PTPN22 variant promotes calpain-mediated Lyp/Pep degradation associated with lymphocyte and dendritic cell hyperresponsiveness. Nature genetics 43: 902–907.

44. Wagenleiter SE, Klein W, Griga T, Schmiegel W, Epplen JT, et al. (2005) A case-control study of tyrosine phosphatase (PTPN22) confirms the lack of association with Crohn's disease. International journal of immunogenetics 32: 323–324.

45. Martin MC, Oliver J, Urcelay E, Orozco G, Gomez-Garcia M, et al. (2005) The functional genetic variation in the PTPN22 gene has a negligible effect on the susceptibility to develop inflammatory bowel disease. Tissue Antigens 66: 314–317.

46. Matesanz F, Rueda B, Orozco G, Fernandez O, Leyva L, et al. (2005) Protein tyrosine phosphatase gene (PTPN22) polymorphism in multiple sclerosis. Journal of neurology 252: 994–995.

47. Wipff J, Allanore Y, Kahan A, Meyer O, Mouthon L, et al. (2006) Lack of association between the protein tyrosine phosphatase non-receptor 22 (PTPN22)*620W allele and systemic sclerosis in the French Caucasian population. Annals of the rheumatic diseases 65: 1230–1232.

48. Orozco G, Garcia-Porrua C, Lopez-Nevot MA, Raya E, Gonzalez-Gay MA, et al. (2006) Lack of association between ankylosing spondylitis and a functional polymorphism of PTPN22 proposed as a general susceptibility marker for autoimmunity. Annals of the rheumatic diseases 65: 687–688.

49. Martin TM, Bye L, Modi N, Stanford MR, Vaughan R, et al. (2009) Genotype analysis of polymorphisms in autoimmune susceptibility genes, CTLA-4 and PTPN22, in an acute anterior uveitis cohort. Molecular vision 15: 208–212.

50. Huang CH, Wei JC, Chen CC, Chuang CS, Chou CH, et al. (2013) Associations of the PTPN22 and CTLA-4 genetic polymorphisms with Taiwanese ankylosing spondylitis. Rheumatol Int.

51. Horie Y, Kitaichi N, Katsuyama Y, Yoshida K, Miura T, et al. (2009) Evaluation of PTPN22 polymorphisms and Vogt-Koyanagi-Harada disease in Japanese patients. Molecular vision 15: 1115–1119.

52. McGonagle D, McDermott MF (2006) A proposed classification of the immunological diseases. PLoS medicine 3: e297.

# 21

# Efficacy of High Intensity Exercise on Disease Activity and Cardiovascular Risk in Active Axial Spondyloarthritis: A Randomized Controlled Pilot Study

Silje Halvorsen Sveaas[1,2]*[¶], Inger Jorid Berg[3][¶], Sella Aarrestad Provan[3], Anne Grete Semb[3], Kåre Birger Hagen[1,2], Nina Vøllestad[2], Camilla Fongen[1], Inge C. Olsen[3], Annika Michelsen[4], Thor Ueland[4,6], Pål Aukrust[4,5,6,7], Tore K. Kvien[3], Hanne Dagfinrud[1,2]

1 National Advisory Unit on Rehabilitation in Rheumatology, Department of Rheumatology, Diakonhjemmet Hospital, Oslo, Norway, 2 Department of Health Sciences, University of Oslo, Oslo, Norway, 3 Department of Rheumatology, Diakonhjemmet Hospital, Oslo, Norway, 4 Research Institute of Internal Medicine, Oslo University Hospital, Rikshospitalet, Oslo, Norway, 5 Section of Clinical Immunology and Infectious Diseases, Oslo University Hospital, Rikshospitalet, Oslo, Norway, 6 Institute of Clinical Medicine, University of Oslo, Oslo, Norway, 7 K.G. Jebsen Inflammatory Research Center, University of Oslo, Oslo, Norway

## Abstract

*Background:* Physical therapy is recommended for the management of axial spondyloarthritis (axSpA) and flexibility exercises have traditionally been the main focus. Cardiovascular (CV) diseases are considered as a major health concern in axSpA and there is strong evidence that endurance and strength exercise protects against CV diseases. Therefore, the aim of this study was to investigate the efficacy of high intensity endurance and strength exercise on disease activity and CV health in patients with active axSpA.

*Methods:* In a single blinded randomized controlled pilot study the exercise group (EG) performed 12 weeks of endurance and strength exercise while the control group (CG) received treatment as usual. The primary outcome was the Ankylosing Spondylitis (AS) Disease Activity Score (ASDAS). Secondary outcomes included patient reported disease activity (Bath AS Disease Activity Index [BASDAI]), physical function (Bath AS Functional Index [BASFI]), and CV risk factors measured by arterial stiffness (Augmentation Index [AIx] and Pulse Wave Velocity [PWV]), cardiorespiratory fitness (VO$_2$ peak) and body composition. ANCOVA on the post intervention values with baseline values as covariates was used to assess group differences, and Mann Whitney U-test was used for outcomes with skewed residuals.

*Results:* Twenty-eight patients were included and 24 (EG, n = 10, CG, n = 14) completed the study. A mean treatment effect of −0.7 (95%CI: −1.4, 0.1) was seen in ASDAS score. Treatment effects were also observed in secondary outcomes (mean group difference [95%CI]): BASDAI: −2.0 (−3.6, −0.4), BASFI: −1.4 (−2.6, −0.3), arterial stiffness (estimated median group differences [95% CI]): AIx (%): −5.3 (−11.0, −0.5), and for PVW (m/s): −0.3 (−0.7, 0.0), VO$_2$ peak (ml/kg/min) (mean group difference [95%CI]: 3.7 (2.1, 5.2) and trunk fat (%): −1.8 (−3.0, −0.6). No adverse events occurred.

*Conclusion:* High intensity exercise improved disease activity and reduced CV risk factors in patients with active axSpA. These effects will be further explored in a larger trial.

*Trial Registration:* ClinicalTrials.gov NCT01436942

**Editor:** Shervin Assassi, University of Texas Health Science Center at Houston, United States of America

**Funding:** The present study was supported by grants from the Norwegian Foundation for Postgraduate Physiotherapist. The funders had no role in study design, data collection and analysis, decision to publish, or preparation of the manuscript.

**Competing Interests:** The authors have declared that no competing interests exist.

* Email: silje.halvorsen@medisin.uio.no

¶ These authors are shared first authors on this work.

## Introduction

Axial spondyloarthritis (axSpA) including ankylosing spondylitis (AS) is characterized by inflammatory back pain and reduced spinal mobility [1]. Over the past decades, the management of many rheumatic diseases has been revolutionized by improve-ments in diagnostic techniques and medication leading to a more active treatment approach for patients with axSpA [2]. Physical therapy with supervised exercise is a cornerstone in the treatment of axSpA together with anti-inflammatory medications such as non-steroidal anti-inflammatory drugs (NSAIDs) and tumor necrosis factor (TNF)-inhibitors [2]. There are no definite recommendations on type of exercise and intensity, and traditionally flexibility exercises at a low intensity level have been recommended [3].

A Cochrane review concluded that physical therapy interventions, mainly consisting of flexibility exercises, have beneficial effects on pain, spinal mobility, physical function and patient global assessment in AS patients, but the effect sizes are small [4]. Additional support for exercise as a part of the treatment repertoire in axSpA is the evidence of increased risk of cardiovascular diseases (CVD) in these patients [5–7]. For healthy adults, cardiorespiratory exercise is recommended in guidelines for CVD prevention [8], and high intensity endurance exercise has been shown to be more effective than low intensity endurance exercise [9]. In addition, the health benefits of strength exercise in CVD prevention are well established [10]. However, the evidence for effects of high intensity endurance and strength exercise on disease activity and cardiovascular (CV) -risk is limited in patients with axSpA.

Therefore, the aim of this study was to investigate the efficacy of high intensive endurance and strength exercise on disease activity and CV-risk in patients with active axSpA.

## Methods

The protocol for this trial and supporting CONSORT checklist are available as supporting information; se Checklist S1 and Protocol S1.

### Design

This study was a single blinded randomized controlled pilot study comparing an exercise group (EG) with a treatment as usual control group (CG). The intervention lasted for 12 weeks, and participants were examined at baseline and post intervention. All the participants provided written informed consent to participate, and all procedures followed the Helsinki declaration. The study was approved by the Regional Committee for medical and health research Ethics of South East Norway (reference: 2011/1468) and is listed in ClinicalTrials.gov (NCT01436942).

### Participants

Patients fulfilling the following criteria were considered eligible: axSpA according to the Assessment of SpA International Society (ASAS) classification criteria [11], age 18–70 years, no change in TNF-inhibitor use during the last 3 months, moderate to high disease activity (Bath AS Disease Activity Index [BASDAI] ≥3.5) and not performed regular endurance or strength exercise during the last year (>1 hour per week). Exclusion criteria were established CVD, other co-morbidity involving reduced exercise capacity, inability to participate in weekly exercise sessions in Oslo and pregnancy. The study was carried out at Diakonhjemmet Hospital in Oslo between October 2011 and June 2012, with recruitment of patients during the first six months. No formal sample size consideration was performed for this intervention due to the exploratory design of the study.

### Intervention

The exercise program followed the American college of sports medicine (ACSM) recommendations for maintenance and improvement of cardiorespiratory- and muscular fitness [10]. Patients in the EG were encouraged to exercise 40–60 minutes three times a week for twelve weeks. Twice a week the exercise sessions were carried out at a fitness center with individual supervision from a physical therapist (SHS). These sessions consisted of both endurance and strength training. The endurance training was high intensity interval training on a treadmill for 40 minutes (four minutes walking/running at 90–95% of maximal heart rate [HR] followed by three minutes of active resting at 70% of maximal HR repeated four times) [12]. The strength training was 20 minutes with external load for major muscle groups (individually adapted, six exercises, eight to ten repetitions maximum, two to three sets). The strength program consisted of the following exercises: bench press with weight manuals or seated in a chest press machine, squat with weight or leg press machine, rowing exercise with weight manuals, exercises for triceps and biceps in a fitness machine and an abdominal stabilization exercise (abdominal bridge).

Once a week the participants exercised individually minimum 40 minutes of endurance training, either an additional session with interval training or a session with long-distance training (above 70% of maximal HR). The exercise program was individually adapted to the participant's fitness level and a physical therapist (SHS) was responsible for an adequate progression of the intensity level during the exercise period.

The maximal HR of each participant was determined during the baseline test and the HR was controlled with a HR monitor to individually tailor the intensity. Attendance at the supervised exercise sessions was recorded by the physical therapist (SHS). The weekly self-imposed exercise session was first recorded in the pulse watch and thereafter weekly reported to the physical therapist. To fulfill the exercise protocol the participants had to attend at least 80% of the planned exercise sessions.

Participants in the CG were asked to not start exercising during the intervention period. The CG was introduced to the exercise program post-intervention to reduce drop out.

### Procedures of assessments

Assessments for efficacy and safety were performed at baseline and after 12 weeks (end of study) and included questionnaires, clinical examinations and laboratory measurements.

Personal characteristics, comorbidities and medication were self-reported in a questionnaire. All physical (spinal mobility, body weight/height, waist circumference and body composition) and performance ($VO_2$ peak) based measures were recorded by an experienced physical therapist (CF). The assessments of blood pressure (BP), HR and arterial stiffness were performed by an experienced rheumatologist (IJB).

### Primary outcome measure

The primary outcome was disease activity assessed by the AS Disease Activity Score (ASDAS) [13]. ASDAS is reported to be a valid measure of disease activity as it has shown acceptable concurrent validity with both patients and physicians global assessments. ASDAS is a composite continuous score consisting of three patient reported items in addition to C-reactive protein (CRP).

### Secondary outcomes measures

**Disease specific measures.** Disease activity was also measured by the patient reported index BASDAI [14]. The BASDAI consists of six items related to major symptoms in AS (fatigue, spinal pain, joint pain, tenderness and degree and length of morning stiffness). BASDAI is reported to be valid as it reflects the entire spectrum of the disease and is sensitive to changes over time [14]. Physical function was measured with Bath AS Functional Index (BASFI) which is a disease specific index that consists of eight questions regarding physical functioning and two questions reflecting the patient's ability to cope with everyday life [15]. For both BASDAI and BASFI each question was answered on a 10 point numeric rating scale, and a sum score was calculated (0–10, 10 = worst). Spinal mobility was measured by Bath AS Metrology Index (BASMI) [16]. BASMI includes five objective measurements of spinal mobility, and the score is 0–10 for each component, and the mean of the five scores produced a BASMI score from 0–10 (10 = worst).

**Cardiorespiratory fitness.** Cardiorespiratory fitness was assessed with a maximal walking treadmill test for estimation of peak oxygen uptake (VO$_2$ peak) as previously described [17]. Resting HR was measured after at least five minutes rest in a supine position and several recordings were made until two measurements differed by ≤5 heart beats, and the mean was then calculated.

**Arterial stiffness.** We measured arterial stiffness after at least five minutes of rest in a supine position, using the Sphygmocor apparatus (AtCor, Sidney, Australia). Several recordings were made from each patient and only those of high quality, according to standardized criteria [18], were chosen for further analyses. Augmentation Index (AIx) was estimated through pulse wave recordings at the radial artery. The pulse waves of the central arteries were derived by applying a validated transfer factor [19]. For measurements of Pulse Wave Velocity (PWV), we recorded the pulse at the carotid artery and the femoral artery. The distance between these points was measured (subtracting the distance between carotid artery and sternal notch from distance between femoral artery and sternal notch). The time of wave travel was simultaneously recorded with electrocardiogram. PWV was calculated by dividing the distance with the time, expressed in m/s.

**Body composition.** Body weight and body height were measured with calculation of body mass index (BMI) (kg/m$^2$). Waist circumference was measured with a measuring tape at the height of umbilicus with the patient lying in supine position. Dual-energy X-ray absorptiometry (DXA) was used to assess body composition (body fat) and DXA is reconized as a validated reference method for assessing body composition [20].

**Blood pressure.** Brachial BP was measured in a supine position after at least five minutes rest using Omron M7 (Kyoto, Japan). Several measurements were performed until two differed by ≤5 mmHg in both systolic and diastolic BP and the average of these two measurements were calculated.

**Inflammatory markers, cytokines and lipids.** Blood samples were drawn after at least four hours fasting, and at least 48 hours after the last exercise session, and then analyzed for CRP, total cholesterol (TC) and high density lipoprotein cholesterol (HDL-c) by COBAS 6000 (Roche Diagnostics, Basel, Switzerland). Low density lipoprotein cholesterol (LDL-c) was calculated from Freidewalds formula [21]. Erythrocyte sedimentation rate (ESR) was measured using the Westergren method. In addition, blood samples were collected in EDTA containing vacutainer tubes, plasma were isolated and frozen at −80°Celsius and batch analyzed by enzyme immunoassays (EIAs). The following were analyzed: interleukin (IL)-6, IL-23 (Abcam, Cambridge, UK), IL-17a (Peprotec, Rocky Hill, NJ, USA), IL-18 and soluble TNF receptor 1 (sTNF-R1) and 2 (sTNF-R2) (RnDsystems, Stillwater, MN) at the end of the study. The inter- and intra-assay coefficients of variation were less than 10% for all EIAs.

**Safety.** Safety was considered as absence of a flare up in disease activity and was defined in terms of stable or decreased self-reported disease activity (ASDAS and BASDAI) and acute phase reactants (CRP and ESR). Further, we included the report of any adverse events in the definition of safety.

## Randomization and blinding

Allocation to EG or CG followed a computer-generated randomization list prepared by a study-independent statistician. Block-randomization with a block-size of four was used. The group assignment was concealed in envelopes and revealed consecutively after baseline testing. The recruiting investigator was unaware of the next participant's allocation. The assessors were blinded for group assignment and participants were instructed not to reveal any information regarding their group attachment or treatment program to the assessors.

## Statistical analyses

Statistical analyses were performed using SPSS version 21. The main statistical analyses were performed on the per-protocol population since this was an explanatory study [22]. The per-protocol population consisted of all randomized patients following the exercise protocol (at least 80% exercise attendance in EG and no exercise in CG). We used analysis of covariance (ANCOVA) on the post-intervention values to assess the group differences with p-values, mean difference and 95% CI. Baseline values were included as covariates. We assessed the normality assumptions of the ANCOVA models by pp-plots of the residuals. The residuals for ESR, CRP, IL-6, AIx and PWV were not normally distributed, and group differences in change from baseline were analyzed using the Mann-Whitney U-test with median and corresponding 95% confidence limits by the Hodges-Lehman estimator. P-values < 0.05 were considered to be statistically significant. We considered all analyses to be exploratory, and did not adjust for multiple testing.

# Results

## Participant flow

Thirty-four patients were assessed for eligibility (Figure 1). Six patients were excluded or withdrawn before randomization. Twenty-eight patients were randomized, 13 in EG, 15 in CG. One patient in the EG withdrew immediately after randomization due to hospitalization. Three patients dropped out during the intervention period (EG = 2, CG = 1). In the EG, one patient dropped out because of a streptococcal infection in the throat and one patient dropped out because the intervention was physically challenging and time consuming. In the CG, one patient did not perform testing after 12 weeks.

All the completing participants in the EG followed ≥80% of the exercise protocol, and reached their targeted HR during the endurance exercise sessions. In the CG, none of the completing participants reported that they had exercised during the intervention period, but one patient in the CG started with TNF-inhibitor four weeks after the baseline assessment. Following this, the per-protocol population consisted of 24 patients, 10 in the EG and 14 in the CG.

## Characteristics

There were significantly more males in the CG compared to the EG (p = 0.01), and the groups differed in weight (p = 0.01) and height (p = 0.01), presumable due to the gender difference (Table 1). Baseline characteristics were similar across the groups for other variables (Table 1).

## Efficacy on disease activity

Although not statistically significant, there was an improvement in the primary outcome ASDAS score in the EG compared to the CG (adjusted mean between group difference −0.66, 95%CI [−1.37, 0.05], p = 0.07) (Table 2), whereas patient reported

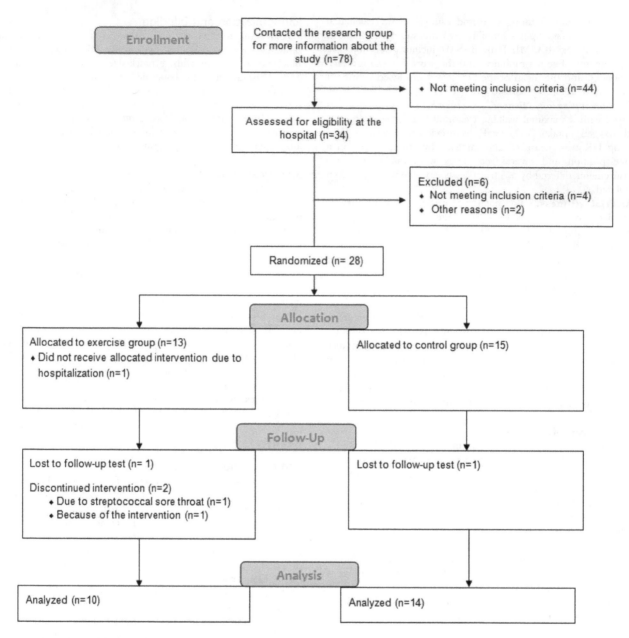

**Figure 1. Flow of participants through the randomized controlled pilot study.** EG: exercise group. CG: control group.

disease activity, BASDAI, improved significantly (adjusted mean between group difference −2.0, 95%CI [−3.6, −0.4], p = 0.02).

### Efficacy on cardiovascular risk factors

Arterial stiffness was significantly reduced in the EG compared to CG. The median changes in AIx and PWV for the EG and CG are presented in Figure 2. All changes were in favor of the EG. Further, significant treatment effects were seen for $VO_2$ peak, resting HR, total body fat and abdominal fat (Table 3). A significant reduction in waist circumference was observed for subjects who had an increased waist circumference at baseline (males ≥94 cm and females ≥80 cm, analyzed: EG n = 6 and CG n = 12) in the EG compared to CG.

### Efficacy on other secondary outcome measures

Significant treatment effects were seen for patient reported physical function, BASFI, but not for spinal mobility (BASMI) (Table 2). In general, there were no differences between the groups in change in inflammatory markers, although there was a trend towards a reduction in IL-17a and IL-23 in the EG compared to the CG (Table 2).

### Safety

Seven of 10 subjects in the EG had decreased disease activity, one had a stable disease activity and two increased their disease activity (+0.2 and +0.5 in ASDAS) from baseline to post intervention. There were no differences in change in inflammatory markers (CRP and ERS) between the groups. Furthermore, no

**Table 1.** Baseline descriptive of all patients, exercise group and control group.

| | All patients, n = 24 | Exercise group, n = 10 | Control group, n = 14 |
|---|---|---|---|
| Age, years, mean (SD) | 48.5 (12.0) | 46.6 (13.6) | 49.9 (11.1) |
| Gender, male, n (%) | 12 (50) | 2 (20)[a] | 10 (71)[a] |
| Current smoking, n (%) | 3 (13) | 1 (10) | 2 (14) |
| Height, m, mean (SD) | 1.75 (0.07) | 1.71 (0.06)[a] | 1.78 (0.07)[a] |
| Weight, kg, mean (SD) | 79.5 (15.7) | 70.0 (12.3)[a] | 86.3 (14.6)[a] |
| Disease duration, years, mean (SD) | 24.9 (15.8) | 19.2 (19.8) | 28.6 (11.9) |
| ASDAS, mean (SD) | 2.6 (0.6) | 2.3 (0.6) | 2.7 (0.8) |
| BASDAI, mean (SD) | 5.3 (1.4) | 5.3 (1.4) | 5.3 (1.4) |
| CRP, median (range) | 2 (1, 23) | 1 (1, 9) | 2 (1, 23) |
| ERS, median (range) | 7(1, 41) | 10 (2, 41) | 6 (1, 24) |
| Diabetes, n (%) | 1 (4) | 1 (10) | 0 (0) |
| Hypertension, n (%) | 4 (17) | 1 (10) | 3 (21) |
| NSAIDs, n (%) | 18 (75) | 8 (80) | 10 (71) |
| TNF-inhibitor, n (%) | 7 (29) | 1 (10) | 6 (43) |
| Anti-hypertensives, n (%) | 4 (17) | 0 (0) | 4 (29) |
| Statins, n (%) | 5 (21) | 2 (20) | 3 (21) |

ASDAS, Ankylosing Spondylitis Disease Activity Score; BASDAI, Bath Ankylosing Spondylitis Disease Activity Index (0–10, 10 = worst); CRP, C-reactiv protein; ESR, erythrocyte sedimentation rate NSAIDs, non-steroidal anti-inflammatory drugs; TNF, tumor necrosis factor, SD; standard deviation.
[a]Statistically significant differences between groups. Analysed with bivariate test as appropriate.

**Table 2.** Effects of high intensity exercise on disease activity, inflammatory markers and cytokines.

| | Exercise group, n = 10 | | Control group, n = 14 | | Estimated mean group difference (95% CI)[a] | p-value |
|---|---|---|---|---|---|---|
| | Baseline | 3 months | Baseline | 3 months | | |
| **Disease activity** | | | | | | |
| ASDAS, mean (SD) | 2.3 (0.6) | 1.8 (0.9) | 2.7 (0.8) | 2.6 (0.8) | −0.7 (−1.4, 0.1)[a] | 0.07 |
| BASDAI, mean (SD) | 5.3 (1.4) | 3.3 (2.0) | 5.3 (1.3) | 5.2 (2.0) | −2.0 (−3.6, −0.4)[a] | 0.02 |
| BASFI, mean (SD) | 2.6 (2.2) | 1.5 (1.5) | 3.1 (1.6) | 3.1 (1.4) | −1.4 (−2.6, −0.3)[a] | 0.02 |
| BASMI, mean (SD) | 2.3 (1.5) | 2.0 (1.6) | 3.0 (1.8) | 2.9 (1.8) | −0.3 (−0.9, 0.3)[a] | 0.32 |
| **Inflammatory markers** | | | | | | |
| ESR (mm/h), median (range) | 10 (2, 41) | 9 (5, 26) | 6 (1, 24) | 7 (1, 46) | −1 (−6, 2)[b] | 0.40[c] |
| CRP (mg/L), median (range) | 1 (1,9) | 1 (1,12) | 2 (1, 23) | 3 (1, 13) | 0 (−1, 2)[b] | 0.89[c] |
| **Cytokines** | | | | | | |
| IL-6 (pg/mL), median (range) | 0.3 (0.2, 5.0) | 0.3 (0.2, 16.2) | 0.4 (0.2, 2.8) | 0.3 (0.2, 2.4) | 0.0 (−0.3, 0.5)[b] | 0.95[c] |
| IL-17a (pg/mL), mean (SD) | 82 (53) | 72 (27) | 103 (90) | 105 (80) | −16 (−34, 2)[a] | 0.08 |
| IL-18 (pg/mL), mean (SD) | 95 (20) | 86 (15) | 97 (37) | 101 (43) | −13 (−30, 4)[a] | 0.12 |
| IL-23 (pg/ml), mean (SD) | 123 (39) | 103 (25) | 95 (47) | 113 (39) | −24 (−49, 1)[a] | 0.06 |
| sTNFr1 (ng/mL), mean (SD) | 0.87 (0.23) | 0.87 (0.16) | 0.98 (0.20) | 1.03 (0.31) | −0.05 (−0.18, 0.09)[a] | 0.46 |
| sTNFr2 (ng/mL), mean (SD) | 3.0 (2.5) | 3.0 (2.5) | 3.9 (3.3) | 4.0 (3.3) | −0.1 (−0.3, 0.2)[a] | 0.64 |

Differences between the groups in post intervention (3 months) values, analyzed with ANCOVA with baseline values as covariates.
All BAS-instruments 0–10, 10 = worst.
ASDAS, Ankylosing Spondylitis Disease Activity Score; BASDAI, Bath Ankylosing Spondylitis Disease Activity Index; BASFI, Bath Ankylosing Spondylitis Functional Index; BASMI, Bath Ankylosing Spondylitis Metrology Index; CRP, C-reactive protein; ESR, erythrocyte sedimentation rate; IL, interleukin; sTNFR, soluble tumor necrosis factor receptor.
[a]Estimated regression coefficients,
[b]Hodges-Lehman median estimator,
[c]Mann-Whitney U-test.

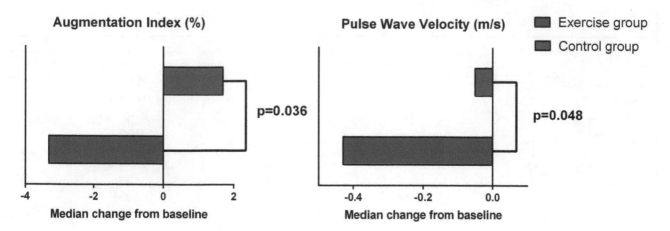

**Figure 2.** Median change in arterial stiffness after 3 months intervention of high intensity exercise, compairsons between control group and exercise group using Mann-Whitney U-test.

**Table 3.** Effects of high intensity exercise on cardiovascular risk.

| | Exercise group, n = 10 | | Control group, n = 14 | | Estimated mean group difference (95% CI)[a] | p-value |
|---|---|---|---|---|---|---|
| | baseline | 3 month | baseline | 3 month | | |
| **Cardiorespiratory fitness** | | | | | | |
| VO$_2$ peak (ml/kg/min) mean (SD) | 36.0 (5.1) | 39.4 (4.5) | 36.8 (4.9) | 36.3 (3.8) | 3.7 (2.1, 5.2)[a] | <0.001 |
| Resting HR, mean (SD) | 64 (7) | 59 (6) | 59 (8) | 62 (9) | −6 (−11, −1)[a] | 0.02 |
| **Body composition** | | | | | | |
| Body weight total (kg), mean (SD) | 70.0 (12.3) | 70.6 (12.5) | 86.3 (14.6) | 86.8 (15.3) | 0.5 (−1.1, 2.1)[a] | 0.49 |
| BMI (kg/m$^2$), mean (SD) | 24.0 (3.8) | 24.2 (3.8) | 27.1 (3.9) | 27.2 (4.0) | 0.0 (−0.6, 0.6)[a] | 0.89 |
| Waist circumference (cm)$^2$, mean (SD) | 94.7 (7.9)[b] | 91.2 (6.8)[b] | 101.3 (9.8)[b] | 101.3 (10.1)[b] | −3.8 (−6.9, −0.8)[a,b] | 0.02[b] |
| Fat, total (%), mean (SD) | 32.2 (7.4) | 30.8 (7.2) | 29.9 (6.2) | 29.8 (6.2) | −1.4 (−2.1, −0.6)[a] | <0.001 |
| Fat, abdominal (%), mean (SD) | 29.8 (8.3) | 27.5 (8.2) | 29.6 (7.2) | 29.2 (7.1) | −1.8 (−3.0, −0.6)[a] | <0.001 |
| **Lipids** | | | | | | |
| TC (mmol/L), mean (SD) | 5.7 (1.2) | 5.4 (1.2) | 5.7 (1.0) | 5.6 (0.7) | −0.2 (−0.8, 0.4)[a] | 0.60 |
| LDL-c, (mmol/L), mean (SD) | 3.1 (1.3) | 2.8 (0.9) | 3.6 (0.9) | 3.6 (0.9) | −0.5 (−1.1, 0.1)[a] | 0.10 |
| HDL-c, (mmol/L), mean (SD) | 2.1 (0.3) | 2.0 (0.5) | 1.3 (0.4) | 1.3 (0.5) | −0.3 (−0.7, 0.1)[a] | 0.11 |
| TC/HDL-c, (mmol/L), mean (SD) | 2.8 (0.9) | 2.9 (1.1) | 4.9 (1.7) | 4.6 (1.5) | −0.1 (−0.8, 0.7)[a] | 0.88 |
| **Blood pressure** | | | | | | |
| Brachial SBP (mmHg), mean (SD) | 126 (17) | 126 (24) | 130 (13) | 124 (9) | 7 (−3, 16)[a] | 0.15 |
| Brachial DBP (mmHg), mean (SD) | 80 (8) | 77 (11) | 81 (7) | 79 (8) | −1 (−8, 6)[a] | 0.68 |
| **Arterial stiffness** | | | | | Estimated median group difference (95%CI)[c] | |
| AIx (%), median (range) | 21.5 (−8.7, 34.5) | 18.5 (−17, 34.5) | 16.4 (−5.0, 29,5) | 15.5 (5, 30) | −5.3 (−11.0, −0.5)[c] | 0.04[d] |
| PWV (m/s), median (range) | 7.2 (5.8, 11.0) | 6.2 (4.4, 10.4) | 7.4 (5.3, 8.8) | 6.6 (5.1, 8.1) | −0.3 (−0.7, 0.0)[c] | 0.048[d] |

Differences between the groups in post intervention (3 months) values, analyzed with ANCOVA with baseline values as covariates.
AIx, Augmentation Index; BMI, body mass index; DBP, diastolic blood pressure; HR, heart rate; HDL-c, high density lipoprotein cholesterol; LDL-c, low density lipoprotein cholesterol; PWV, Pulse Wave Velocity; SBP, systolic blood pressure; TC, total cholesterol; VO$_2$ peak, peak oxygen uptake.
[a]Estimated regression coefficients;
[b]analyzing only subjects with an increased waist circumference at baseline (males ≥94 cm and females ≥80 cm, EG n = 6, CG n = 12),
[c]Hodges-Lehman median estimator,
[d]Mann-Whitney U-test.

adverse events were reported during the intervention, indicating that high intensity exercise was safe and well tolerated in patients with active axSpA.

## Discussion

This pilot study showed that high intensity endurance and strength exercise improved disease activity and reduced CV-risk factors in axSpA patients with active disease.

To our knowledge this is the first study aiming to examine whether patients with active axSpA could participate in a high intensity exercise program without a flare up in disease activity. Given the treatment effect of improved patient reported disease activity and stable inflammatory markers, the concept of high intensity exercise for axSpA-patients with active disease seems to be applicable. Our results are in accordance with a recently published case matched study by Stavropoulos-Kalinoglou et al. reporting that high intensity exercise significantly improved disease activity in patient with rheumatoid arthritis (RA) [23].

BASDAI has commonly been used as disease activity outcome measure in studies of effects of medication or exercise in patients with AS. Systematic reviews have reported treatment effects of TNF-inhibitors with effect size (ES) between 0.3 and 1.5 [24], and ES of exercise therapy (mainly flexibility exercises) to be between 0 and 0.8 in BASDAI [25]. In comparison, we found an ES of 1.4, suggesting that the intervention may have beneficial effects on patient reported disease symptoms. Thus, the improvement in BASDAI in our study supports that high intensity exercise may serve as an effective supplement to a pharmacological intervention.

Increased CV risk is an important factor for increased morbidity and mortality in patients with rheumatic diseases including those with axSpA. In the present study we found improvements in several CV risk factors. Central arterial stiffness measured as PWV is a validated marker of CV risk and has been used as a surrogate endpoint of CVD [26]. AIx is an estimation of central arterial pressure and has also been shown to predict CV mortality [27]. This is the first study to demonstrate improvements of arterial stiffness after exercise intervention in patients with axSpA, and in rheumatic diseases in general. However, improvement in arterial stiffness after an exercise intervention has been reported in young and middle aged healthy men [28,29], and a cross-sectional study on RA patients reported that a higher level of self-reported physical activity was associated with lower arterial stiffness [30]. The magnitude of the reduction in arterial stiffness in the exercise group was AIx 3% and PWV 0.4 m/s, which is comparable to the reduction reported in studies on other populations [28,29,31]. A population study has shown that in young men, 10 years of vascular aging corresponds to an increase in PWV of 0.48 m/s and AIx of 9%, and in elderly men an increase in PWV of 1.36 m/s and AIx 1% [32]. Thus, the improvement in arterial stiffness in our study seems to be clinically meaningful in reducing CV risk. Arterial stiffness is determined by elastic properties of the artery wall (composition of elastin and collagen) and vasoconstrictor tone exerted by the smooth muscle cells [33]. The structural composition of elastin and collagen is believed to develop over years, and thus it seems unlikely that this would change after a short term intervention. Exercise can however alter arterial stiffness over a short period by modulation of the sympathetic-adrenergic tone either directly or through nitric oxide [29,33,34]. In addition, arterial stiffness can be affected by alterations of CV risk factors such as lipids, inflammation and especially BP [26]. In the present study these parameters showed no significant treatment effects. Our findings are supported by a study on

healthy men, demonstrating favorable effects of exercise on arterial stiffness without changes in traditional CV risk factors, thus indicating a direct effect of exercise on the arterial stiffness [29].

In addition to arterial stiffness, the EG group improved $VO_2$ peak and reduced resting HR, and hereby confirm that the exercise intervention was effective in improving cardiorespiratory fitness. In the exercise study by Stavropoulos-Kalinoglou et al., the RA patients showed similar improvements in $VO_2$ peak [35]. Physical fitness is inversely related to CV risk in the general population [36]. Even small improvements in cardiorespiratory fitness are recognized as significant in reducing CV morbidity and mortality [37], and a prospective study reported that an increase in $VO_2$ peak of 3.5 ml/kg/min corresponded to a substantial decrease in cardiac events in a broad heterogeneous cohort of middle-aged men [38]. We found a mean 3.7 ml/kg/min difference in change in $VO_2$ peak in favor of the EG, thus indicating that the improvement in cardiorespiratory fitness seen in this study is of clinically importance in preventing CVD.

In addition, this study demonstrated significant treatment effects on total body fat and abdominal fat, although there were no differences in change in total body weight between the groups. Abdominal fat is associated with CV risk [39], and adipose tissue is described as an endocrine organ secreting inflammatory mediators like adipokines which play relevant roles in the pathophysiology of both CVD and inflammatory diseases [40]. Thus, the significant treatment effect on abdominal fat underline the potential of intensive exercise as a disease modifying treatment modality in patients with axSpA.

In contrast to these effects, and as mentioned above, we found no differences between the groups in change the plasma lipids and brachial BP. Two different meta-analyses concluded that exercise interventions have beneficial effects on BP, HDL-c and to some extend TC in the general population [41,42]. Furthermore, Stavropoulos-Kalinoglou et al. found significant reductions in BP and improvement of lipid profile after three months and six months of exercise in RA patients [35]. In contrast and in line with our results, a recent RCT on a 12 week moderate intensity exercise intervention in AS did not show any significant reductions in TC [43]. The lack of effect on lipids and brachial BP in our study might be due to a small sample size, a short intervention period and that most patients were within the normal range of BP and lipids at baseline.

Enhanced inflammation is an important pathogenic mediator in various rheumatic disorders including axSpA. For healthy adults, an anti-inflammatory effect of exercise is reported [44], but to our knowledge, this has not been investigated in patients with axSpA. We found no significant effects of high intensity endurance and strengths exercise on plasma levels of a wide range of cytokines or cytokine modulators. However, the EG showed a trend towards a decrease in IL-17a and IL-23 as compared with the CG, and notably both these cytokines have recently been suggested to be major players in the pathogenesis of axSpA [45]. Interestingly, treatment with inhibitors of IL-17 [46] and IL-23/IL-12 [47] has recently shown promising results in reducing disease activity in patients with active AS. In order to obtain more insight in the effects of exercise on the inflammatory process in axSpA patients, exercise-response of relevant inflammatory markers should be further explored.

Our findings support a favourable effect of exercise on CV risk in an axSpA population. Whether these results may be extrapolated to other inflammatory diseases with increased CV risk, e.g. suchs as HIV infections [48], should be investigated.

A strength of the present study was the randomized controlled design. Further, the intervention was in accordance with the ASCMs exercise recommendations, was individualized and the patients were supervised in order to obtain the optimal dose of exercise as prescribed in the protocol. The intervention was individually adapted and the intensity was controlled, ensuring that the intended physiological goals were met. Thus, the results of this study may be considered as measures of efficacy, and the adherence to the program was confirmed by the physiological response in terms of increased cardiorespiratory fitness. The main limitation is that this was a small explanatory study carried out under close to optimal conditions. Further, the participants and the therapist were not blinded to treatment allocation, and lack of blinding is likely to exaggerate treatment effects on subjective outcomes [49]. The sample size is small, and negative results may not be true negative due to the insufficient power to show significant differences. Moreover, based on its explorative nature, a large number of parameters were compared in a relative small study population without correcting for multiple comparisons further underscoring that secondary outcomes should be interpreted with some caution.

## Conclusions

The results of the present study showed that high intensity cardiorespiratory and strength exercises improved disease activity and reduced CV risk factors in patients with active axSpA. The promising results of this pilot study will be further explored in a larger randomized controlled trial.

## Author Contributions

Conceived and designed the experiments: SHS IJB KB NV AGS SAP HD CF. Performed the experiments: SHS IJB CF. Analyzed the data: SHS IJB SAP AGS ICO TU PA AM TKK HD KB. Contributed reagents/materials/analysis tools: SHS IJB SAP AGS AM TU PA TKK HD. Wrote the paper: SHS IJB SAP AGS KBH NV CF ICO AM TU PA TKK HD. Final approval of the manuscript to be published: SHS IJB SAP AGS KBH NV CF ICO AM TU PA TKK HD.

## References

1. Dougados M, Baeten D (2011) Spondyloarthritis. Lancet 377: 2127–2137.
2. Braun J, van den Berg, Baraliakos X, Boehm H, Burgos-Vargas R, et al. (2011) 2010 update of the ASAS/EULAR recommendations for the management of ankylosing spondylitis. Ann Rheum Dis 70: 896–904.
3. Corrigan B, Kannangra S (1978) Rheumatic disease: exercise or immobilization? Aust Fam Physician 7: 1007–1014.
4. Dagfinrud H, Kvien TK, Hagen KB (2008) Physiotherapy interventions for ankylosing spondylitis. Cochrane Database Syst Rev CD002822.
5. Szabo SM, Levy AR, Rao SR, Kirbach SE, Lacaille D, et al. (2011) Increased risk of cardiovascular and cerebrovascular disease in individuals with ankylosing spondylitis: A population-based study. Arthritis Rheum 63: 3294–304.
6. Bremander A, Petersson IF, Bergman S, Englund M (2011) Population-based estimates of common comorbidities and cardiovascular disease in ankylosing spondylitis. Arthritis Care Res (Hoboken) 63: 550–556.
7. Mathieu S, Gossec L, Dougados M, Soubrier M (2011) Cardiovascular profile in ankylosing spondylitis: A systematic review and meta-analysis. Arthritis Care Res (Hoboken) 63: 557–563.
8. Perk J, De BG, Gohlke H, Graham I, Reiner Z, et al. (2012) European Guidelines on cardiovascular disease prevention in clinical practice (version 2012): The Fifth Joint Task Force of the European Society of Cardiology and Other Societies on Cardiovascular Disease Prevention in Clinical Practice (constituted by representatives of nine societies and by invited experts). Atherosclerosis 223: 1–68.
9. Rehn TA, Winett RA, Wisloff U, Rognmo O (2013) Increasing physical activity of high intensity to reduce the prevalence of chronic diseases and improve public health. Open Cardiovasc Med J 7: 1–8.
10. Garber CE, Blissmer B, Deschenes MR, Franklin BA, LaMonte MJ, et al. (2011) American College of Sports Medicine position stand. Quantity and quality of exercise for developing and maintaining cardiorespiratory, musculoskeletal, and neuromotor fitness in apparently healthy adults: guidance for prescribing exercise. Med Sci Sports Exerc 43: 1334–1359.
11. Rudwaleit M, van der Heijde D, Landewe R, Listing J, Akkoc N, et al. (2009) The development of Assessment of SpondyloArthritis international Society classification criteria for axial spondyloarthritis (part II): validation and final selection. Ann Rheum Dis 68: 777–783.
12. Helgerud J, Høydal K, Wang E, Karlsen T, Berg P, et al. (2007) Aerobic high-intensity intervals improve VO2max more than moderate training. Med Sci Sports Exerc 39: 665–671.
13. van der Heijde D, Lie E, Kvien TK, Sieper J, Van den Bosch F, et al. (2009) ASDAS, a highly discriminatory ASAS-endorsed disease activity score in patients with ankylosing spondylitis. Ann Rheum Dis 68: 1811–1818.
14. Garrett S, Jenkinson T, Kennedy LG, Whitelock H, Gaisford P, et al. (1994) A new approach to defining disease status in ankylosing spondylitis: the Bath Ankylosing Spondylitis Disease Activity Index. J Rheumatol 21: 2286–2291.
15. Calin A, Garrett S, Whitelock H, Kennedy LG, O'Hea J, et al. (1994) A new approach to defining functional ability in ankylosing spondylitis: the development of the Bath Ankylosing Spondylitis Functional Index. J Rheumatol 21: 2281–2285.
16. van der Heijde D, Landewe R, Feldtkeller E (2008) Proposal of a linear definition of the Bath Ankylosing Spondylitis Metrology Index (BASMI) and comparison with the 2-step and 10-step definitions. Ann Rheum Dis 67: 489–493.
17. Halvorsen S, Vøllestad NK, Fongen C, Provan SA, Semb AG, et al. (2012) Physical fitness in patients with ankylosing spondylitis: comparison with population controls. Phys Ther 92: 298–309.
18. AtCor Medical (2013) Available: http://atcormedical.com/technical_notes.html. Accessed December.
19. Pauca AL, O'Rourke MF, Kon ND (2001) Prospective evaluation of a method for estimating ascending aortic pressure from the radial artery pressure waveform. Hypertension 38: 932–937.
20. Andreoli A, Scalzo G, Masala S, Tarantino U, Guglielmi G (2009) Body composition assessment by dual-energy X-ray absorptiometry (DXA). Radiol Med 114: 286–300.
21. Friedewald WT, Levy RI, Fredrickson DS (1972) Estimation of the concentration of low-density lipoprotein cholesterol in plasma, without use of the preparative ultracentrifuge. Clin Chem 18: 499–502.
22. Armijo-Olivo S WS, Magee D (2009) Intention to treat analysis, compliance, drop-outs an how to deal with missing data in clinical research: a review. Physical Therapy Reviews 14: 36–49.
23. Stavropoulos-Kalinoglou A, Metsios GS, Veldhuijzen van Zanten JJ, Nightingale P, Kitas GD, et al. (2012) Individualised aerobic and resistance exercise training improves cardiorespiratory fitness and reduces cardiovascular risk in patients with rheumatoid arthritis. Ann Rheum Dis 72: 1819–25.
24. Baraliakos X, van den Berg R, Braun J, van der Heijde D (2012) Update of the literature review on treatment with biologics as a basis for the first update of the ASAS/EULAR management recommendations of ankylosing spondylitis. Rheumatology (Oxford) 51: 1378–1387.
25. van den Berg R, Baraliakos X, Braun J, van der Heijde D (2012) First update of the current evidence for the management of ankylosing spondylitis with non-pharmacological treatment and non-biologic drugs: a systematic literature review for the ASAS/EULAR management recommendations in ankylosing spondylitis. Rheumatology (Oxford) 51: 1388–1396.
26. Laurent S, Cockcroft J, Van BL, Boutouyrie P, Giannattasio C, et al. (2006) Expert consensus document on arterial stiffness: methodological issues and clinical applications. Eur Heart J 27: 2588–2605.
27. Vlachopoulos C, Aznaouridis K, O'Rourke MF, Safar ME, Baou K, et al. (2010) Prediction of cardiovascular events and all-cause mortality with central haemodynamics: a systematic review and meta-analysis. Eur Heart J 31: 1865–1871.
28. Heydari M, Boutcher YN, Boutcher SH (2013) High-intensity intermittent exercise and cardiovascular and autonomic function. Clin Auton Res 23: 57–65.
29. Tanaka H, Dinenno FA, Monahan KD, Clevenger CM, DeSouza CA, et al. (2000) Aging, habitual exercise, and dynamic arterial compliance. Circulation 102: 1270–1275.
30. Crilly MA, Wallace A (2013) Physical inactivity and arterial dysfunction in patients with rheumatoid arthritis. Scand J Rheumatol 42: 27–33.
31. Edwards DG, Schofield RS, Magyari PM, Nichols WW, Braith RW (2004) Effect of exercise training on central aortic pressure wave reflection in coronary artery disease. Am J Hypertens 17: 540–543.
32. McEniery CM, Yasmin, Hall IR, Qasem A, Wilkinson IB, et al. (2005) Normal vascular aging: differential effects on wave reflection and aortic pulse wave

velocity: the Anglo-Cardiff Collaborative Trial (ACCT). J Am Coll Cardiol 46: 1753–1760.

33. Zieman SJ, Melenovsky V, Kass DA (2005) Mechanisms, pathophysiology, and therapy of arterial stiffness. Arterioscler Thromb Vasc Biol 25: 932–943.

34. Schuler G, Adams V, Goto Y (2013) Role of exercise in the prevention of cardiovascular disease: results, mechanisms, and new perspectives. Eur Heart J 34: 1790–1799.

35. Stavropoulos-Kalinoglou A, Metsios GS, Veldhuijzen van Zanten JJ, Nightingale P, Kitas GD, et al. (2012) Individualised aerobic and resistance exercise training improves cardiorespiratory fitness and reduces cardiovascular risk in patients with rheumatoid arthritis. Ann Rheum Dis.

36. Kodama S, Saito K, Tanaka S, Maki M, Yachi Y, et al. (2009) Cardiorespiratory fitness as a quantitative predictor of all-cause mortality and cardiovascular events in healthy men and women: a meta-analysis. JAMA 301: 2024–2035.

37. Aspenes ST, Nilsen TI, Skaug EA, Bertheussen GF, Ellingsen O, et al. (2011) Peak oxygen uptake and cardiovascular risk factors in 4631 healthy women and men. Med Sci Sports Exerc 43: 1465–1473.

38. Laukkanen JA, Kurl S, Salonen R, Rauramaa R, Salonen JT (2004) The predictive value of cardiorespiratory fitness for cardiovascular events in men with various risk profiles: a prospective population-based cohort study. Eur Heart J 25: 1428–1437.

39. Pischon T, Boeing H, Hoffmann K, Bergmann M, Schulze MB, et al. (2008) General and abdominal adiposity and risk of death in Europe. N Engl J Med 359: 2105–2120.

40. Scotece M, Conde J, Gomez R, Lopez V, Pino J, et al. (2012) Role of adipokines in atherosclerosis: interferences with cardiovascular complications in rheumatic diseases. Mediators Inflamm 2012: 125458.

41. Cornelissen VA, Fagard RH (2005) Effects of endurance training on blood pressure, blood pressure-regulating mechanisms, and cardiovascular risk factors. Hypertension 46: 667–675.

42. Leon AS, Sanchez OA (2001) Response of blood lipids to exercise training alone or combined with dietary intervention. Med Sci Sports Exerc 33: S502–S515.

43. Niedermann K, Sidelnikov E, Muggli C, Dagfinrud H, Hermann M, et al. (2013) Cardiovascular training improves fitness in patients with ankylosing spondylitis. Arthritis Care Res (Hoboken).

44. Walsh NP, Gleeson M, Shephard RJ, Gleeson M, Woods JA, et al. (2011) Position statement. Part one: Immune function and exercise. Exerc Immunol Rev 17: 6–63.

45. Sherlock JP, Joyce-Shaikh B, Turner SP, Chao CC, Sathe M, et al. (2012) IL-23 induces spondyloarthropathy by acting on ROR-gammat+ CD3+CD4-CD8-entheseal resident T cells. Nat Med 18: 1069–1076.

46. Baeten D, Baraliakos X, Braun J, Sieper J, Emery P, et al. (2013) Anti-interleukin-17A monoclonal antibody secukinumab in treatment of ankylosing spondylitis: a randomised, double-blind, placebo-controlled trial. Lancet 382: 1705–1713.

47. Poddubnyy D, Hermann KG, Callhoff J, Listing J, Sieper J (2014) Ustekinumab for the treatment of patients with active ankylosing spondylitis: results of a 28-week, prospective, open-label, proof-of-concept study (TOPAS). Ann Rheum Dis 73: 817–823.

48. D'Ascenzo F, Cerrato E, Biondi-Zoccai G, Moretti C, Omede P, et al. (2012) Acute coronary syndromes in human immunodeficiency virus patients: a meta-analysis investigating adverse event rates and the role of antiretroviral therapy. Eur Heart J 33: 875–880.

49. Wood L, Egger M, Gluud LL, Schulz KF, Juni P, et al. (2008) Empirical evidence of bias in treatment effect estimates in controlled trials with different interventions and outcomes: meta-epidemiological study. BMJ 336: 601–605.

# 22

# Decreased Frequencies of Circulating Follicular Helper T Cell Counterparts and Plasmablasts in Ankylosing Spondylitis Patients Naïve for TNF Blockers

**María-Belén Bautista-Caro[1], Irene Arroyo-Villa[1], Concepción Castillo-Gallego[1], Eugenio de Miguel[1], Diana Peiteado[1], Chamaida Plasencia-Rodríguez[1], Alejandro Villalba[1], Paloma Sánchez-Mateos[2], Amaya Puig-Kröger[2], Emilio Martín-Mola[1], María-Eugenia Miranda-Carús[1]***

1 Department of Rheumatology, Hospital Universitario La Paz-IdiPAZ, Madrid, Spain, 2 Laboratorio de Inmuno-Oncología, Hospital General Universitario Gregorio Marañón, Madrid, Spain

## Abstract

Follicular helper T cells (Tfh), localized in lymphoid organs, promote B cell differentiation and function. Circulating CD4 T cells expressing CXCR5, ICOS and/or PD-1 are counterparts of Tfh. Three subpopulations of circulating CD4+CXCR5+ cells have been described: CXCR3+CCR6- (Tfh-Th1), CXCR3-CCR6+ (Tfh-Th17), and CXCR3-CCR6- (Tfh-Th2). Only Tfh-Th17 and Tfh-Th2 function as B cell helpers. Our objective was to study the frequencies of circulating Tfh (cTfh), cTfh subsets and plasmablasts (CD19+CD20-CD27+CD38$^{high}$ cells), and the function of cTfh cells, in patients with Ankylosing Spondylitis (AS). To this end, peripheral blood was drawn from healthy controls (HC) (n = 50), AS patients naïve for TNF blockers (AS/nb) (n = 25) and AS patients treated with TNF blockers (AS/b) (n = 25). The frequencies of cTfh and plasmablasts were determined by flow cytometry. Cocultures of magnetically sorted CD4+CXCR5+ T cells with autologous CD19+CD27- naïve B cells were established from 3 AS/nb patients and 3 HC, and concentrations of IgG, A and M were measured in supernatants. We obseved that AS/nb but not AS/b patients, demonstrated decreased frequencies of circulating CD4+CXCR5+ICOS+PD-1+ cells and plasmablasts, together with a decreased (Tfh-Th17+Tfh-Th2)/Tfh-Th1 ratio. The amounts of IgG and IgA produced in cocultures of CD4+CXCR5+ T cells with CD19+CD27- B cells of AS/nb patients were significantly lower than observed in cocultures established from HC. In summary, AS/nb but not AS/b patients, demonstrate a decreased frequency of cTfh and plasmablasts, and an underrepresentation of cTfh subsets bearing a B helper phenotype. In addition, peripheral blood CD4+ CXCR5+ T cells of AS/nb patients showed a decreased capacity to help B cells ex vivo.

**Editor:** Peter Szodoray, Institute of Immunology, Rikshospitalet, Norway

**Funding:** This work was supported by Fondo de Investigación Sanitaria grant PI-13/00084 from Ministerio de Economía y Competitividad/Instituto de Salud Carlos III (MINECO/ISCIII) (www.isciii.es), by RETICS Program RD12/0009/0012 (Red de Investigación en Inflamación y enfermedades Reumáticas - RIER) from MINECO/ISCIII (www.isciii.es), and by Comunidad Autónoma de Madrid/Fondo Europeo de Desarrollo Regional RAPHYME (http://www.madrimasd.org). The funders had no role in study design, data collection and analysis, decision to publish, or preparation of the manuscript.

**Competing Interests:** The authors have declared that no competing interests exist.

* Email: mariaeugenia.miranda@salud.madrid.org

## Introduction

Ankylosing spondylitis (AS) is the prototype of Spondyloarthritis (SpA) [1,2], a group of diseases sharing clinical, radiographic and genetic features [1,2]. Despite intensive research, the pathogenesis of SpA is not well understood, and evidence suggesting the implication of either autoinflammatory or autoimmune mechanisms has been reported [3].

The role of B cells and of humoral immunity in SpA is not clear. Several autoantibodies have been observed in patients with SpA [4–7], but their poor sensitivity or specificity have not allowed to establish a clear pathogenic association. More recently, reactivity against CD74 has been proposed as a marker for SpA [8,9]. Also, increased numbers of CD5+ B lymphocytes have been described in SpA [10]. Furthermore, it has been reported that some patients with AS seem to benefit from B cell depleting therapeutic strategies [11].

Follicular helper T cells (Tfh) are a major subset of effector T lymphocytes specialized in the provision of help to B cells [12–17], and characterized by their surface phenotype (CD4+CXCR5+ ICOS+PD-1+), cytokine profile (IL-21, IL-10, IL-17) and transcriptional program (BCL-6) [12–17]. Tfh cells seem to be implicated in autoimmunity [18], and increased numbers are found in murine models of Systemic Lupus Erythematosus (SLE) [18–20] and inflammatory arthritis [21]; furthermore, strategies directed at reducing Tfh cell generation ameliorate disease manifestations in these animal models [20,22].

The initial definition of Tfh cells was based on both their phenotype and their characteristic location in secondary lymphoid organs [12–17]. Several reports have subsequently described circulating populations of CD4 T cells that express CXCR5 and share both phenotypical and functional properties of classical Tfh cells [23–26]. Increased frequencies of circulating Tfh cell counterparts (cTfh), have been associated with autoimmune diseases such as SLE [23], Rheumatoid Arthritis (RA) [27], Sjögren's Syndrome [28], autoimmune thyroiditis [29], chronic active hepatitis [30] and myasthenia gravis [31]. More recently, three subpopulations of cTfh cells have been described, based on their differential expression of the chemokine receptors CXCR3 and CCR6 and on their distinct functional capacities [24]. An altered balance of these cTfh subsets has been associated with autoimmunity in juvenile dermatomyositis and SLE [24,32].

The features of cTfh cells or their subsets in SpA have not been fully characterized, and to our knowledge only two articles with discordant results have been published on this matter [33,34]. Therefore, our objective was to study the frequency and function of cTfh cells, together with the frequency of cTfh subsets and plasmablasts (CD19+CD20-CD27+CD38$^{high}$ B cells), in patients with Ankylosing Spondylitis (AS). We observed that AS patients naïve for TNF blockers (AS/nb) but not those receiving TNF blocking agents (AS/b), demonstrate a decreased frequency of cTfh and plasmablasts, and an underrepresentation of cTfh subsets bearing a B helper phenotype. In addition, peripheral blood CD4+CXCR5+ T cells of AS/nb patients showed a decreased capacity to help B cells ex vivo.

## Patients and Methods

### Ethics Statement

The study was approved by the Hospital La Paz - IdiPAZ Ethics Committee, and all subjects provided written informed consent according to the Declaration of Helsinki.

### Patients

Peripheral blood was obtained from 25 AS patients who had never received TNF blockers (AS/nb), 25 AS patients treated with TNF blockers (AS/b) and from 50 age and gender-matched healthy controls (HC). AS was diagnosed according to the 1984 modified New York criteria [35]. For patients receiving TNF blockers, blood was drawn immediately before the infusion/administration of the drug. All subjects were of Western European descent.

Among AS/nb patients, 16 were taking non-steroidal anti-inflammatory drugs (NSAIDs) and 4 were receiving sulfasalazine (SSZ); 5 of them did not take any medication regularly. Among AS/b patients, 20 were receiving infliximab, 4 etanercept and 1 adalimumab. In addition to TNF blockers, 7 patients were taking NSAIDs, and 8 were taking SSZ. Clinical characteristics of all patients are shown in Tables 1 and 2.

### Isolation of CD4+ T cells and B cells from human peripheral blood

Peripheral blood mononuclear cells (PBMCs) were separated immediately after blood sample collection, by Ficoll-Hypaque (GE Healthcare Biosciences AB, Uppsala, Sweden) density gradient centrifugation. CD4+ T or B cells were purifed from freshly isolated PBMCs by exhaustive immunomagnetic negative selection in an Automacs (Miltenyi Biotec, Bergisch Gladbach, Germany), using the "CD4+ T Cell Isolation Kit" or the "B Cell Isolation Kit II" from Miltenyi Biotec. Isolated CD4+ T cells or CD19+ B cells were >98% pure. CXCR5+ and CXCR5- subpopulations were subsequently isolated from total CD4+ T cells using PE-labeled CXCR5 microbeads (Miltenyi Biotec). Naïve (CD19+CD27-) and memory (CD19+CD27+) B cells were selected from total CD19+ B cells using CD27+ microbeads (Miltenyi Biotec). T and B cell subpopulations were >98% pure and used immediately after isolation.

### B cell/T cell cocultures

To assess the functional capacity of circulating CD4+CXCR5+ T cells, sorted CXCR5+ cells ($2 \times 10^5$ cells/well) were cocultured for 13 days with autologous naïve B (CD19+CD27-) cells ($1 \times 10^5$ cells/well) in U-bottom 96-well plates containing RPMI 1640 medium (Lonza, Alendale, NJ, USA) with 10% FCS, 2 mM L-glutamine, 50 U/ml penicillin, 50 µg/ml streptomycin and 50 µM 2-mercapto-ethanol. Endotoxin-reduced staphylococcal enterotoxin B (SEB) (1 mg/ml) (Sigma-Aldrich) was also added to the cultures, since the production of immunoglobulins in Tfh/B cell cocultures has been shown to depend on cognate T/B cell interactions [24]. For comparison, autologous cocultures of CD4+CXCR5+ T cells with CD19+CD27+ memory B cells and cocultures of CD4+CXCR5- T cells with naïve or memory B cells were also established. Concentrations of IgG, IgA and IgM were measured in coculture supernatants at different time points by ELISA.

### Cell Surface Staining and Flow Cytometry

The frequency and phenotype of Tfh-like cells and of plasmablasts present in the peripheral blood of AS patients and HC was assessed by flow cytometry after staining freshly isolated PBMCs with antibodies directed against surface phenotypical markers. Fluorochrome-conjugated mAbs from BD Pharmingen (San Diego, CA, USA) were used to examine the expression of CD3, CD4, CD8, CXCR5, ICOS, PD-1, CCR6, CXCR3, CD19, CD20, CD27 and CD38 in a FACSCalibur flow cytometer with CellQuest software (BD Biosciences).

### ELISAs

Cell-free coculture supernatants were collected and stored at −80°C. The concentrations of immunoglobulins were measured by ELISA. In brief, 96-well plates (MaxiSorp, Thermo Fisher Scientific, Waltham, MA, USA) were coated overnight at 4°C with 10 µg/ml mouse monoclonal anti-human IgG, IgA or IgM (AbD Serotec, Munich, Germany), and subseqently blocked with 2% BSA/PBS. Standard curves of human IgG, IgA or IgM (Sigma-Aldrich) together with culture supernatants diluted in 2% BSA/PBS were incubated for 3 hours at room temperature, washed and developed with HRP-conjugated goat anti-human IgG, IgA or IgM (ABD serotec) followed by TMB substrate solution (BD-Pharmingen). Absorbance was measured at 450 nm in a Synergy H4 Hybrid Multi-Mode Microplate Reader (BioTec Instruments, Inc., Winoosi, VT, USA).

### Determination of serum IgG, IgA and IgM concentrations

Sera from all studied subjects were collected on the day when phenotypical studies were done, and stored at −80°C. Concentrations of IgG, IgA and IgM were subsequently examined in sera of AS/nb, AS/b patients and HC by nephelometry in an Immage 800 Immunochemistry System (Beckman Coulter, Brea, CA, U.S.A). For AS/b patients, determinations of Igs were also performed in serum that had been collected just before initiation of treatment with TNF blockers.

### Statistical Analysis

Comparison between groups was by Mann-Whitney or Kruskal-Wallis test. When appropriate, Bonferroni correction for multiple comparisons was applied. Correlations were analyzed using Spearman's rank correlation coefficients. All analyses were performed using Prism version 5.0 software (GraphPad Software, San Diego, CA, USA).

**Table 1.** Clinical characteristics of AS/nb and AS/b patients.

| | AS/nb (n = 25) | AS/b (n = 25) |
|---|---|---|
| Age (years); median (IQR) | 56 (45.5–65.5) | 53 (45–61.5) |
| Male; n° (%) | 12 (48) | 16 (64) |
| HLA-B27+; n° (%) | 22 (88) | 23 (92) |
| Duration of symptoms (yrs); median (IQR) | 25.5 (17.5–35) | 24.5 (14–36) |
| Time since diagnosis (yrs); median (IQR) | 11.5 (5.5–20) | 15 (9–22.5) |
| Time on TNF blockers (yrs); median (IQR) | - | 7 (5–9) |
| BASDAI; median (IQR) | 3.9 (2.8–4.8) | 2.6 (1.3–6.1) |
| BASFI; median (IQR) | 1.8 (0.5–4.9) | 3 (0.6–5.8) |
| ASDAS-ESR; median (IQR) | 2.14 (1.89–2.72) | 2.22 (1.41–3.15) |
| ASDAS-CRP; median (IQR) | 2.55 (1.9–3.13) | 2.34 (1.07–3.02) |
| CRP; median (IQR) | 7.37 (2.51–11.1) | 4.52 (1.44–15.4) |
| Pt. global assessment; median (IQR) | 3 (2–6) | 3 (2–6.5) |

AS/nb: AS patients naïve for TNF blockers; AS/b: AS patients treated with TNF blockers.

## Results

### Patients with AS naïve for TNF blockers demonstrate decreased numbers of circulating Tfh counterparts

We first sought to examine the expression of Tfh phenotypical surface markers on peripheral blood CD4+ T cells. The frequency of CXCR5+ cells contained in circulating CD4+ T lymphocytes was not different among the three groups of studied subjects: 18.3±5.8 % in HC, 18.6±7.6 % in AS patients naïve for TNF blockers (AS/nb) and 18.1±5.6 % in AS patients treated with TNF blockers (AS/b) (mean ± SD). However, the frequencies of circulating total CD4+CXCR5+ICOS+ and of CD4+CXCR5+ICOS$^{high}$, together with the frequencies of total CD4+CXCR5+ICOS+ PD-1+ and of CD4+CXCR5+ICOS$^{high}$PD-1$^{high}$ T cells, that are currently considered as circulating counterparts of classical Tfh cells (cTfh) [23,25,26], were significantly decreased in AS/nb patients (Figure 1, A, B) but were not different from controls in AS/b patients (Figure 1, A, B). In parallel, the absolute numbers of cTfh were also decreased in AS/nb patients (Figure 1 C).

### Patients with AS naïve for TNF blockers demonstrate an altered balance of circulating Tfh subsets

We then examined the frequency of cTfh cell subsets as described by Morita et al. [24], based on the combined expression on CD4+ T cells of CXCR5 with CCR6 or CXCR3, that are characteristic chemokine receptors expressed on Th17 or Th1 cells, respectively. AS/nb patients demonstrated an increased frequency of circulating CD4+CXCR5+CXCR3+CCR6- (Tfh-Th1) cells together with a decreased frequency of CD4+CXCR5+CXCR3-CCR6+ (Tfh-Th17) cells, whereas the frequency of CD4+CXCR5+CXCR3-CCR6- (Tfh-Th2) cells was not different from controls (Figure 2A). Furthermore, the sum of %Tfh-Th2

plus %Tfh-Th17 cells and the ratio (%Tfh-Th2+%Tfh-Th17)/%Tfh-Th1, were decreased in AS/nb patients (Figure 2B). That is, AS/nb but not AS/b patients demonstrated a relative deficiency of cTfh cell subsets bearing a phenotype associated with B cell helping capacity [24].

### Patients with AS naïve for TNF blockers demonstrate decreased numbers of circulating plasmablasts

The frequency of circulating plasmablasts among CD19+ cells, defined as CD19+CD20-CD27+CD38$^{high}$ B cells, was decreased in AS/nb but not in AS/b patients (Figure 3, A, B). In parallel, the absolute number of circulating plasmablasts was also decreased in AS/nb (Figure 3C).

Interestingly, in AS/nb patients, the frequency of circulating plasmablasts was positively correlated not only with the frequency of cTfh counterparts, but also with the sum %Tfh-Th2+%Tfh-Th17 and with the ratio (%Tfh-Th2+%Tfh-Th17)/%Tfh-Th1 cells (Figure 3D). Conversely, the frequency of circulating plasmablasts was negatively correlated with the frequency of Tfh-Th1 cells in AS/nb (Figure 3D).

In addition, the absolute number of circulating plasmablasts was positively correlated with the absolute numbers of CD4+CXCR5+ICOS+ (r = 0.40, p<0.05), CD4+CXCR5+ICOS$^{high}$ (r = 0.46, p<0.05) and CD4+CXCR5+ICOS$^{high}$PD-1$^{high}$ T cells (r = 0.41, p<0.05).

### Functional capacity of circulating CD4+CXCR5+ T cells

We then went on to examine the functional capacity of circulating total CD4+CXCR5+ T cells, which in AS/nb patients contain decreased proportions of cTfh, together with decreased proportions of cTfh cell subsets bearing a phenotype associated

**Table 2.** Number of patients according to disease activity state based on ASDAS-CRP values [38].

| ASDAS-CRP = => | < 1.3 (inactive disease) | 1.3-2.1 (moderate activity) | 2.1-3.5 (high activity) | >3.5 (very high activity) |
|---|---|---|---|---|
| AS/nb (# of patients) | 2 | 7 | 13 | 3 |
| AS/b (# of patients) | 7 | 1 | 13 | 4 |

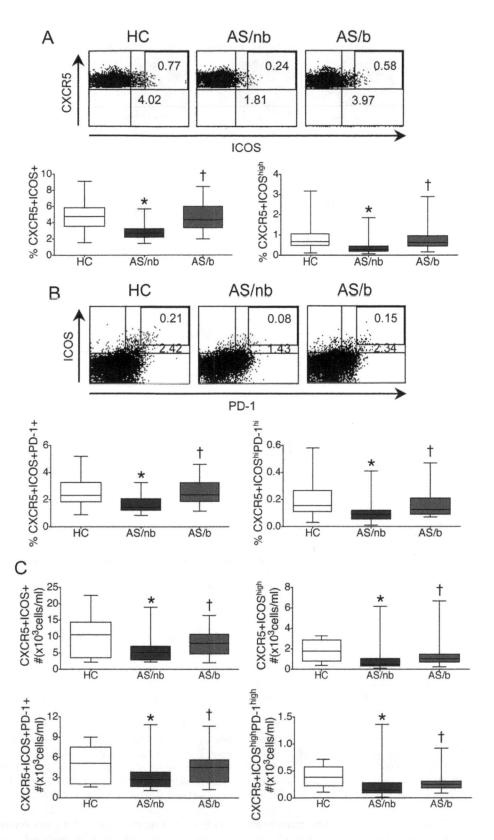

**Figure 1. Numbers of circulating Tfh counterparts (cTfh) in patients with AS.** AS/nb but not AS/b patients demonstrate decreased frequencies and absolute numbers of cTfh. A, B. Frequency of cTfh in HC, AS/nb and AS/b patients. Representative dot plots demonstrate ICOS and CXCR5 expression (A) or ICOS and PD-1 expression (B) in cells gated for CD3, CD4 and CXCR5. C. Absolute numbers of circulating Tfh counterparts (cTfh) in HC, AS/nb and AS/b patients. Box and whiskers plots represent the median, interquartile range, maximum and minimum values calculated from 25 AS/nb patients, 25 AS/b patients and 50 HC. *p<0.0001 vs HC; † p<0.01 vs AS/nb patients.

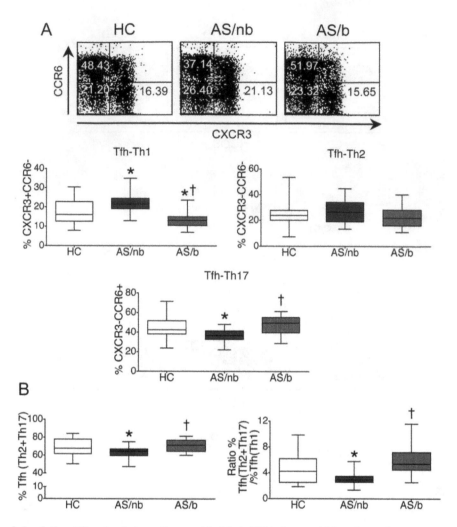

**Figure 2. Frequency of circulating Tfh subsets in patients with AS.** A. AS/nb, but not AS/b patients, demonstrate an increased frequency of circulating CD4+CXCR5+CXCR3+CCR6- (Tfh-Th1) cells and a decreased frequency of CD4+CXCR5+CXCR3-CCR6+ (Tfh-Th17) cells as compared with HC, whereas the frequency of CD4+CXCR5+CXCR3-CCR6- (Tfh-Th2) cells is not different among the three groups. Representative dot plots demonstrate CXCR3 and CCR6 expression in cells gated for CD3, CD4 and CXCR5. B. Underrepresentation of cTfh subsets with a B cell helper phenotype (Tfh-Th17 plus Tfh-Th2 cells) in AS/nb but not in AS/b patients. Box and whiskers plots represent the median, interquartile range, maximum and minimum values calculated from 25 AS/nb patients, 25 AS/b patients and 50 HC. *p<0.05 vs HC, †p<0.005 vs AS/nb.

with B cell helping capacity. To this end, cocultures of sorted CD4+CXCR5+ T cells from 3 AS/nb patients and 3 age and gender-matched healthy controls were established with autologous naïve CD19+CD27- B cells; secretion of IgG and IgA in supernatants were measured as a readout of B cell maturation. All three patients were male, aged 45, 51 and 57 years and were taking NSAIDs. Two of them were HLA B27+ and one was HLA B27-. Duration of symptoms was 28, 33 and 36 years and time since diagnosis was 25, 27 and 13 years, respectively. Their ASDAS-CRPs were 3.4, 2.75 and 2.05.

In cocultures of naïve B cells with CD4+CXCR5+ T cells, increased proportions of CD19+CD20-CD38$^{high}$ plasmablasts (Figure 4A) were observed; in addition, IgG and IgA were detected in supernatants from the 6th day on, with increasing concentrations up to the 13th day (Figure 4B,C). Interestingly, in cocultures established with T and B cells of AS/nb patients, lower proportions of CD19+CD20-CD38$^{high}$ plasmablasts and lower concentrations of both IgG and IgA were observed as compared with with HC (Figure 4, A-C). In contrast, the amount of secreted IgM was not different in cocultures of naïve B cells with CD4+

CXCR5+ T cells established from HC or AS/nb patients (Figure 4B, C). Of note, the number of recovered viable B cells was not different in cocultures established from HC or AS/nb patients (Figure 4D).

No IgG or IgA could be detected in coculture supernatants of naïve B cells with CD4+ CXCR5- T cells from either AS/nb patients or healthy controls (Figure 4B,C), which only produced low amounts of IgM (Figure 4B, C). This was not attributable to poor T cell survival since the amount of recovered viable T cells was comparable in cocultures of naïve B cells established with either CXCR5+ or CXCR5- CD4+ T cells (Figure 4D).

In addition, isolated CD4+CXCR5+ of HC or AS/nb patients were more efficient than CD4+CXCR5- T cells at helping memory CD19+CD27+ B cells to secrete IgG, IgA and IgM. No differences between HC and AS/nb were observed when measuring the secreted amounts of IgG, IgA or IgM in these CD4+CXCR5+/ CD19+CD27+ or CD4+CXCR5-/CD19+CD27+ cocultures (data not shown).

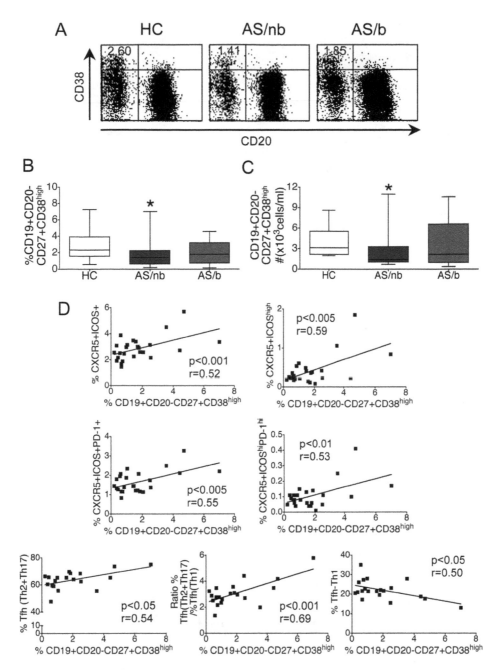

**Figure 3. Numbers of circulating plasmablasts in patients with AS.** A, B. AS/nb but not AS/b patients demonstrate a decreased frequency of circulating plasmablasts. Shown are representative dot plots of CD20 and CD38 expression on CD19+ cells (A). C. Decreased absolute numbers of circulating plasmablasts in AS/nb patients. B and C represent box and whiskers plots from 25 AS/nb patients, 25 AS/b patients and 50 HC; * p <0.005 vs HC. D. The frequency of circulating plasmablasts in AS/nb patients is positively correlated with the frequency of circulating Tfh counterparts, with the frequency of Tfh(Th2+Th17) and with the ratio [%Tfh(Th2+Th17)]/%Tfh(Th1) cells, and negatively correlated with the frequency of Tfh-Th1 cells.

## Serum levels of IgG, IgA and IgM in AS/nb and AS/b patients, and their relation with disease activity and cTfh numbers

As previously described [36,37], serum IgA levels were elevated in AS patients (Figure 5A, B). Interestingly, among our AS/nb patients, serum IgA was ony increased in those who had high or very high activity as determined by an ASDAS-CRP > 2.1 [38] (Figure 5B). In contrast, all of our AS/b patients demonstrated elevated serum IgA, even those with inactive disease or moderate activity, as determined by an ASDAS-CRP < 2.1 [38], although

levels were higher in patients with high or very high activity (Figure 5B). In addition, AS/b patients had elevated serum IgG and IgM levels, that were more marked in subjects with high or very high activity (Figure 5B). Importantly, increased serum IgA and IgM levels in this group were already present in sera taken just before initiation of treatment with TNF blockers (Figure 5A). This is consistent with previous observations indicating that AS patients with severe disease can demonstrate increased levels of all three IgG, IgA and IgM [39]. Interestingly, the above described normal or increased Ig levels did not parallel the decreased or normal cTfh and plasmablast numbers observed in AS/nb or AS/b subjects,

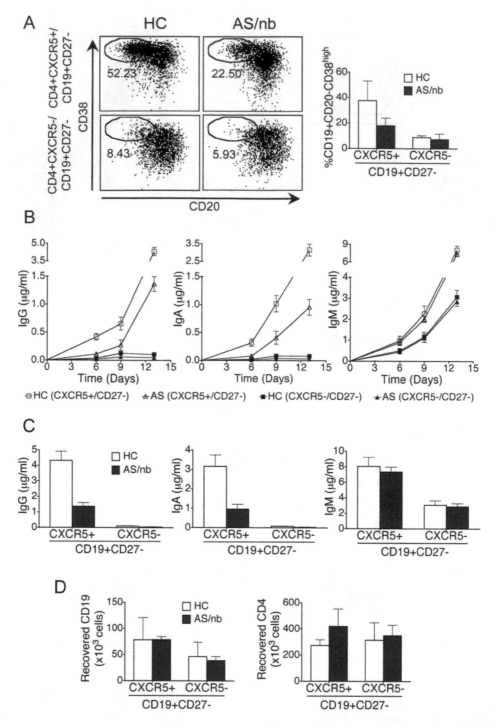

**Figure 4. Functional capacity of circulating CD4+CXCR5+ T cells.** CD4+CXCR5+ T cells isolated from peripheral blood of HC are more efficient than cells from AS/nb patients at inducing maturation of cocultured autologous naïve B cells. A. CD19+CD20-CD38^high plasmablasts in 9-day cocultures of naïve B cells from AS/nb patients or HC with autologous CXCR5+ or CXCR5- CD4+ T cells. B, C. Concentrations of IgG, A and M at different time points (B) or at 13 days (C) in cocultures of naïve B cells from AS/nb patients or HC with autologous CXCR5+ or CXCR5- CD4+ T cells. D. Recovered viable B and T cells in 9-day cocultures of naïve B cells from AS/nb patients or HC with autologous CXCR5+ or CXCR5- CD4+ T cells. Line and bar graphs represent the mean and SD of 3 independent experiments.

respectively (Figure 5B). That is, AS/nb patients showed normal or increased IgA levels in the presence of decreased cTfh and plasmablasts and altered cTfh subset ratio (Figure 5B). In addition, AS/b patients demonstrated increased Ig levels in the presence of cTfh, cTfh subset ratio and plasmablast values that were not

different from HC (Figure 5B). Furthermore, whereas serum Ig concentrations paralleled disease activity, cTfh and plasmablast numbers did not (Figure 5B).

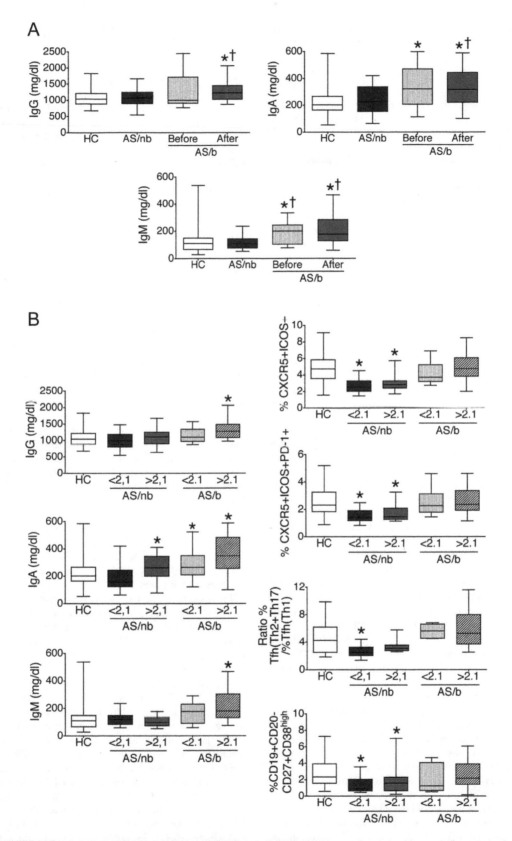

**Figure 5. Serum levels of IgG, IgA and IgM in patients with AS.** A. IgG, IgA and IgM were determined by nephelometry in the serum of AS/nb and AS/b patients. For AS/b patients, determinations were not only done in sera collected on the day when phenotypical studies were done, but also on sera that had been taken just before initiation of treatment with TNF blockers. B. Relation of serum Ig concentrations with cTfh, circulating plasmablasts and disease activity. Shown are cTfh proportions, cTfh subset ratio and circulating plasmablast proportions together with serum IgG, IgA and IgM concentrations in HC, AS patients with inactive disease or moderate disease activity (ASDAS-CRP < 2.1) [38] and AS patients with high or very high disease activity (ASDAS-CRP > 2.1) [38]. Normal or elevated serum Ig levels are observed despite the presence of decreased or normal cTfh

and plasmablasts, respectively. Note that serum Ig concentrations vary with disease activity whereas cTfh and plasmablast numbers do not. Box and whiskers plots represent the median, interquartile range, maximum and minimum values. *p<0.05 vs HC, $^\dagger$p<0.05 vs AS/nb.

## Discussion

Spondyloarthritis (SpA) and their prototype disease, AS, are typically not associated with circulating autoantibodies [1–3] and therefore, the role of B cells or B-helper T cells (Tfh) in their pathogenesis has not been thoroughly investigated. There is more recent evidence indicating that B cells may indeed be implicated in SpA [8–11], and we deemed it interesting to study the frequency of cTfh cells and plasmablasts in AS.

We have herein described that AS/nb patients demonstrate a decreased frequency of cTfh cells, together with a decreased frequency of circulating plasmablasts. Furthermore, an altered proportion of cTfh subpopulations is observed: AS/nb patients showed a predominance of Tfh-Th1 cells, that lack B cell helping capacity in healthy subjects [24], over Tfh-Th17 and Tfh-Th2 cells, that do have B cell helping capacity as described by Morita et al. [24]. In contrast, AS/b patients do not display these alterations. Discordance with previously published observations [33,34] may be attributable to different treatment, ethnicity, disease duration or activity.

Because AS/nb patients were not receiving methotrexate or other drugs that may interfere with the cell cycle, the observed alterations in cTfh and plasmablasts in this patient group are not attributable to a drug effect. Conversely, the finding of normal frequencies of cTfh and plasmablasts in AS patients receiving TNF blockers suggests that these drugs may restore the initial immune alteration. Because the ASDAS-CRP and ASDAS-ESR indexes were comparable beween AS/nb and AS/b patients, the observed differences in cTfh numbers and cTfh subset balance do not seem related with different disease activity. In addition, there was no correlation of cTfh cell numbers or subsets with disease activity in either group; this parallels the observation that increased numbers of cTfh in SLE do not associate with disease activity [23] but are related to the pathogenesis of the disease [23].

Of note, the ex vivo functional studies herein described demonstrated that isolated peripheral blood CD4+CXCR5+ T cells are indeed able to provide B cell help as previously reported [24–26]: CD4+CXCR5+ but not CD4+CXCR5- T cells, induced IgG and IgA secretion in cocultured CD19+CD27- B cells. In the presence of CD4+CXCR5- T cells, CD19+CD27- B cells only produced low amounts of IgM as expected [24,25]. In addition, CD4+CXCR5+ T cells were more efficient than CD4+CXCR5- T cells at helping memory CD19+CD27+ B cells to produce Igs. Interestingly, we observed that total CD4+CXCR5+ T cells from AS/nb patients, containing decreased proportions of cTfh and an altered balance of cTfh subpopulations, do have a reduced capacity to promote maturation of naïve B cells, as indicated by a lower induced secretion of IgG and IgA from naïve B cells when compared with HC. In contrast, the amount of IgM produced in cocultures of CD4+CXCR5+ T with autologous naïve B cells of AS/nb patients or HC was comparable. To our knowledge, this is the first functional study directed to assessing the B cell helping capacity of cTfh cells in patients with a rheumatic disease.

Our findings in AS/nb patients are in contrast with the elevated frequency of cTfh and plasmablasts described in autoimmune diseases characterized by autoantibody production [23,27–31]. In fact, it has been proposed that increased numbers of cTfh can be a signature of human immune-mediated diseases [26]. Specifically, a causal relation between accumulation of Tfh cells, autoantibody production and lupus nephritis has been demonstrated in mice

[20], and augmented numbers of Tfh counterparts in the peripheral blood of patients with SLE have been associated with disease severity [23]. Conversely, patients with deficiency of CD40-ligand or ICOS demonstrate a severely impaired generation of GC together with decreased circulating CD4+CXCR5+ T cells [40], suggesting that the numbers of cTfh are a reflection of the pool of typical Tfh in lymphoid organs.

The lower frequency of cTfh and plasmablasts in AS/nb might be related with a predominant contribution of innate versus acquired immune mechanisms to the pathogenesis of the disease [3] or with a lower capacity of AS/nb patients to produce T-dependent antibodies. However, AS has not been associated with immunodeficiency, and AS/nb patients are able to mount good antibody responses to vaccination with T-dependent antigens [41]. Alternatively, Tfh could be sequestered in the gut-associated lymphoid tissue (GALT) of AS/nb patients. In fact, subclinical gut inflammation has been described in up to 65% of AS patients [42], and is associated with increased numbers of lymphoid follicles in the ileum and colon [43]; furthermore, increased intestinal permeability has been observed not only in AS patients but also in their relatives [44]. In this context, normal numbers of cTfh cells and plasmablasts in our AS/b patients, the majority of which were receiving infliximab or adalimumab, could parallel an improvement of subclinical gut inflammation induced by these drugs. This would be consistent with studies indicating the leading role of TNF-α in intestinal homeostasis, gut barrier integrity, and pathogenesis of inflammatory bowel disease [45]. However, the levels of serum IgG, IgA and IgM in AS/nb or AS/b patients were discordant with the numbers of cTfh, cTfh subset ratio or plasmablasts: AS/nb patients, with decreased cTfh and plasmablasts, demonstrated normal or high serum IgA concentrations whereas AS/b patients, with normal cTfh and plasmablast numbers, demonstrated increased Ig concentrations. In addition, whereas numbers of cTfh or plasmablasts did not parallel disease activity parameters in AS/nb or AS/b patients, serum IgA in AS/nb or serum IgG, IgA and IgM levels in AS/b patients did, which is consistent with previous observations [36,37,39].

Interestingly, patients with AS/b demonstrated increased IgA and IgM concentrations before TNF blockade was started, which did not return to normal levels with treatment, even in patients who achieved a state of inactive or moderate disease activity as determined by ASDAS-CRP values. This suggests that AS/b patients do have a more severe disease as compared with AS/nb subjects, and that increased Ig concentrations in this group are not a side effect of treatment with TNF blockers. In addition, this observation reflects the difficulty in assessing disease activity and severity in AS with the currently available tools [38].

The lack of parallelism of cTfh and plasmablast numbers with serum Ig levels may be explained by two different mechanisms. First, Tfh and plamablasts may be sequestered in the GALT as mentioned above. Also, the altered cTfh subset ratio of AS/nb patients could result from preferential accumulation of Tfh-Th17 over Tfh-Th1 cells in the gut: whereas CCL20, the ligand for CCR6, is normally expressed in the GALT and intestinal epithelium [46,47], its expression level significantly increases in states of gut inflammation, which conditions local accumulation of CCR6 expressing cells [46,47]. Local sequestration would lead to decreased cTfh and circulating plasmablast numbers, together with altered cTfh subset ratio, in AS/nb patients. In turn, AS/b patients, with a more severe disease and a more marked alteration of intestinal permeability, would have an even higher accumulation of Tfh and plasmablasts in the GALT, with a higher rate of local Ig production and an increased number of lymphocytes available for recirculation, resulting not only in elevated serum Ig levels [48] but also in apparently normal numbers of cTfh and plasmablasts.

Of note, and as mentioned above, local Tfh sequestration at the inflammatory sites does not seem to occur in autoimmune diseases such as SLE, where increased numbers of total classical Tfh in lymphoid organs are associated with increased numbers of cTfh and autoantibody production [23]. Therefore, local sequestration of Tfh in the gut would be a mechanism operating differentially in AS. An alternative explanation for our findings would be that the number of cTfh does indeed parallel the number of true Tfh in lymphoid organs of AS patients: that is, decreased cTfh in AS/nb or normal cTfh numbers in AS/b patients would be a reflection of a decreased or "normal" pool of classsical Tfh. In this setting, innate immunity with T cell independent class switch recombination, would have a pivotal contribution to Ig production in both AS/nb and AS/b [49–51]; in turn, normal numbers of cTfh in AS/b patients would reflect activation of the acquired immune system in patients with a more severe disease [51,52]. In fact, it has been proposed that the role of innate immunity is predominant at initial stages of bowel inflammation in SpA [51], and as disease progresses or advances in severity, the contribution of acquired immunity tends to become more prominent [51,52].

Finally, both mechanisms, local Tfh sequestration and increased Ig production by innate mechanisms, may operate simultaneously in AS.

In summary, we have herein described decreased circulating Tfh and plasmablast numbers in AS/nb but not in AS/b patients, in the presence of normal or augmented serum levels of Igs. This observation sheds new light into the pathogenesis of AS and suggests that Tfh cells and plasmablasts may be sequestered in the GALT and/or innate immune mechanisms in the gut have a leading role in the pathogenesis of the disease.

## Acknowledgments

We wish to thank Dr. Margarita López Trascasa (Immunology Department, Hospital Universitario La Paz, IdiPAZ, Madrid, Spain) and Dr. Joaquín Navarro Caspistegui (Hospital Universitarion Gregorio Marañón, Madrid, Spain) for their invaluable help in determinining serum Ig concentrations.

## Author Contributions

Conceived and designed the experiments: MEMC. Performed the experiments: MBBC IAV. Analyzed the data: MEMC IAV MBBC PSM APK EDM CCG EMM. Contributed reagents/materials/analysis tools: IAV MBBC CCG EDM DP CPR AV EMM PSM APK. Contributed to the writing of the manuscript: MEMC.

## References

1. Rudwaleit M, van der Heijde D, Landewé R, Akkoc N, Brandt J, et al. (2011) The Assessment of SpondyloArthritis International Society classification criteria for peripheral spondyloarthritis and for spondyloarthritis in general. Ann Rheum Dis 70: 25–31.

2. Rudwaleit M, van der Heijde D, Landewé R, Listing J, Akkoc N, et al. (2009) The development of Assessment of SpondyloArthritis international Society classification criteria for axial spondyloarthritis (part II): validation and final selection. Ann Rheum Dis 68: 777–783.

3. Ambarus C, Yeremenko N, Tak PP, Baeten D (2012) Pathogenesis of spondyloarthritis: autoimmune or autoinflammatory? Curr Opin Rheumatol 24: 351–358.

4. Chou CL, Wu MJ, Yu CL, Lu MC, Hsieh SC, et al. (2010) Anti-agalactosyl IgG antibody in ankylosing spondylitis and psoriatic arthritis. Clin Rheumatol 29: 875–881.

5. Wang M, Li X, Chen J, Zhou Y, Cao H, et al. (2011) Screening and evaluating the mimic peptides as a useful serum biomarker of ankylosing spondylitis using a phage display technique. Rheumatol Int 31: 1009–1016.

6. Duftner C, Dejaco C, Klauser A, Falkenbach A, Lakomek HJ, et al. (2006) High positive predictive value of specific antibodies cross-reacting with a 28-kDa Drosophila antigen for diagnosis of ankylosing spondylitis. Rheumatology (Oxford) 45: 38–42.

7. Georgopoulos K, Dick WC, Goodacre JA, Pain RH (1985) A reinvestigation of the cross-reactivity between Klebsiella and HLA-B27 in the aetiology of ankylosing spondylitis. Clin Exp Immunol 62: 662–671.

8. Baerlecken NT, Nothdorft S, Stummvoll GH, Sieper J, Rudwaleit M, et al. (2014) Autoantibodies against CD74 in spondyloarthritis. Ann Rheum Dis 73: 1211–1214.

9. Baraliakos X, Baerlecken N, Witte T, Heldmann F, Braun J (2014) High prevalence of anti-CD74 antibodies specific for the HLA class II-associated invariant chain peptide (CLIP) in patients with axial spondyloarthritis. Ann Rheum Dis 73:1079–1082.

10. Cantaert T, Doorenspleet ME, Francosalinas G, Paramarta JE, Klarenbeek PL, et al. (2012) Increased numbers of CD5+ B lymphocytes with a regulatory phenotype in spondylarthritis. Arthritis Rheum 64:1859–1868.

11. Song IH, Heldmann F, Rudwaleit M, Listing J, Appel H, et al. (2010) Different response to rituximab in tumor necrosis factor blocker-naive patients with active ankylosing spondylitis and in patients in whom tumor necrosis factor blockers have failed: a twenty-four-week clinical trial. Arthritis Rheum 62:1290–1297.

12. Craft JE (2012) Follicular helper T cells in immunity and systemic autoimmunity. Nat Rev Rheumatol 8:337–347.

13. Fazilleau N, Mark L, McHeyzer-Williams LJ, McHeyzer-Williams MG (2009) Follicular helper T cells: lineage and location. Immunity 30: 324–335.

14. Breitfeld D, Ohl L, Kremmer E, Ellwart J, Sallusto F, et al. (2000) J Exp Med 192:1545–1552.

15. Schaerli P, Willimann K, Lang AB, Lipp M, Loetscher P, et al. (2000) CXC chemokine receptor 5 expression defines follicular homing T cells with B cell helper function. J Exp Med 192:1553–1562.

16. Kim CH, Rott LS, Clark-Lewis I, Campbell DJ, Wu L, et al. (2001) Subspecialization of CXCR5+ T cells: B helper activity is focused in a germinal center-localized subset of CXCR5+ T cells. J Exp Med 193:1373–1381.

17. Crotty S (2011) Follicular helper CD4 T cells (TFH). Annu Rev Immunol 29: 621–663.

18. Vinuesa CG, Cook MC, Angelucci C, Athanasopoulos V, Rui L, et al. (2005) A RING-type ubiquitin ligase family member required to repress follicular helper T cells and autoimmunity. Nature 435(7041): 452–458.

19. Subramanian S, Tus K, Li QZ, Wang A, Tian XH, et al. (2006) A Tlr7 translocation accelerates systemic autoimmunity in murine lupus. Proc Natl Acad Sci U S A 103: 9970–9975.

20. Linterman MA, Rigby RJ, Wong RK, Yu D, Brink R, et al. (2009) Follicular helper T cells are required for systemic autoimmunity. J Exp Med 206: 561–576.

21. Ji YR, Kim HJ, Yu DH, Bae KB, Park SJ, et al. (2012) Enforced expression of roquin protein in T cells exacerbates the incidence and severity of experimental arthritis. J Biol Chem 287: 42269–42277.

22. Hron JD, Caplan L, Gerth AJ, Schwartzberg PL, Peng SL (2004) SH2D1A regulates T-dependent humoral autoimmunity. J Exp Med 200: 261–266.

23. Simpson N, Gatenby PA, Wilson A, Malik S, Fulcher DA, et al. (2010) Expansion of circulating T cells resembling follicular helper T cells is a fixed phenotype that identifies a subset of severe systemic lupus erythematosus. Arthritis Rheum 62: 234–244.

24. Morita R, Schmitt N, Bentebibel SE, Ranganathan R, Bourdery L, et al. (2011) Human blood CXCR5(+)CD4(+) T cells are counterparts of T follicular cells and contain specific subsets that differentially support antibody secretion. Immunity 34: 108–121.

25. Chevalier N, Jarrossay D, Ho E, Avery DT, Ma CS, et al. (2011) CXCR5 expressing human central memory CD4 T cells and their relevance for humoral immune responses. J Immunol 186: 5556–5568.

26. Vinuesa CG, Cook MC (2011) Blood relatives of follicular helper T cells. Immunity 34: 10–12.

27. Wang J, Shan Y, Jiang Z, Feng J, Li C, et al. (2013) High frequencies of activated B cells and T follicular helper cells are correlated with disease activity in patients with new-onset rheumatoid arthritis. Clin Exp Immunol 174: 212–220.

28. Szabo K, Papp G, Barath S, Gyimesi E, Szanto A, et al. (2013) Follicular helper T cells may play an important role in the severity of primary Sjögren's syndrome. Clin Immunol 147: 95–104.

29. Zhu C, Ma J, Liu Y, Tong J, Tian J, et al. (2012) Increased frequency of follicular helper T cells in patients with autoimmune thyroid disease. J Clin Endocrinol Metab 97: 943–950.

30. Feng J, Lu L, Hua C, Qin L, Zhao P, et al. (2011) High frequency of CD4+ CXCR5+ TFH cells in patients with immune-active chronic hepatitis B. PLoS One 6(7): e21698.

31. Luo C, Li Y, Liu W, Feng H, Wang H, et al. (2013) Expansion of circulating counterparts of follicular helper T cells in patients with myasthenia gravis. J Neuroimmunol 256: 55–61.

32. Le Coz C, Joublin A, Pasquali JL, Korganow AS, Dumortier H, et al. (2013) Circulating TFH subset distribution is strongly affected in lupus patients with an active disease. PLoS One 8(9): e75319.

33. Xiao F, Zhang HY, Liu YJ, Zhao D, Shan YX, et al. (2013) Higher frequency of peripheral blood interleukin 21 positive follicular helper T cells in patients with ankylosing spondylitis. J Rheumatol 40: 2029–2037.

34. Wu S, Yang T, Pan F, Xia G, Hu Y, et al. (2014) Increased frequency of circulating follicular helper T cells in patients with ankylosing spondylitis. Mod Rheumatol [Epub ahead of print] PMID: 24716597.

35. van der Linden S, Valkenburg HA, Cats A (1984) Evaluation of diagnostic criteria for ankylosing spondylitis. A proposal for modification of the New York criteria. Arthritis Rheum 27: 361–368.

36. Trull A, Ebringer A, Panayi G, Ebringer R, James DC (1984) HLA-B27 and the immune response to enterobacterial antigens in ankylosing spondylitis. Clin Exp Immunol 55: 74–80.

37. Franssen MJ, van de Putte LB, Gribnau FW (1985) IgA serum levels and disease activity in ankylosing spondylitis: a prospective study. Ann Rheum Dis 44: 766–771.

38. Machado P, Landewé R, Lie E, Kvien TK, Braun J, et al. (2011) Assessment of SpondyloArthritis international Society. Ankylosing Spondylitis Disease Activity Score (ASDAS): defining cut-off values for disease activity states and improvement scores. Ann Rheum Dis 70: 47–53.

39. Richter MB, Woo P, Panayi GS, Trull A, Unger A, et al. (1983) The effects of intravenous pulse methylprednisolone on immunological and inflammatory processes in ankylosing spondylitis. Clin Exp Immunol 53:51–59.

40. Bossaller L, Burger J, Draeger R, Grimbacher B, Knoth R, et al. (2006) ICOS deficiency is associated with a severe reduction of CXCR5+CD4 germinal center Th cells. J Immunol 177: 4927–4932.

41. Salinas GF, De Rycke L, Barendregt B, Paramarta JE, Hreggvidsdottir H, et al. (2013) Anti-TNF treatment blocks the induction of T cell-dependent humoral responses. Ann Rheum Dis 72:1037–1043.

42. Mielants H, Veys EM, Goemaere S, Goethals K, Cuvelier C, et al. (1991) Gut inflammation in the spondyloarthropathies: clinical, radiologic, biologic and genetic features in relation to the type of histology. A prospective study. J Rheumatol 18:1542–1551.

43. Demetter P, Van Huysse JA, De Keyser F, Van Damme N, Verbruggen G, et al. (2002) Increase in lymphoid follicles and leukocyte adhesion molecules emphasizes a role for the gut in spondyloarthropathy pathogenesis. J Pathol 198: 517–522.

44. Martínez-González O, Cantero-Hinojosa J, Paule-Sastre P, Gómez-Magán JC, Salvatierra-Ríos D (1994) Intestinal permeability in patients with ankylosing spondylitis and their healthy relatives. Br J Rheumatol 33:644–647.

45. Gibson PR (2004) Increased gut permeability in Crohn's disease: is TNF the link? Gut 53:1724–1725.

46. Wang C, Kang SG, Lee J, Sun Z, Kim CH (2009) The roles of CCR6 in migration of Th17 cells and regulation of effector T-cell balance in the gut. Mucosal Immunol 2: 173–183.

47. Izadpanah A, Dwinell MB, Eckmann L, Varki NM, Kagnoff MF (2001) Regulated MIP-3alpha/CCL20 production by human intestinal epithelium: mechanism for modulating mucosal immunity. Am J Physiol Gastrointest Liver Physiol 280: G710–719.

48. Zimmermann K, Haas A, Oxenius A (2012) Systemic antibody responses to gut microbes in health and disease. Gut Microbes 3:42–47.

49. Macpherson AJ, Gatto D, Sainsbury E, Harriman GR, Hengartner H, et al. (2000) A primitive T cell-independent mechanism of intestinal mucosal IgA responses to commensal bacteria. Science 288(5474): 2222–2226.

50. Bergqvist P, Stensson A, Lycke NY, Bemark M (2010) T cell-independent IgA class switch recombination is restricted to the GALT and occurs prior to manifest germinal center formation. J Immunol 184: 3545–3553.

51. Van Praet L, Jacques P, Van den Bosch F, Elewaut D (2012) The transition of acute to chronic bowel inflammation in spondyloarthritis. Nat Rev Rheumatol 8:288–295.

52. Iwasaki A, Medzhitov R (2010) Regulation of adaptive immunity by the innate immune system. Science 327(5963): 291–295.

# Permissions

All chapters in this book were first published in PLOS ONE, by The Public Library of Science; hereby published with permission under the Creative Commons Attribution License or equivalent. Every chapter published in this book has been scrutinized by our experts. Their significance has been extensively debated. The topics covered herein carry significant findings which will fuel the growth of the discipline. They may even be implemented as practical applications or may be referred to as a beginning point for another development.

The contributors of this book come from diverse backgrounds, making this book a truly international effort. This book will bring forth new frontiers with its revolutionizing research information and detailed analysis of the nascent developments around the world.

We would like to thank all the contributing authors for lending their expertise to make the book truly unique. They have played a crucial role in the development of this book. Without their invaluable contributions this book wouldn't have been possible. They have made vital efforts to compile up to date information on the varied aspects of this subject to make this book a valuable addition to the collection of many professionals and students.

This book was conceptualized with the vision of imparting up-to-date information and advanced data in this field. To ensure the same, a matchless editorial board was set up. Every individual on the board went through rigorous rounds of assessment to prove their worth. After which they invested a large part of their time researching and compiling the most relevant data for our readers.

The editorial board has been involved in producing this book since its inception. They have spent rigorous hours researching and exploring the diverse topics which have resulted in the successful publishing of this book. They have passed on their knowledge of decades through this book. To expedite this challenging task, the publisher supported the team at every step. A small team of assistant editors was also appointed to further simplify the editing procedure and attain best results for the readers.

Apart from the editorial board, the designing team has also invested a significant amount of their time in understanding the subject and creating the most relevant covers. They scrutinized every image to scout for the most suitable representation of the subject and create an appropriate cover for the book.

The publishing team has been an ardent support to the editorial, designing and production team. Their endless efforts to recruit the best for this project, has resulted in the accomplishment of this book. They are a veteran in the field of academics and their pool of knowledge is as vast as their experience in printing. Their expertise and guidance has proved useful at every step. Their uncompromising quality standards have made this book an exceptional effort. Their encouragement from time to time has been an inspiration for everyone.

The publisher and the editorial board hope that this book will prove to be a valuable piece of knowledge for researchers, students, practitioners and scholars across the globe.

# List of Contributors

**Sooah Kim, Jinhua Xuan, Young Hoon Jung and Kyoung Heon Kim**
Department of Biotechnology, Korea University Graduate School, Seoul, Republic of Korea

**Jiwon Hwang and Hoon-Suk Cha**
Samsung Medical Center, Sungkyunkwan University School of Medicine, Seoul, Republic of Korea

**Lei Zhang, Yong-gang Li, Lei Qi, Zhen-feng Li, Qiang Yang and Jian-min Li**
Department of Orthopedics, Qilu Hospital, Shandong University, Jinan, China

**Yu-hua Li**
Department of Emergency, Qilu Hospital, Shandong University, Jinan, China

**Xin-guang Liu and Daoxin Ma**
Department of Hematology, Qilu Hospital, Shandong University, Jinan, China

**Cun-zhong Yuan**
Department of Obstetrics and Gynecology, Qilu Hospital, Shandong University, Jinan, China

**Nai-wen Hu**
Department of Rheumatology, Provincial Hospital affiliated to Shandong University, Jinan, China

**Wei Li**
Department of Clinical Laboratory, Qilu Hospital, Shandong University, Jinan, China

**Ruxandra Schiotis**
Department of Pharmacology, "Iuliu Hatieganu" University of Medicine and Pharmacy and SCBI-Rheumatology Department, Cluj-Napoca, Romania
Department of Rheumatology, University Hospital "Reina Sofía"/IMIBIC, Córdoba, Spain

**Eduardo Collantes Estevez**
Department of Rheumatology, University Hospital "Reina Sofía"/IMIBIC, Córdoba, Spain

**Nerea Bartolomé, Magdalena Szczypiorska, Antonio Martínez, Diego Tejedor and Marta Artieda**
Department of R+D, Progenika Biopharma SA, Derio-Vizcaya, Spain

**Juan Mulero, Alejandra Sánchez and Jesús Sanz**
Department of Rheumatology, "Puerta de Hierro Majadahonda", University Hospital, Madrid, Spain

**Eduardo Cuende**
Department of Rheumatology, University Hospital "Pri´ncipe de Asturias", Alcalá de Henares, Madrid, Spain

**Anca Buzoianu**
Department of Pharmacology, "Iuliu Hatieganu" University of Medicine and Pharmacy, Cluj-Napoca, Romania

**James Cheng-Chung Wei, Chun-Huang Huang and Ruey-Hong Wong**
Division of Allergy, Immunology and Rheumatology, Department of Medicine, Chung Shan Medical University Hospital, Institute of Medicine, Chung Shan Medical University, Graduate Institute of Integrated Medicine, China Medical University, Taichung, Taiwan

**Wei-Chiao Chen, Yu-Shiuan Wang, Yi-Ching Chiu, Tusty-Jiuan Hsieh and Edward Hsi**
Department of Medical Genetics, College of Medicine, Kaohsiung Medical University, Kaohsiung, Taiwan

**Suh-Hang Hank Juo and Wei-Chiao Chang**
Department of Medical Genetics, College of Medicine, Kaohsiung Medical University, Kaohsiung, Taiwan
Cancer Center, Kaohsiung Medical University Hospital, Kaohsiung, Taiwan

**Jeng-Hsien Yen**
Division of Rheumatology, Department of Internal Medicine, Kaohsiung Medical University Hospital, Kaohsiung, Taiwan, Graduate Institute of Medicine, Kaohsiung Medical University, Kaohsiung, Taiwan

**Hsueh-Wei Chang**
Department of Biomedical Science and Environmental Biology, Kaohsiung, Taiwan

**Wei-Pin Chang**
Department of Healthcare Management, Yuanpei University, HsinChu, Taiwan

**Yuh-Cherng Guo**
Department of Neurology, Kaohsiung Municipal Hsiao-Kang Hospital, Kaohsiung Medical University, Kaohsiung, Taiwan

**Ke-Li Tsai**
Department of Physiology, College of Medicine, Kaohsiung Medical University, Kaohsiung, Taiwan

**Hui-Po Wang**
Department of Pharmacy, Taipei Medical University, Taipei, Taiwan

**Yang-Chang Wu**
Graduate Institute of Integrated Medicine, China Medical University, Taichung, Taiwan

**Gernot Steinwender, Martin Weger and Navid Ardjomand**
Department of Ophthalmology, Auenbrugger University Graz, Graz, Austria

**Ewald Lindner, Sophie Plainer and Yosuf El-Shabrawi**
Department of Ophthalmology, Klinikum Klagenfurt, Klagenfurt, Austria

**Wilfried Renner**
Clinical Institute of Medical and Chemical Laboratory Diagnostics, Medical University Graz, Graz, Austria

**Astrid Hjelholt**
Department of Biomedicine – Medical Microbiology and Immunology, Aarhus University, Aarhus, Denmark

**Thomas Carlsen**
Department of Health Science and Technology, Aalborg University, Aalborg, Denmark

**Bent Deleuran**
Department of Biomedicine – Medical Microbiology and Immunology, Aarhus University, Aarhus, Denmark
Department of Rheumatology, Aarhus University Hospital, Aarhus, Denmark

**Anne Grethe Jurik**
Department of Radiology, Aarhus University Hospital, Aarhus, Denmark

**Berit Schiøttz-Christensen**
Aarhus Clinic for Rheumatic Diseases, Aarhus, Denmark

**Gunna Christiansen**
Department of Biomedicine – Medical Microbiology and Immunology, Aarhus University, Aarhus, Denmark
Loke Diagnostics, Risskov, Denmark

**Svend Birkelund**
Department of Health Science and Technology, Aalborg University, Aalborg, Denmark
Loke Diagnostics, Risskov, Denmark

**Anne C. Bay-Jensen, Inger Byrjalsen, Diana J. Leeming, Claus Christiansen and Morten A. Karsdal**
Rheumatology, Nordic Bioscience, Herlev, Denmark

**Stephanie Wichuk, Nathalie Morency and Walter P. Maksymowych**
Division of Rheumatology, University of Alberta, Edmonton, Alberta, Canada

**James Cheng-Chung Wei**
Division of Allergy, Immunology and Rheumatology, Department of Medicine, Chung Shan Medical University Hospital, Taichung, Taiwan
Institute of Medicine, Chung Shan Medical University, Taichung, Taiwan

**Chun-Huang Huang**
Institute of Medicine, Chung Shan Medical University, Taichung, Taiwan

**Kuo-Sheng Hung**
Department of Neurosurgery, Center of Excellence for Clinical Trial and Research, Graduate Institute of Injury Prevention and Control, Taipei Medical University, Wan Fang Medical Center, Taipei, Taiwan

**Yu-Wen Hsu**
Department of Clinical Pharmacy, School of Pharmacy, Taipei Medical University, Taipei, Taiwan

**Ruey-Hong Wong**
Department of Public Health, Chung Shan Medical University, Taichung, Taiwan

**Ming-Shiou Jan**
Institute of Microbiology and Immunology, Chung Shan Medical University, Taichung, Taiwan

**Shyh-Jong Wu**
Department of Medical Laboratory Science and Biotechnology, College of Health Sciences, Kaohsiung Medical University, Kaohsiung, Taiwan

**Yung-Shun Juan**
Department of Urology, Kaohsiung municipal Hsiao-Kang Hospital and College of Medicine, Kaohsiung Medical University, Kaohsiung, Taiwan

**Wei-Chiao Chang**
Department of Clinical Pharmacy, School of Pharmacy, Taipei Medical University, Taipei, Taiwan
Department of Pharmacy, Taipei Medical University-Wanfang Hospital, Taipei, Taiwan

**Wen-Yi Tseng**
Division of Rheumatology, Allergy and Immunology, Chang Gung Memorial Hospital at Keelung, Keelung, Taiwan
Graduate Institute of Clinical Medicine, Chang GungUniversity, Tao-Yuan, Taiwan

**Yi-Shu Huang and Nien-Yi Chiang**
Graduate Institute of Biomedical Sciences, Chang Gung University, Tao-Yuan, Taiwan

**Yeong-Jian Jan Wu**
Division of Rheumatology, Allergy and Immunology, Chang Gung Memorial Hospital at Keelung, Keelung, Taiwan
Department of Medicine, College of Medicine, Chang Gung University, Tao-Yuan, Taiwan

**Yeh-Pin Chou**
Department of Medicine, College of Medicine, Chang Gung University, Tao-Yuan, Taiwan
Division of Hepato-Gastroenterology, Department of Internal Medicine, Chang Gung Memorial Hospital at Kaohsiung, Kaohsiung, Taiwan

**Shue-Fen Luo**
Department of Medicine, College of Medicine, Chang Gung University, Tao-Yuan, Taiwan
Division of Rheumatology, Allergy and Immunology, Chang Gung Memorial Hospital at Linkou, Linkou, Taiwan

**Chang-Fu Kuo**
Division of Rheumatology, Allergy and Immunology, Chang Gung Memorial Hospital at Linkou, Linkou, Taiwan

**Ko-Ming Lin**
Division of Rheumatology, Allergy and Immunology, Chang Gung Memorial Hospital at Chiayi, Chiayi, Taiwan

**Hsi-Hsien Lin**
Graduate Institute of Biomedical Sciences, Chang Gung University, Tao-Yuan, Taiwan
Department of Microbiology and Immunology, College of Medicine, Chang Gung University,Tao-Yuan, Taiwan

**Wei Chai**
Department of Orthopaedics, Chinese People's Liberation Army General Hospital, Beijing, China

**Yan Wang**
Department of Orthopaedics, Chinese People's Liberation Army General Hospital, Beijing, China
Medical School of Nankai University, Tianjin, China

**Jingyi Liu**
Medical School of Nankai University, Tianjin, China

**Zijian Lian**
Department of Orthopaedics, Chinese People's Liberation Army General Hospital, Beijing, China
Medical School of Nankai University, Tianjin, China
Department of Orthopaedics, Tianjin Hospital, Tianjin, China

**Chao Chen**
Department of Orthopaedics, Chinese People's Liberation Army General Hospital, Beijing, China
Department of Orthopaedics, Tianjin Hospital, Tianjin, China

**Lewis L. Shi**
Department of Orthopaedics, University of Chicago Hospital, Maryland Avenue, Chicago, Illinois, United States of America

**Elisa Nurzia, Valentina Tedeschi, Silvana Caristi and Maria Teresa Fiorillo**
Department of Biology and Biotechnology "C. Darwin", Sapienza University, Rome, Italy

**Rainer A. Böckmann and Daniele Narzi**
Computational Biology, Department of Biology, University of Erlangen-Nürnberg, Erlangen, Germany

**Alberto Cauli and Alessandro Mathieu**
2nd Chair of Rheumatology, Department of Medical Sciences, University of Cagliari, Cagliari, Italy

**Rosa Sorrentino**
Istituto Pasteur-Fondazione Cenci Bolognetti, Department of Biology and Biotechnology "C. Darwin", Sapienza University, Rome, Italy

**Zheng Li, Jianxiong Shen, Guixing Qiu, Haiquan Yu, Yipeng Wang, Jianguo Zhang, Hong Zhao, Yu Zhao, Shugang Li, Xisheng Weng, Jinqian Liang and Lijuan Zhao**
Department of Orthopaedic Surgery, Peking Union Medical College Hospital, Chinese Academy of Medical Sciences & Peking Union Medical College, Beijing, China

**Hongtao Dong and Qiuming Li**
Department of Ophthalmology, the First Affiliated Hospital of Zhengzhou University, Zhengzhou, China

**Ying Zhang and Wei Tan**
Department of Ophthalmology, The First People's Hospital of Zunyi, The Third Affiliated Hospital of Zunyi Medical University, Zunyi, China

**Zhengxuan Jiang**
Department of Ophthalmology, the Second Affiliated Hospital of Anhui Medical University, Hefei, China

**Ya-Ping Huang**
Department of Physical Medicine and Rehabilitation, National Taiwan University Hospital Yun-Lin Branch, Yunlin, Taiwan

**Yen-Ho Wang and Shin-Liang Pan**
Department of Physical Medicine and Rehabilitation, National Taiwan University Hospital, Taipei, Taiwan
Department of Physical Medicine and Rehabilitation, National Taiwan University College of Medicine, Taipei, Taiwan

**Thijs Willem Swinnen**
Rheumatology, University Hospitals Leuven, Leuven, Belgium
Department of Development and Regeneration, KU Leuven, Leuven, Belgium
Department of Rehabilitation Sciences, KU Leuven, Heverlee, Belgium

**Rene Westhovens and Kurt de Vlam**
Rheumatology, University Hospitals Leuven, Leuven, Belgium
Department of Development and Regeneration, KU Leuven, Leuven, Belgium

**Wim Dankaerts**
Department of Rehabilitation Sciences, KU Leuven, Heverlee, Belgium

**Johan Lefevre**
Department of Kinesiology, KU Leuven, Heverlee, Belgium

**Tineke Scheers**
Department of Kinesiology, KU Leuven, Heverlee, Belgium
Research Foundation Flanders, Brussel, Belgium

**Anneke Spoorenberg, Martha K. Leijsma, Hendrika Bootsma and Elisabeth Brouwer**
Rheumatology and Clinical Immunology, University of Groningen, University Medical Center Groningen, Groningen, The Netherlands

**Suzanne Arends**
Rheumatology and Clinical Immunology, University of Groningen, University Medical Center Groningen, Groningen, The Netherlands
Rheumatology, Medical Center Leeuwarden, Leeuwarden, The Netherlands

**Monique Efde and Reinhard Bos**
Rheumatology, Medical Center Leeuwarden, Leeuwarden, The Netherlands

**Nic J. G. M. Veeger**
Epidemiology, University of Groningen, University Medical Center Groningen, Groningen, The Netherlands

**Eveline van der Veer**
Laboratory Medicine, University of Groningen, University Medical Center Groningen, Groningen, The Netherlands

**Chia-Wei Lin and Yu-Tsun Ho**
Department of Physical Medicine and Rehabilitation, National Taiwan University Hospital, Taipei, Taiwan

**Ya-Ping Huang**
Department of Physical Medicine and Rehabilitation, National Taiwan University Hospital Yu-Lin Branch, Yunlin, Taiwan

**Yueh-Hsia Chiu**
Department and Graduate Institute of Health Care Management, Chang Gung University, Tao-Yuan, Taiwan

**Shin-Liang Pan**
Department of Physical Medicine and Rehabilitation, National Taiwan University Hospital, Taipei, Taiwan
Department of Physical Medicine and Rehabilitation, National Taiwan University College of Medicine, Taipei, Taiwan

**James Cheng-Chung Wei**
Division of Allergy, Immunology and Rheumatology, Department of Medicine, Chung Shan Medical University Hospital, Taichung, Taiwan
Institute of Medicine, Chung Shan Medical University, Taichung, Taiwan

**Hung-Yi Chiou**
School of Public Health, Taipei Medical University, Taipei, Taiwan
Master Program for Clinical Pharmacogenomics and Pharmacoproteomics, School of Pharmacy, Taipei Medical University, Taipei, Taiwan

**Ruey-Hong Wong**
Department of Public Health, Chung Shan Medical University, Taichung, Taiwan

**Wei-Chiao Chang**
Department of Clinical Pharmacy, School of Pharmacy, Taipei Medical University, Taipei, Taiwan
Department of Pharmacy, Taipei Medical University-Wanfang Hospital, Taipei, Taiwan
Master Program for Clinical Pharmacogenomics and Pharmacoproteomics, School of Pharmacy, Taipei Medical University, Taipei, Taiwan

**Ya-Feng Wen and Yu-Wen Hsu**
Department of Clinical Pharmacy, School of Pharmacy, Taipei Medical University, Taipei, Taiwan
Master Program for Clinical Pharmacogenomics and Pharmacoproteomics, School of Pharmacy, Taipei Medical University, Taipei, Taiwan

**Henry Sung-Ching Wong**
Master Program for Clinical Pharmacogenomics and Pharmacoproteomics, School of Pharmacy, Taipei Medical University, Taipei, Taiwan

**Shiro Ikegawa**
Master Program for Clinical Pharmacogenomics and Pharmacoproteomics, School of Pharmacy, Taipei Medical University, Taipei, Taiwan
Laboratory for Bone and Joint Diseases, RIKEN Center for Integrative Medical Science, Yokohama, Japan

**Young Bin Joo, So-Young Bang and Tae-Hwan Kim**
Department of Rheumatology, Hanyang University Hospital for Rheumatic Diseases, Seoul, Republic of Korea

**Seung-Cheol Shim**
Division of Rheumatology, Daejeon Rheumatoid & Degenerative Arthritis Center, Chungnam National University Hospital, Daejeon, Republic of Korea

**Seunghun Lee and Kyung Bin Joo**
Department of Radiology, Hanyang University Hospital for Rheumatic Diseases, Seoul, Republic of Korea

**Jong Heon Kim**
Department of Orthopedics, Hanyang University Hospital for Rheumatic Diseases, Seoul, Republic of Korea

**Hye Joon Min**
Department ofanthropology, Cornell University, Ithaca, New York, United States of America

**Proton Rahman**
Department of Rheumatology, Memorial University, St. Clare's Mercy Hospital, St. John's Newfoundland, Canada

**Robert D. Inman**
Division of Rheumatology, University of Toronto, Toronto Western Hospital, Toronto, Ontario, Canada

**Qi Zhang, Jian Qi, Shengping Hou, Liping Du, Hongsong Yu, Qingfeng Cao, Yan Zhou, Dan Liao and Peizeng Yang**
The First Affiliated Hospital of Chongqing Medical University, Chongqing Key Laboratory of Ophthalmology and Chongqing Eye Institute, Chongqing, P. R. China

**Aize Kijlstra**
University Eye Clinic Maastricht, Maastricht, The Netherlands

**Silje Halvorsen Sveaas, Kåre Birger Hagen and Hanne Dagfinrud**
National Advisory Unit on Rehabilitation in Rheumatology, Department of Rheumatology, Diakonhjemmet Hospital, Oslo, Norway
Department of Health Sciences, University of Oslo, Oslo, Norway

**Camilla Fongen**
National Advisory Unit on Rehabilitation in Rheumatology, Department of Rheumatology, Diakonhjemmet Hospital, Oslo, Norway

**Nina Vøllestad**
Department of Health Sciences, University of Oslo, Oslo, Norway

**Inger Jorid Berg, Sella Aarrestad Provan, Anne Grete Semb, Tore K. Kvien and Inge C. Olsen**
Department of Rheumatology, Diakonhjemmet Hospital, Oslo, Norway

**Annika Michelsen**
Research Institute of Internal Medicine, Oslo University Hospital, Rikshospitalet, Oslo, Norway

**Thor Ueland**
Research Institute of Internal Medicine, Oslo University Hospital, Rikshospitalet, Oslo, Norway
Institute of Clinical Medicine, University of Oslo, Oslo, Norway

**Pål Aukrust**
Research Institute of Internal Medicine, Oslo University Hospital, Rikshospitalet, Oslo, Norway
Section of Clinical Immunology and Infectious Diseases, Oslo University Hospital, Rikshospitalet, Oslo, Norway
Institute of Clinical Medicine, University of Oslo, Oslo, Norway
K.G. Jebsen Inflammatory Research Center, University of Oslo, Oslo, Norway

**María-Belén Bautista-Caro, Irene Arroyo-Villa, Concepción Castillo-Gallego, Eugenio de Miguel, Diana Peiteado, Chamaida Plasencia-Rodríguez, Alejandro Villalba, Emilio Martín-Mola and María-Eugenia Miranda-Carús**
Department of Rheumatology, Hospital Universitario La Paz-IdiPAZ, Madrid, Spain

**Paloma Sánchez-Mateos and Amaya Puig-Kröger**
Laboratorio de Inmuno-Oncología, Hospital General Universitario Gregorio Marañón, Madrid, Spain

# Index